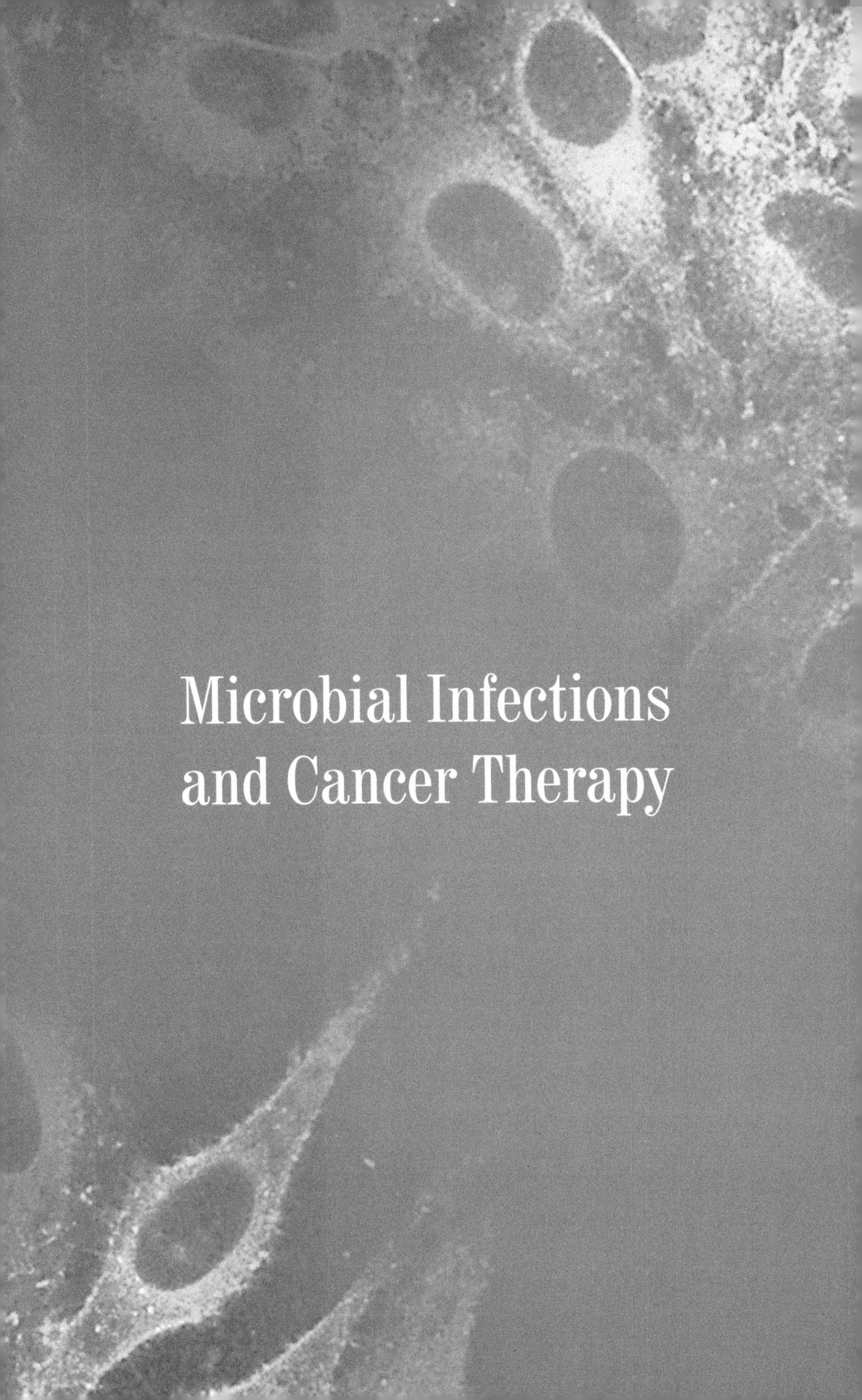

Microbial Infections and Cancer Therapy

Microbial Infections and Cancer Therapy

Recent Advances

edited by

Ananda M. Chakrabarty
Arsénio M. Fialho

PAN STANFORD PUBLISHING

Published by

Pan Stanford Publishing Pte. Ltd.
Penthouse Level, Suntec Tower 3
8 Temasek Boulevard
Singapore 038988

Email: editorial@panstanford.com
Web: www.panstanford.com

British Library Cataloguing-in-Publication Data
A catalogue record for this book is available from the British Library.

Microbial Infections and Cancer Therapy: Recent Advances

ISBN 978-981-4774-86-4 (Hardcover)
ISBN 978-1-351-04190-4 (eBook)

Contents

Preface

The bacterial world is extremely diversified, evidencing the existence of bacteria able to successfully colonize the most varied environments, that is, from inhospitable places on the planet to their coexistence with humans. Such nature is based on the existence of unique and complex genetic systems, which is seen to be the key for the great success of their ubiquity. Nowadays, microbial biotechnology makes use of live microorganisms or derived products to find various industrial applications, particularly in health, food, and environment. Among those, in recent years, the use of pathogenic (attenuated) or non-pathogenic live bacteria and their purified products as new anticancer agents have gained prominence. In fact, based on a significant number of scientific publications, human clinical trials, and even clinical practice, it is found that bacteria can be successfully used as agents capable of stimulating the immune system and fight cancer. Furthermore, through genetic intervention, it is possible to modify bacteria and use them as gene delivery vehicles for anticancer proposals. In addition, it also deserves mentioning the fact that bacteria harboring this additional genetic information are able to show tropism, preferentially colonizing the tumor microenvironment. Besides live bacteria, the use of purified bacterial products as anticancer agents, namely proteins, peptides, and compounds derived from secondary metabolism, has also gained relevance. In this book, twelve chapters address the most recent developments regarding the success and limitations of the use of bacteria and their products as cancer therapeutic agents. Considering that we now face an era where the resistance of cancer cells to chemotherapy has become a global burden, the establishment of alternative anticancer therapies may add value in the definition of more efficient therapeutic protocols. As editors, we hope to be able to bring together in this book the most relevant and up-to-date information on this subject.

Ananda M. Chakrabarty
Arsénio M. Fialho
Autumn 2018

Chapter 1

Bifidobacterium as a Delivery System of Functional Genes for Cancer Therapy

Chao Han,[a] Yu-Qing Dai,[b] Zi-Chun Hua,[a] Geng-Feng Fu,[c] Yan Yin,[a] Bi Hu,[a] and Gen-Xing Xu[a]

[a]*The State Key Laboratory of Pharmaceutical Biotechnology, College of Life Science, Nanjing University, Nanjing 210046, China*
[b]*College of Pharmacy, Nanjing University of Chinese Medicine, Nanjing 210029, China*
[c]*Jiangsu Provincial Center for Disease Prevention and Control, Nanjing, China*

genxingxu@nju.edu.cn

Bifidobacteria were first discovered in 1899 by Henri Tissier, a French pediatrician at the Pasteur Institute in Paris. They are gram-positive, anaerobic, catalase-negative, fermentative rods, which are often Y- or V-shaped. As an anaerobe, *Bifidobacteria* can germinate and proliferate in the hypoxic regions of solid tumors. Plasmids of *Bifidobacterium* encode many specific characteristics of *Bifidobacterium*, and they can also establish shuttle vectors to express exogenous genes. Previous studies exhibited anticancer effects of *Bifidobacteria* on many kinds of tumors. To date, only a few plasmids were found to replicate and express exogenous proteins in *Bifidobacterium;* besides the transformation efficiency and expression level were low in all cases. It can be foreseen that the *Bifidobacterium* will be the most important and perfect vector

Microbial Infections and Cancer Therapy: Recent Advances
Edited by Ananda M. Chakrabarty and Arsénio M. Fialho

ISBN 978-981-4774-86-4 (Hardcover), 978-1-351-04190-4 (eBook)
www.panstanford.com

of anticancer gene in cancer gene therapy. The study on related plasmids of *Bifidobacterium* expression plasmids in *Bifidobacterium* for cancer gene therapy is summarized in this chapter, and the advantages and disadvantages of the use of *Bifidobacterium* as a delivery system of functional genes for cancer gene therapy are also discussed.

1.1 The Potential Superiority of *Bifidobacterium* as a Delivery System for Cancer Gene Therapy

1.1.1 The Biological Features of *Bifidobacterium* Associated with Cancer Gene Therapy

As a delivery system and compared with other bacterial genera, *Bifidobacterium* represents a promising biological tool for cancer therapy. *Bifidobacterium* is gram-positive, a strictly anaerobic bacterium with bifid morphology. Its anaerobic specialty is important for cancer therapy. Tissue oxygen electrode measurements taken in cancer patients show a median range of oxygen partial pressure of 10–30 mm Hg in tumors, with a significant proportion of readings below 2.5 mm Hg, whereas those in normal tissues range from 24 to 66 mm Hg [1]. Early in 1980, Kimura and colleagues showed that genus *Bifidobacterium* could germinate and grow in the hypoxic regions of solid tumors after intravenous injection. Contrastingly, the number of *Bifidobacterium* in normal tissues decreased and then disappeared [2]. Later, Yazawa *et al.* showed that wild-type and genetically engineered *B. longum* has the tumor specificity to localize and germinate in tumor regions [3]. Besides its anaerobic specialty, *Bifidobacterium* is known as a health-promoting and probiotic agent, playing an important role in the maintenance of a proper balance of normal intestinal flora [4]. Some bifidobacterial species are frequently used as the probiotic element in many functional foods, which means a high safety in administration. In early studies, *Bifidobacterium* itself also indicated the effect of cancer prevention [5, 6]. Jagveer *et al.* found that oral administration of *B. longum* exerted strong antitumor activity, as showed by modulation of the intermediate biomarkers of colon cancer, and reduced tumor outcome [7].

1.1.2 Endogenous Plasmids and Cloning Vectors in *Bifidobacterium*

To develop a cloning vector of *Bifidobacterium*, a comprehensive understanding of the replication mechanism and characterization of natural bifidobacterial plasmids is necessary. Plasmids in *Bifidobacterium* attracted great interest because they encode many special characters and play an important role in the research on genetics and construction of engineering strains for *Bifidobacterium*. *Bifidobacterium* with related plasmids not only revealed its own characteristics but also gained characters encoded by the plasmids, such as lactose catabolism, generation of bacteriocin, drug resistance and antibiotic resistance [8–10].

The majority of bifidobacterial strains do not harbor any plasmid. But if they do, they rarely contain more than one, which range in size from 1 to 19 kb [11]. Several plasmids have been isolated from 9 of the 32 species and 44 plasmids have been fully sequenced and annotated (Table 1.1). The majority of the sequenced plasmids were isolated from *B. longum*. Other sources are *B. asteroides*, *B. bifidum*, *B. breve*, *B. catenulatum*, *B. kashiwanohense*, *B. pseudocatenulatum*, *B. pseudolongum* subsp. *globosum* and *B. sp. A 24* (Table 1.1). Analysis of their replication (Rep) proteins has indicated that the majority of identifying bifidobacterial plasmids replicate by means of the so-called rolling circle mechanism (RCR), while other functions if encoded, remain to a large degree unknown [11, 12].

Several cloning vectors have been constructed with plasmids from *Bifidobacterium* and *Escherichia coli* and transformed into both of them by electroporation. In all cases, electroporation efficiency in *Bifidobacterium* was very low, and numerous attempts have been made to optimize it.

The nucleotide sequence of the *B. longum B2577* cryptic plasmid pMB1 was sequenced in 1996. Recombinant plasmids containing the pMB1 replicon could replicate in *B. animalis* MB209 [13]. Later, another pMB1-based vector pNC7 was successfully transformed into 10 bifidobacterial species [14]. In 1999, plasmid pKJ50 was isolated from *B. longum* KJ and a shuttle vector constructed by cloning pKJ50 and a chloramphenicol resistance gene into pBR322 [15].

Table 1.1 Completely sequenced plasmids found in *Bifidobacterium* species

Species	Plasmid	Size (bp)	Accession no.
B. asteroides	pCIBA089	2,111	NC_010908.1
B. bifidum	pB80	4,898	NC_011332.1
B. breve	pCIBb1	5,750	NC_002133.1
	pB21a	5,206	NC_010930.1
	pMP7017	190,178	GI:704484592
	pBR3	4,891	NZ_CP010414.1
B. catenulatum	pBC1	2,540	NC_007068.1
B. kashiwanohense	pBBKW-1	7,716	NC_021875.1
	pBBKW-2	2,920	NC_021876.1
B. longum	pKJ36	3,625	NC_002635.1
	pB44	3,624	NC_004443.1
	pNAC3	10,224	NC_004768.1
	PNAC2	3,684	NC_004769.1
	pNAC1	3,538	NC_004770.1
	pKJ50	4,960	NC_004978.1
	pMG1	3,682	NC_006997.1
	pTB6	3,624	NC_006843.1
	pBIF10	9,275	GI:73665544
	pFI2576	2,197	NC_011139.1
	p6043A	4,896	NC_010857.1
	p6043B	3,680	NC_010861.1
	pSP02	4,896	NC_019200.1
	pNAL8M	4,910	NC_025161.1
	pNAL8L	3,489	NC_025162.1
	pRY68	2,638	NZ_CP010454.1
	pDOJH10L	10,073	NC_004252.1
	pDOJH10S	3,661	NC_004253.1
	pBLO1	3,626	NC_004943.1

	p157F-NC1	4,895	NC_015053.1
	p157F-NC2	3,624	NC_015066.1
	p1-5B2	3,624	GI:822874551
	p1-5B1	3,919	GI:822874554
	p1-6B2	3,624	GI:822874529
	p1-6B1	3,919	GI:822874532
	p17-1B	3,919	GI:822874562
	p2-2B	3,624	GI:822874523
	p35B	3,624	GI:822874526
	p72B	3,624	GI:822874548
	pEK13	7,050	GI:822874540
	BLNIAS_P1	4,233	NC_017220.1
	BLNIAS_P2	6,230	NC_017222.1
B. pseudocatenulatum	p4M	4,488	NC_003527.1
B. pseudolongum subsp. Globosum	pASV479	4,815	NC_010877.1
B. sp. A24	pBIFA24	4,892	NC_010164.1

Most *Bifidobacterium* are resistant to a wide range of antibiotics, including vancomycin, gentamicin, kanamycin, streptomycin and nalidixic acid [16]. The used selection markers in *Bifidobacterium* are genes conferring resistance to spectinomycin, erythromycin, chloramphenicol, or ampicillin [17–19].

1.1.3 Expression Plasmids in *Bifidobacterium* for Cancer Gene Therapy

Based on the research of the endogenous plasmids and cloning vectors in *Bifidobacterium*, many shuttle vectors encoding target genes were constructed. Efforts are focused mainly on the following three representatives: *B. longum, B. infantis,* and *B. adolescentis* [20]. The main expression plasmids used in *Bifidobacterium* for cancer gene therapy are discussed in the following text.

1.1.3.1 Plasmid pBLES100

pBLES100, which was constructed by cloning with a *B. longum* plasmid, pTB6, and an *E. coli* vector, pBR322, has been used as an expression vector for several genes in cancer gene therapy. Yazawa *et al.* cloned a gene-encoding spectinomycin adenyltransferase AAD and the pBLES100 constructs were transferred directly into *B. longum*105-A or 108-A by electroporation. When these genetically engineered *Bifidobacterium* were introduced into tumor-bearing mice, bacteria were found only in the tumor environments [1]. Later, transformed *B. longum*105-A carrying pBLES100-AAD was also used in the gene therapy of chemically induced 7,12-dimethylbenz[a]anthracene (DMBA) rat mammary tumors. Consistent results were obtained demonstrating that transformed *B. longum* selectively colonize the tumors [2, 3].

In another study, Nakamura and colleagues constructed the plasmid pBLES100-S-eCD, which included the HU gene promoter and the gene encoding the cytosine deaminase from *E. coli* (converts the prodrug 5-fluorocytosine (5-FC) to the drug 5-fluorouracil (5-FU)). The results obtained suggest that the *B. longum* plasmid is an excellent gene delivery system and an effective candidate for enzyme/prodrug therapy [21, 22].

1.1.3.2 Plasmid pGEX-1LamdaT

Yi *et al.* successfully constructed a *B. infantis*/CD targeting the gene therapy system with a recombinant CD/pGEX-1LamdaT plasmid [23]. Experiments on the mice melanoma model showed that the tumor volume was significantly inhibited compared with controls after treatment with a combination of transfected *B. infantis* and 5-FC [24]. The engineered *B. infantis* containing the Herpes simplex virus—thymidine kinase (HSV-TK) gene was constructed by transformation of recombinant plasmid PGEX-1LamdaT [25]. Using the rat model of bladder tumors, Xiao *et al.* found that the rats treated with BI-TK/GCV group enhanced the efficacy of tumor growth compared with the normal saline control group [26]. Later, Zhou *et al.* demonstrated the efficacy and safety of the TK/GCV system for cancer therapy by intravenous administration [27].

1.1.3.3 Plasmids pBV220 and pBV22210

In our laboratory, a shuttle pBV220 was used to construct pBV220-endostatin and transformed the recombinant plasmid into *B. adolescentis* and *B. longum*. *B. adolescentis* with endostatin gene was injected into the mice bearing Heps liver cancer. After determination of the expression of endostatin, the distribution and antitumor effect of transfected *B. adolescentis* were examined. At 168 hours after the third injection of *B. adolescentis* with endostatin gene, *B. adolescentis* cells were only found in the tumor tissues (Fig. 1.1). Our research group utilized a strain of *B. longum* as a delivery system to transport an endostatin gene that can inhibit growth of a tumor. The *B. longum* strain with the endostatin gene (*B. longum*-endostatin) was taken orally by tumor-bearing nude mice through drencher preparation. The results showed that *B. longum*-endostatin could strongly inhibit the growth of solid liver tumor in nude mice and prolong the survival time of such tumor-bearing mice. Furthermore, tumor growth was inhibited more efficiently when the *B. longum*-endostatin treatment included selenium (Se-*B. longum*-En) (Fig. 1.2). Se-*B. longum*-En also could improve the activities of NK and T cells and stimulate the activity of IL-2 and TNF-α in BALB/c mice [20]. Xu *et al.* constructed a new vector pBV22210-endostatin combining a chloramphenicol resistance gene and a cryptic plasmid pMB1 from a wild type *B. longum* strain, and *B. longum*-pBV22210-endostatin exhibited higher stability and stronger inhibitory effect on H22 liver tumor growth in xenografts models than the *B. longum*-pBV220-endostatin. Our results also indicated that the plasmid electroporated into *B. longum* was maintained stable in the absence of selective antibiotics and did not significantly affect biological characteristics of *B. longum*. These results suggested that pBV22210 may be a stable vector in *B. longum* for transporting anticancer genes in cancer gene therapy [28]. Besides the above, other genes were also successfully expressed by shuttle vectors in *Bifidobacterium*.

In addition, Cronin *et al.* constructed a reporter vector pLuxMC1, which is based on the plasmid pBC1 and the *luxABCDE* operon from pPL2lux. Later, they found it stably replicated in *B. breve* UCC2003. Thus, it can track the colonization potential and persistence of this probiotic species in real time [29]. Further studies showed that the *B. breve* harboring the plasmid expressing lux fed to mice bearing tumors were readily detected specifically in tumors, by live whole-body imaging, at levels equal to administration. The reporter gene expression was visible for at least two weeks in tumors [30]. Recently, this team revealed the evidence, which furthermore underlined the significance of bioluminescent imaging and micro-computed tomography as tools to advance the application of vectors [31].

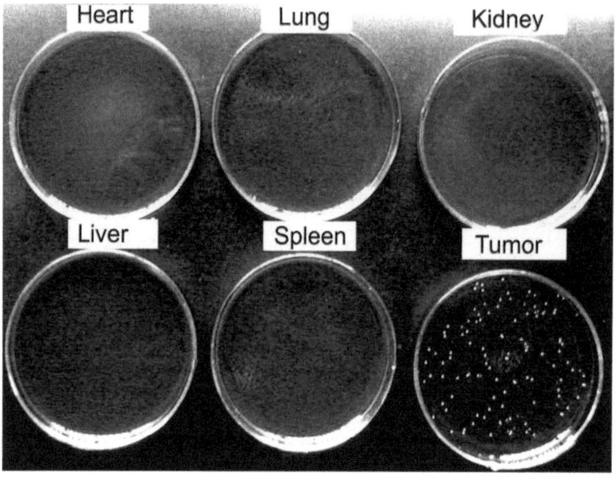

Figure 1.1 Comparison of the number of *B. adolescentis* carrying pBV220/endostatin plasmid in both tumors and normal tissues, after 68 hours of the third administration of 1 × 10^8 viable bacilli into tumor-bearing mice through tail vein for each time. After 72 hours of anaerobic cultivation, many colonies of *B. adolescentis* carrying pBV220/endostatin plasmid were observed in the tumor, but no colonies were found in normal tissues. Adapted from Ref. [52].

In another report, Guglielmetti *et al.* transformed the human intestinal bacterium *B. longum* with a vector (pGBL8b) containing the insect luciferase gene. The bioluminescent *B. longum* was used to test the efficacy of different carbohydrates to preserve cell physiology under acidic conditions. The results showed that bioluminescent *B. longum* harboring the pGBL8b plasmid is a valuable tool to study the physiological state of anaerobic bacterial cells under different environmental conditions [32].

Many studies have successfully constructed expression plasmids in *Bifidobacterium*, including those not for anticancer [33, 34]. But the accumulating evidence indicates the stability and expression level of these shuttle vectors, and the vectors were useful for further research and application of *Bifidobacterium* in cancer gene therapy.

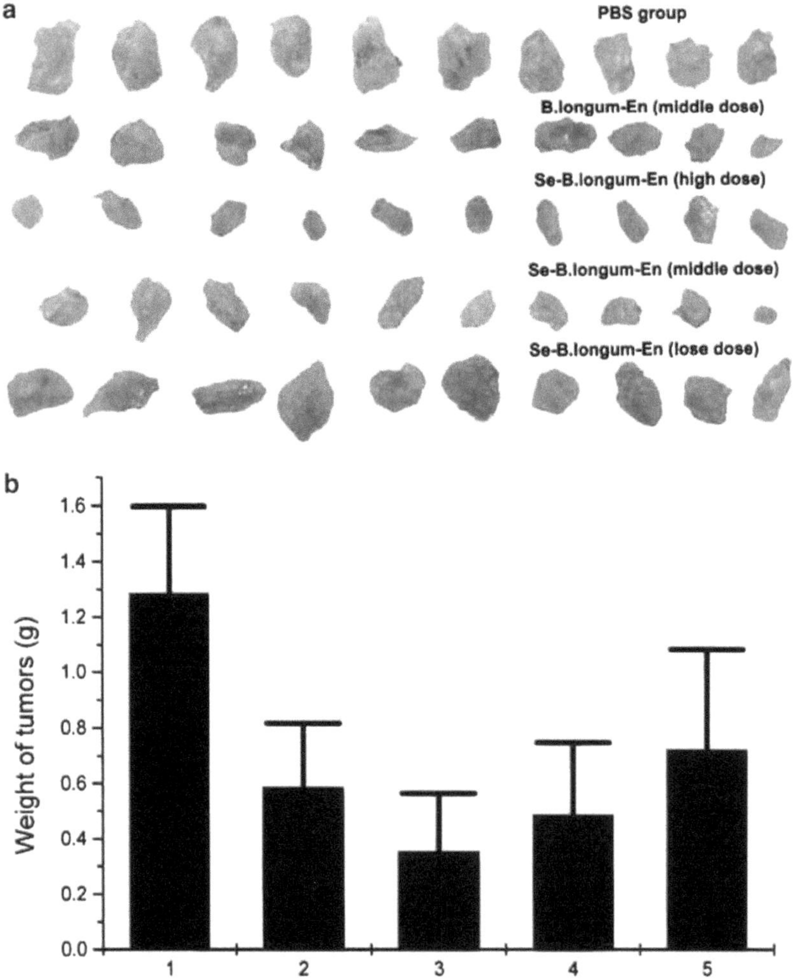

Figure 1.2 (a) Photograph of tumors excised from the mice of a control group (top row), *B. longum*-endostatin group (middle dose, second row), Se-*B. longum*-endostatin (high dose, third row), Se-*B. longum*-endostatin (middle dose, fourth row) and with Se-*B. longum*-endostatin (low dose, bottom row). (b) Average tumor weights in different treatment groups. Bar 1 was weight of control group, bars 2–5 were the weight of tumors orally treated with *B. longum*-endostatin (middle dose), Se-*B. longum*-endostatin (high dose, $p < 0.001$), Se-*B. longum*-endostatin (middle dose, $p < 0.01$), and Se-*B. longum*-endostatin (low dose, $p < 0.01$), respectively. Adapted from Ref. [20].

1.2 The Anticancer Mechanism of *Bifidobacterium* as an Oral Delivery System for Cancer Gene Therapy

1.2.1 Oral Administration of *Bifidobacterium* Affects the Immune System

The relationship between the immune system and human cancer is dynamic and extremely complex [35, 36]. Sivan *et al.* provided strong evidence in the role of *Bifidobacterium* in driving antitumor immune responses in a mouse model of melanoma [37]. Oral administration of a mixture of *Bifidobacterium* species to mice displayed reduced tumor growth in comparison with their non-*Bifidobacterium* treated counterparts, which was accompanied by increasing tumor-infiltrating SIY-specific CD8+ T cells. Further investigations revealed that signals from *Bifidobacterium* improve dendritic cell (DC) activation, which leads to improved antigen presentation to, and activation of, CD8+ T cells [38]. Moreover, cell wall preparation (whole peptidoglycan, or WPG) and exopolysaccharides derived from *Bifidobacterium* strains have been shown to exert anticancer effects attributed to the increased expression of several cytokines, such as IL-1β, IL-6, IL-10, IFN-α, and TNF-α [39, 40].

1.2.2 Oral Administration of *Bifidobacterium* Modulates Gut Microbial Community

Recent research has discovered that commensal bacteria affect optimal response to cancer therapy through modulating the tumor microenvironment, which emphasizes the importance of the microbiota in the outcome of cancer treatment [41]. Sivan *et al.* have shown that mice from two vendors tend to exhibit different tumor growth. This difference was abrogated upon a cohousing period, suggesting that differential gut microbiota may contribute to this difference. In fact, a fecal microbiota transplantation has been shown to protect the mice by delaying the growth of the tumors [37]. Other studies showed that supplementation with the *B. longum* BB536 strain altered gut luminal biotin and butyrate metabolism through a modification of the gut microbial community [42].

What in the preceding information indicates that the commensal bacteria, specifically *Bifidobacterium*, may affect cancer treatment in a positive way through modulating the gut microbial community?

1.2.3 Oral Administration of *Bifidobacterium* Affects Cancer Cell Signal Transduction

The growth factors relating to cancers can regulate cancer cell growth, differentiation, death, apoptosis and blood vessel formation. Overall, these factors promote different biological functions through connection and activation of specific ligands in the surface of the cancer cells [23, 43]. Jiang *et al.* found that the WPG of *Bifidobacterium* regulates the concentration of Ca^{2+} in Lovo cancer cells, thereby inhibiting cancer cell growth and inducing cancer cell differentiation to mature cells [44]. In another study, Kim *et al.* found that *B. lactis* decreased AOM-induced carcinogenesis by the inhibition of I*k*B-*α* degradation *in vivo* and a suppression of NF-*k*B activation, including NF-*k*B binding activity and NF-*k*B-dependent reporter gene expression [45].

1.3 The Application of *Bifidobacterium* as a Delivery System of Functional Genes for Cancer Therapy

1.3.1 *Bifidobacterium* as a Delivery System of Functional Genes for Cancer Gene Therapy

In recent years, gene therapy in solid tumors that targets gene expression to hypoxic tumor cells is currently being investigated [46]. However, a crucial obstacle in cancer gene therapy is the specific targeting of therapy directly to a solid tumor, and lack of specificity of current delivery systems. As already mentioned, *Bifidobacterium* can selectively germinate and grow in the hypoxic regions of solid tumors after intravenous injection. In view of the tumor specificity of *Bifidobacterium*, it could be used as a specific gene delivery vector for anticancer gene therapy. Until now, many efforts have made to apply *Bifidobacterium* to carry different anticancer genes for better cancer gene therapy (Table 1.2).

Table 1.2 Expression plasmids of vector-mediated cancer gene therapies in *Bifidobacterium*

Function genes	Strain	Plasmid	Replicon	Promoter	Model	Ref.
Tumstatin	*B. longum*	pBBADs	—	—	CT26 mouse colon cancer	[47]
HSV-TK/GCV suicide gene	*B. infantis*	pGEX-1λT	—	—	Bladder cancer	[25]
Soluble kinase insert domain receptor (sKDR)	*B. infantis*	pTRKH2-PsT	—	—	Lewis lung cancer	[48]
soluble Flt (sFlt-1)	*B. infantis*	pTRKH2-PsT	—	—	Lewis lung cancer	[49]
Granulocyte colony stimulating factor (GCSF)	*B. longum*	pBV22210	pMB1	$\lambda P_R P_L$	H22 and S180	[50]
TRAIL	*B. longum*	pBV22210	pMB1	$\lambda P_R P_L$	S180	[51]
Endostatin	*B. longum*	pBV22210	pMB1	$\lambda P_R P_L$	Heps mouse Liver cancer	[52]
Cytosine deaminase/ 5-fluorocyto-sine (CD/5-FC)	*B. infantis*	pBLES100	pTB6	P_{hup}	Melanoma	[22]
Spectin omycin Adenyltransferase (AAD)	*B. longum*	pBLES100	pTB6	P_{hup}	Mammary cancer	[3]

In our lab, pBV22210 encoding the extracellular domain of tumor necrosis factor-related apoptosis-inducing ligand (TRAIL) was electroporated into *B. longum* (*B. longum*-TRAIL) [51, 53]. The growth curve of *B. longum*-TRAIL and wild-type *B. longum* was similar in TPY medium without selective pressure while the lag phase of *B. longum*-TRAIL in selective medium was statistically longer than that in the nonselective medium as shown in Fig. 1.3. Both *B. longum* in TPY medium without chloramphenicol grew to an exponential phase after 6 h and stationary phase (OD 600 = 1.1) after 10 h of incubation. However, *B. longum*-TRAIL cells in TPY medium with chloramphenicol (5 μg/ml) grew to an exponential phase after 15 h and stationary phase after 18 h of incubation (Fig. 1.4).

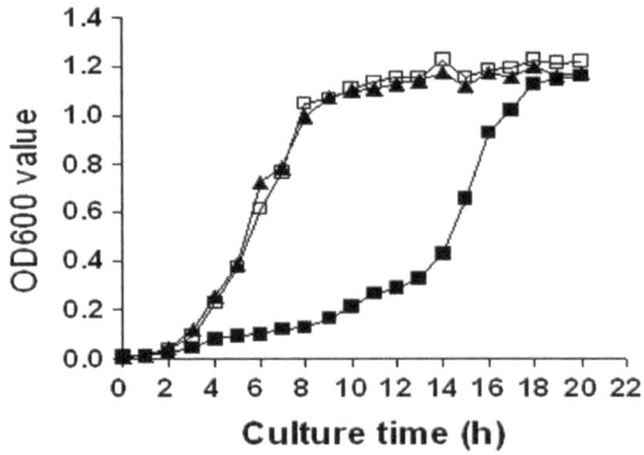

Figure 1.3 The growth curves of *B. longum*-TRAIL and wild-type *B. longum* cells. *B. longum*-TRAIL cells were incubated anaerobically at 37°C in TPY medium with 5 μg/ml chloramphenicol (filled squares) or without chloramphenicol (filled triangles). Wild-type *B. longum* was incubated anaerobically in TPY medium without selective pressure (open squares). (OD 600, optical density at 600 nm). Adapted from Ref. [51].

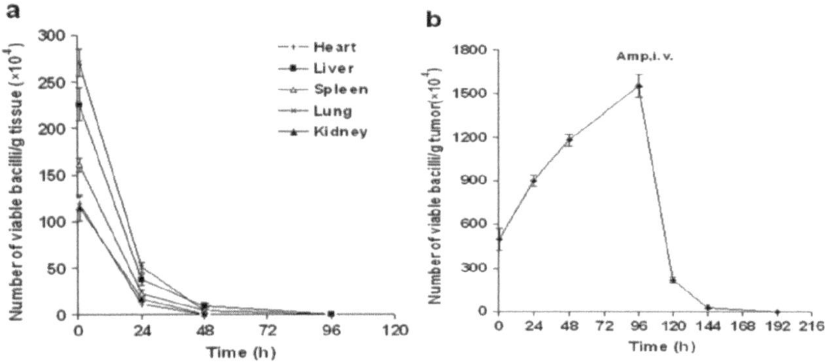

Figure 1.4 Viable bacilli number of *B. longum*-TRAIL in tumors and normal organs of treated mice. (a) shows the distribution of *B. longum*-TRAIL in different normal organs at different times after the third injection of 1 × 10^8 viable bacilli. (b) shows the viable bacilli number in tumors after administration of ampicillin (50 mg/kg) following the treatment of *B. longum*-TRAIL cells. Adapted from Ref. [51].

After 72 h of subcutaneous inoculation with S180 cells, tumor-bearing mice were intravenously injected with *B. longum*-TRAIL cells. Tumor-bearing mice were sacrificed at 1, 24, 48, and 96 hours after the third injection of *B. longum*-TRAIL cells and the location of transformed *B. longum* in tumors and several normal tissues were detected. Other mice were sacrificed at 24, 48, and 96 h after an additional injection of ampicillin at 96 h following the treatment of *B. longum*-TRAIL cells and the presence of transformed *B. longum* in tumors was detected. At 96 h, about 1.55×10^7 bacilli/g tumor tissue was found, but few bacilli were detected in normal tissues such as the heart, liver, spleen, lung, and kidney from the tumor-bearing mice. The increasing number of bacilli in tumor suggested that the transformed *B. longum* selectively proliferated in the tumor tissue. In contrast, the number of transformed *B. longum* in normal tissues decreased rapidly 24 h after injection, indicating that transformed *B. longum* did not germinate in normal tissues. Interestingly, the number of transformed *B. longum* located in the tumor decreased rapidly after an additional treatment of ampicillin, and few viable bacilli were detected in tumor 96 h after the administration of ampicillin (Fig. 1.4) [51].

Compared to the dextrose-saline solution group, combined treatment with *B. longum*-TRAIL and *B. longum*-endostatin significantly suppressed tumor in weight by 79.6% ($p = 0.0034$) and in volume by 82.6% ($p = 0.001$); *B. longum*-TRAIL alone by 58.0% ($p = 0.006$) and by 60.9% ($p = 0.0038$); *B. longum*-endostatin alone by 55.3% ($p = 0.0074$) and by 58.1% ($p = 0.0037$), and CTX by 63.4% ($p = 0.0051$) and by 65.1% ($p = 0.0026$), respectively. Compared with wild-type *B. longum*, the combination group inhibited the tumor growth in tumor weight by 73.6% ($p = 0.0077$) and in tumor volume by 76.7% ($p = 0.0006$) while *B. longum*-TRAIL alone respectively by 45.6% ($p = 0.0229$) and by 47.7% ($p = 0.0059$) and *B. longum*-endostatin alone respectively by 42.1% ($p = 0.0299$) and by 40.0% ($p = 0.0074$) [50, 53]. Based on these results, we could conclude that the combination of *B. longum*-TRAIL and *B. longum*-endostatin showed synergistic interactions and had a stronger inhibitive effect on tumor growth than either *B. longum*-TRAIL or *B. longum*-endostatin alone (Fig. 1.5). In addition, when low dosage of Adriamycin (5 mg/kg) or *B. longum*-endostatin was combined, the antitumor effect was significantly enhanced. The successful inhibition of S180 tumor growth suggests a stable vector in *B. longum* for transporting anticancer genes and combined with low dose chemotherapeutic drugs or other target genes is a promising approach in cancer gene therapy [51].

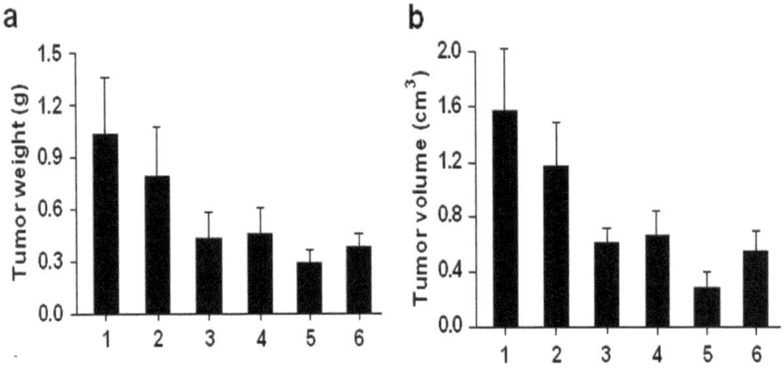

Figure 1.5 The inhibition effects on S180 tumor growth by *B. longum*-TRAIL cells and/or *B. longum*-endostatin cells in tumor-bearing mice. The tumor weights and tumor volumes were measured for each mouse. (a) shows tumor weights in different treatment groups. Row 1, dextrose-saline solution group; row 2, wide-type *B. longum* cells group; row 3, *B. longum*-endostatin cells group; row 4, *B. longum*-TRAIL cells group; row 5, *B. longum*-TRAIL cells combined with *B. longum*-endostatin cells group; row 6, CTX group. (b) shows the average tumor volume. Both tumor weights and tumor volumes were significantly reduced in *B. longum*-TRAIL cells combined with *B. longum*-endostatin cells group. Adapted from Ref. [50].

1.3.2 *Bifidobacterium* Combination with Other Factors for Synergy

Though *Bifidobacterium* is effective for tumor therapy, it can only delay the progress of cancer rather than cure the tumor completely. So in order to improve the curative effect, *Bifidobacterium* should be combined with other factors to treat the tumor together. Many combined strategies can be adopted.

1.3.2.1 Combination with radiation and chemotherapeutic drugs

Presently, the surgical treatment combined with radiation and chemotherapy is still the major approach to treat malignancies.

Chemotherapeutic approaches for cancer are in part limited by the inability of drugs to destroy neoplastic cells within poorly vascularized compartments of tumors. The poorly vascularized regions are less sensitive to ionizing radiation because its cell-killing effects depend on oxygen and they are less sensitive to chemotherapeutic drugs because drug delivery to these regions is suboptimal [54]. Radiation and chemotherapeutic drugs can kill tumor cells around the necrotic and hypoxic areas which the application of *Bifidobacterium* cannot have an effect on.

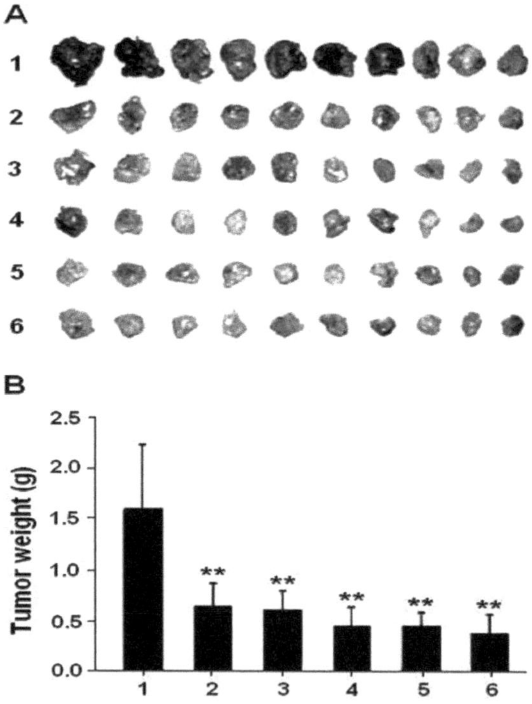

Figure 1.6 Inhibition of S180 osteosarcoma growth by combining CTX and *B. longum*-pBV22210-GCSF and/or *B. longum*-pBV22210-endostatin. Tumors excised from different groups (A). Rows 1–6 represented tumors in dextrose–saline solution, CTX, CTX + WT *B. longum*, CTX + *B. longum*-pBV22210-GCSF, CTX + *B. longum*-pBV22210-endostatin, and CTX + *B. longum*-pBV22210-GCSF + *B. longum*-pBV22210-endostatin, respectively. Tumor weights of different groups (B). Bars 1–6 showed the corresponding average weight of tumors in rows 1–6. The tumor weights were presented as mean ± S.D. (n = 10). ** indicates p < 0.01. Adapted from Ref. [50].

Besides, high dosage of many antitumor agents would have side effects. Evidence has showed that a high dose of cyclophosphamide (CTX) often leads to severe neutropenia, which greatly affect the quality of a patient's life [55]. In our previous study, *B. longum*-IL-2 could lessen the tumor size and prolong the survival time of the H22 tumor-bearing mice. In addition, when CTX or *B. longum*-endostatin, or *B. longum*-TRAIL was combined with *B. longum*-IL-2, the antitumor effect was significantly enhanced (Fig. 1.6). The survival time of mice in the combined groups of *B. longum*-endostatin or *B. longum*-TRAIL was even longer (Fig. 1.7). These results suggested that *B. longum*-IL-2 had potent antitumor effects which could be enhanced when combined with chemotherapeutic drugs or other antitumor genes [50].

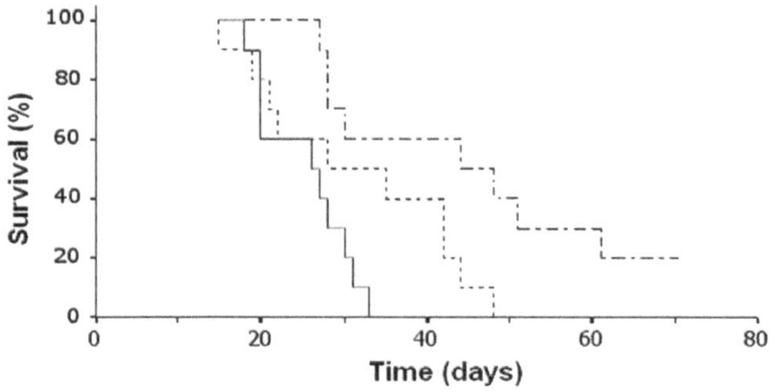

	Median	95% Confidence Interval	p
—— Control	26.00	(18.25, 33.75)	
····· CTX	28.00	(4.76, 51.24)	>0.01
–·– CTX + GCSF + Endo	44.00	(16.11, 71.89)	<0.01

Figure 1.7 Kaplan–Meier curves of survival of mice treated with CTX and two transformed *B. longums*. Mice in three groups received 5% dextrose-saline solution, CTX, and CTX + *B. longum*-pBV22210-GCSF + *B. longum*-pBV22210-endostatin, respectively. *p* values were from the Mann–Whitney test.

Bifidobacterium with functional genes can reduce the side effects and is propitious to cancer therapy. Therefore, the combination of *Bifidobacterium* with conventional chemotherapy drugs and radiation is a potential tool to destroy tumor cells more drastically [50, 53].

1.3.2.2 Combination with prebiotics

Prebiotics are those known as "a non-digestible food ingredient that beneficially affects the host by selectively stimulating the growth or activity of one or limited number of bacteria in the colon" [56]. Many studies showed that *Bifidobacterium* together with prebiotics could more effectively protect against cancer development in rats than by the administration of the two separately. Anjana Challa demonstrated that *Bifidobacterium* combined with lactulose highly suppressed azoxymethane-induced colonic aberrant crypt foci in rats [57]. Rowland *et al.* also found a synergistic antitumorigenic effect when *B. longum* was combined with inulin [58]. Besides, other combinations such as inulin-type fructans, resistant starch, lycopene, and oligofructose have inhibition effects in a synergistic manner [59–62].

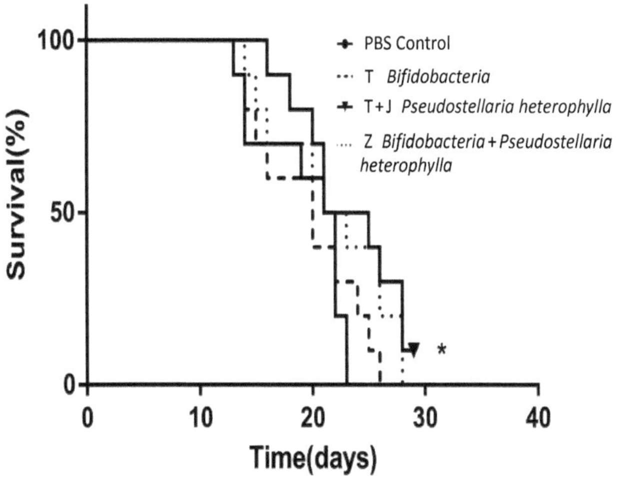

Figure 1.8 Survival curves of melanoma-bearing mice in different treatment groups. Mice in four groups received phosphate-buffered saline, *Bifidobacteria*, *Pseudostellaria heterophylla*, and *Bifidobacteria* + *Pseudostellaria heterophylla*, respectively. *p* values were from the log-rank test.

Most prebiotics mentioned above mainly belong to carbohydrates, but evidence showed that the composition of intestinal bacteria could also be regulated by traditional Chinese medicine [63]. Thus, here a potential combination is introduced, which is the extract of nature plants. Talib *et al.* have demonstrated that a combination of *Ononis hirta* and *B. longum* decreases the syngeneic mouse mammary tumor burden and enhances immune response [64]. Otherwise, our laboratory acquired the water extract of *Pseudostellaria heterophylla*, a kind of Chinese medicine, which indicates an obvious promotion of the growth of *Bifidobacterium* in the MRS medium. *B. longum* combined water extract of *Pseudostellaria heterophylla* could lessen the tumor size and prolong the survival time of melanoma-bearing mice (Fig. 1.8).

All these results indicated that combined treatment with prebiotics is more effective and safer in cancer therapy. Furthermore, the combination with extracts of nature plants, such as in Chinese medicine, may represent a new and promising synergetic combination.

1.3.2.3 Combination with trace element selenium

Selenium (Se) is an essential trace element with antioxidant properties. It has reported that it can inhibit the proliferation and invasion of tumor cells in different tumor models [65, 66]. *B. longum* has the ability to accumulate and biotransform inorganic selenium to elemental and organic forms (Se-*B. longum*) [67]. Our previous work measured the inorganic and organic Se content in a Se-*B. longum* sample. We detected SeMet in Se-*B. longum*, whereas SeCys were not detected, based on the HPLC–ICP–MS data (Fig. 1.9). SeMet was the major Se species in the Se-*B. longum* sample. The percentage of inorganic Se (IV) and Se (VI) in total Se of Se-*B. longum* was only 0.144%, whereas the percentage of SeMet was 59.55%.

Thus, enrichment of *Bifidobacterium* supplements with Se could be a way to improve the positive antitumor effect. Our laboratory found that Se-enriched *B. longum* can significantly inhibit tumor growth in a dose-effect related manner compared with the normal strain as well as stimulate the immune function more efficiently [68]. Other studies showed that selenium could be absorbed adequately by tumor-bearing mice and *B. longum* carrying pBV22210-endostatin and, enriched with selenium, have a much better antitumor effect [69]. Moreover, engineered *Bifidobacterium* with different genes can be used together for cancer treatment and the inhibition of tumors.

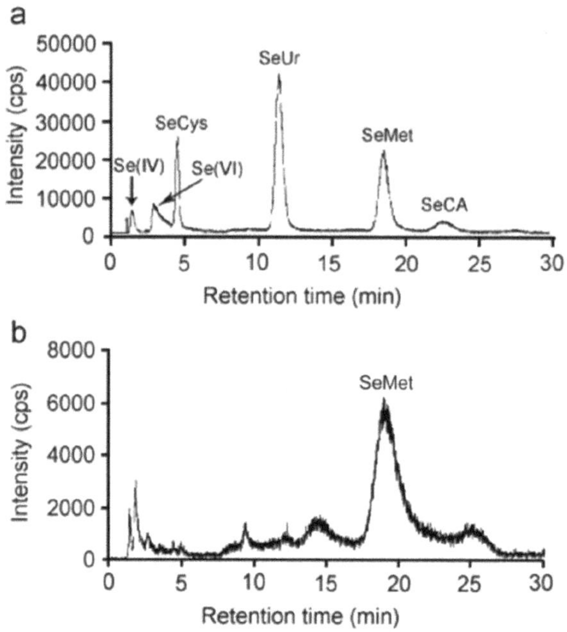

Figure 1.9 Chromatographic profiles obtained by HPLC-ICP-MS of mixture of Se standards (a) and enzymatic extraction of Se-*B. longum* (b). Isotope ^{80}Se was monitored. A peak that matched with the retention time 18 min of SeMet standard was detected, suggesting that SeMet is the major Se specie in the Se-*B. longum* sample. Adapted from Ref. [68].

In summary, the combined treatment results in the conspicuous inhibition of tumor growth more efficiently and provides a novel, selective location for advancing the treatment of cancer.

1.3.3 The New Mutagenesis Strategies for Genetic Modification of *Bifidobacterium*

There are a few reports on targeted gene inactivation in *Bifidobacterium*, although in recent years a number of techniques have been developed resulting in the successful inactivation of genes in other bacterium Table 1.3 [70]. The gold standard approach to study the role of a single gene and its products is through site-directed mutagenesis and subsequent phenotypic analysis of the generated mutants [17].

Table 1.3 Reports on Targeted Gene Inactivation in *Bifidobacterium*

Strain	Gene	Plasmid	Ref.
Single-Crossover Plasmid Insertion			
B. breve UCC2003	*galA* and *apuB*	pORI19-tet	[73]
Double-Crossover Gene Deletion			
B. longum subsp. longum NCC 2705	*BL0033*		[81]
Double Crossover Markerless Gene Deletion			
B. longum 105-A	*aga*		[83]
Temperature-Sensitive (Ts) Plasmid for Gene Disruption			
B. breve UCC2003	*apuB*		[71]
B. longum 105-A	*pyrE/BL0033*		[84]

1.3.3.1 Single-crossover plasmid insertion

This method involves the use of a non-replicative plasmid to select homologous recombination events. The first successful mutation created in a bifidobacterial strain was in the gene *apuB* using this single-crossover plasmid insertion approach whereby a combination of plasmids facilitated the conditional replication of the non-replicative plasmid pORI19 [71]. By-pass of native restriction/modification (R-M) systems and the single-crossover plasmid insertion approach, using a non-replicating plasmid, has been successfully and repeatedly employed for mutagenesis [72–80].

1.3.3.2 Double-crossover and double-crossover markerless gene deletion

Double-crossover gene disruption was first applied in *Bifidobacterium* for inactivation of an ABC-type carbohydrate transporter gene, BL0033, in *B. longum* NCC2705 [81, 82]. The non-replicative vector harbors two homologous regions of the target gene between which an antibiotic resistance gene is inserted [82].

The first two strategies leave the vector DNA or a marker gene in the mutated gene allele. Maintenance of these exogenous

DNA regions occasionally affects the gene expression of the surrounding genes of the target locus, leading to confusing results in phenotype analysis of the mutant. It also restricts the introduction of multiple mutations in the same strain due to the limited availability of the antibiotic resistance genes in *Bifidobacterium*.

The double-crossover markerless strategy's successful knock-outs were left without the antibiotic marker. Like the previous approach, a non-replicative plasmid was used for the first crossover. However, in this case the antibiotic marker was located beside the mutated targeted gene. The second crossover event occurs during long-term sub-culturing of the first crossover integrants [83].

1.3.3.3 Homologous recombination mediated by a temperature-sensitive plasmid

The temperature-sensitive (Ts) plasmid does not require high transformation efficiencies. Therefore, this would be an ideal and widely applicable approach for bifidobacterial strains [84]. The successful creation of insertion mutants using a Ts plasmid has been achieved in *B. breve* UCC2003, *B. longum* 105-A and *B. longum* NCC2705 [71, 84].

Moreover, efficient genome editing in some Gram-positive bacteria (*Clostridium cellulolyticum* [85–87], *Lactobacillus reuteri* [88], and *Streptomyces coelicolor* [89–91]) via CRISPR-Cas9 have been reported, proving the potential application value of CRISPR for genetic modification of *Bifidobacterium.*

1.4 Future Prospects

Bifidobacterium as a delivery system of functional genes for cancer gene therapy has shown immense promise over the past few years. In fact, several researchers have demonstrated encouraging results and even a human clinical trial is underway (https://clinicaltrials.gov/ct2/show/NCT01562626). However, it is still a long way from achieving the commercial use of *Bifidobacterium* as a vector for anticancer gene therapies [92].

Only a small number of *Bifidobacterium* natural plasmids have so far been characterized. There is a strong need for work with other vectors that can transfect *Bifidobacterium* with high efficiency and generate target proteins in *Bifidobacterium* with a high level. Thus, one avenue for future work is the construction of new shuttle vectors with high stability and expression levels in *Bifidobacterium*. As more and more advantages of *Bifidobacterium* have been discovered, the inborn characterization, especially molecular characterization of different *Bifidobacterium* strains, should be elucidated to select the most suitable delivery system.

Another avenue that should be explored is the combination of transformed *Bifidobacterium* carrying target genes with different anticancer mechanisms. These agents may have had cross-talk that resulted in a synergistic effect, causing massive vascular shutdowns and tumor cell apoptosis because the selective location of *Bifidobacterium* in tumors maintained a persistent expression of anticancer genes. Further work is needed to explore the potential of such combinations.

The identification of suitable selection markers and *Bifidobacterium* hosts will also be pursued. If the host-vector system is to be used in the dairy industry, it must eventually have food-grade selection markers, such as genes related to lactose metabolism and/or bacteriocin resistance.

Another strategy that can be used implies the insertion of the genes of interest into the *Bifidobacterium* chromosome. This strategy has already proved successful and has both advantages and disadvantages. One of the major advantages is the overcoming of the segregational instability of plasmids. On the other hand, one of the main drawbacks of generating such recombinant strains is the low level of expression of the genes inserted into the genome.

References

1. Yazawa K., Fujimori M., Amano J., Kano Y., Taniguchi S. *Bifidobacterium longum* as a delivery system for cancer gene therapy: Selective localization and growth in hypoxic tumors. *Cancer Gene Therapy*, 7(2) (2000) 269–274.
2. Kimura N. T., Taniguchi S., Aoki K., Baba T. Selective localization and growth of *Bifidobacterium bifidum* in mouse tumors following intravenous administration. *Cancer Research*, 40(6) (1980) 2061–2068.

3. Yazawa K., Fujimori M., Nakamura T., Sasaki T., Amano J., Kano Y., Taniguchi S. *Bifidobacterium longum* as a delivery system for gene therapy of chemically induced rat mammary tumors. *Breast Cancer Research and Treatment*, 66(2) (2001) 165–170.

4. Leahy S. C., Higgins D. G., Fitzgerald G. F., van Sinderen D. Getting better with *Bifidobacteria*. *Journal of Applied Microbiology*, 98(6) (2005) 1303–1315.

5. Reddy B. S., Rivenson A. Inhibitory effect of *Bifidobacterium longum* on colon, mammary, and liver carcinogenesis induced by 2-amino-3-methylimidazo[4,5-F]quinoline., a food mutagen. *Cancer Research*, 53(17) (1993) 3914–3918.

6. Pool-Zobel B. L., Neudecker C., Domizlaff I., Ji S., Schillinger U., Rumney C., *et al.* *Lactobacillus*- and *Bifidobacterium*-mediated antigenotoxicity in the colon of rats. *Nutrition and Cancer*, 26(3) (1996) 365–380.

7. Singh J., Rivenson A., Tomita M., Shimamura S., Ishibashi N., Reddy B. S. *Bifidobacterium longum*, a lactic acid-producing intestinal bacterium inhibits colon cancer and modulates the intermediate biomarkers of colon carcinogenesis. *Carcinogenesis*, 18(4) (1997) 833–841.

8. Klijn A., Mercenier A., Arigoni F. Lessons from the genomes of *Bifidobacteria*. *FEMS Microbiology Reviews*, 29(3) (2005) 491–509.

9. McKay L. L., Baldwin K. A., Zottola E A. Loss of lactose metabolism in lactic streptococci. *Applied Microbiology*, 23(6) (1972) 1090–1096.

10. Sgorbati B., Scardovi V., Leblanc D. J. Plasmids in the genus *Bifidobacterium*. *Journal of General Microbiology*, 128(9) (1982) 2121–2131.

11. Bottacini F., Ventura M., van Sinderen D., O'Connell Motherway M. Diversity, ecology and intestinal function of *Bifidobacteria*. *Microbial Cell Factories*, 13(Suppl 1) (2014) S4.

12. Lee J. H., O'Sullivan D. J. Genomic insights into *Bifidobacteria*. *Microbiology and Molecular Biology Reviews*, 74(3) (2010) 378.

13. Rossi M., Brigidi P., Rodriguez A. G. V. Y., Matteuzzi D. Characterization of the plasmid pMB1 from *Bifidobacterium longum* and its use for shuttle vector construction. *Research in Microbiology*, 147(3) (1996) 133–143.

14. Rossi M., Brigidi P., Matteuzzi D. An efficient transformation system for *Bifidobacterium* spp. *Letters in Applied Microbiology*, 24(1) (1997) 33–36.

15. Park M. S., Shin D. W., Lee K. H., Ji G. E. Sequence analysis of plasmid pKJ50 from *Bifidobacterium longum*. *Microbiology*, 145(Pt 3) (1999) 585–592.

16. Charteris W. P., Kelly P. M., Morelli L., Collins J. K. Antibiotic susceptibility of potentially probiotic *Bifidobacterium* isolates from the human gastrointestinal tract. *Letters in Applied Microbiology*, 26(5) (1998) 333–337.

17. Sun Z., Baur A., Zhurina D., Yuan J., Riedel C. U. Accessing the inaccessible: Molecular tools for *Bifidobacteria*. *Applied and Environmental Microbiology*, 78(15) (2012) 5035–5042.

18. Delgado S., Florez A. B., Mayo B. Antibiotic susceptibility of *Lactobacillus* and *Bifidobacterium* species from the human gastrointestinal tract. *Current Microbiology*, 50(4) (2005) 202–207.

19. Kheadr E., Dabour N., Le Lay C., Lacroix C., Fliss I. Antibiotic susceptibility profile of *Bifidobacteria* as affected by oxgall, acid, and hydrogen peroxide stress. *Antimicrobial Agents and Chemotherapy*, 51(1) (2007) 169–174.

20. Fu G. F., Li X., Hou Y. Y., *et al.* Bifidobacterium longum as an oral delivery system of endostatin for gene therapy on solid liver cancer. *Cancer Gene Therapy*, 12 (2005) 133–140.

21. Nakamura T., Sasaki T., Fujimori M., Yazawa K., Kano Y., Amano J., *et al.* Cloned cytosine deaminase gene expression of *Bifidobacterium longum* and application to enzyme/pro-drug therapy of hypoxic solid tumors. *Bioscience, Biotechnology, and Biochemistry*, 66(11) (2002) 2362–2366.

22. Sasaki T., Fujimori M., Hamaji Y., Hama Y., Ito K., Amano J., *et al.* Genetically engineered *Bifidobacterium longum* for tumor-targeting enzyme-prodrug therapy of autochthonous mammary tumors in rats. *Cancer Science*, 97(7) (2006) 649–657.

23. Ma Y. P., Luo Y. L., Huang X. P., Song F. Z., Liu G. L. Construction of *Bifidobacterium infantis* as a live oral vaccine that expresses antigens of the major fimbrial subunit (CfaB) and the b subunit of heat-labile enterotoxin (LTB) from enterotoxigenic *Escherichia coli*. *Microbiology*, 158 (2012) 498–504.

24. Yi C., Huang Y., Guo Z. Y., Wang S. R. Antitumor effect of cytosine deaminase/5-fluorocytosine suicide gene therapy system mediated by *Bifidobacterium infantis* on melanoma. *Acta Pharmacologica Sinica*, 26(5) (2005) 629–634.

25. Tang W., He Y., Zhou S., Ma Y., Liu G. A novel *Bifidobacterium infantis*–mediated TK/GCV suicide gene therapy system exhibits antitumor

activity in a rat model of bladder cancer. *Journal of Experimental & Clinical Cancer Research*, 28 (2009) 155–162.

26. Xiao X., Jin R., Li J., Bei Y., Wei T. The antitumor effect of suicide gene therapy using *Bifidobacterium infantis*-mediated herpes simplex virus thymidine kinase/ganciclovir in a nude mice model of renal cell carcinoma. *Urology*, 84(4) (2014) 982.e15–e20.
27. Yin X., Yu B., Tang Z., He B., Ren J., Xiao X., *et al.* *Bifidobacterium infantis*-mediated HSV-TK/GCV suicide gene therapy induces both extrinsic and intrinsic apoptosis in a rat model of bladder cancer. *Cancer Gene Therapy*, 20(2) (2013) 77–81.
28. Xu Y. F., Zhu L. P., Hu B., Fu G. F., Zhang H. Y., Wang J. J., *et al.* A new expression plasmid in *Bifidobacterium longum* as a delivery system of endostatin for cancer gene therapy. *Cancer Gene Therapy*, 14(2) (2007) 151–157.
29. Cronin M., Sleator R. D., Hill C., Fitzgerald G. F., van Sinderen D. Development of a luciferase-based reporter system to monitor *Bifidobacterium breve* UCC2003 persistence in mice. *BMC Microbiology*, 8 (2008) 161.
30. Cronin M., Morrissey D., Rajendran S., El MashadS. M., van Sinderen D., O'Sullivan G. C., *et al.* Orally administered *Bifidobacteria* as vehicles for delivery of agents to systemic tumors. *Molecular Therapy*, 18(7) (2010) 1397–1407.
31. Cronin M., Akin A. R., Collins S. A., Meganck J., Kim J. B., Baban C. K., *et al.* High resolution *in vivo* bioluminescent imaging for the study of bacterial tumour targeting. *PLOS One*, 7(1) (2012) e30940.
32. Guglielmetti S., Ciranna A., Mora D., Parini C., Karp M. Construction, characterization and exemplificative application of bioluminescent *Bifidobacterium longum* biovar longum. *International Journal of Food Microbiology*, 124(3) (2008) 285–290.
33. Park M. S., Kwon B., Shim J. J., Huh C. S., Ji G. E. Heterologous expression of cholesterol oxidase in *Bifidobacterium longum* under the control of 16s rRNA gene promoter of *Bifidobacteria*. *Biotechnology Letters*, 30(1) (2008) 165–172.
34. Reyes Escogido M. L., De Leon Rodriguez A., Barba de la Rosa A. P. A novel binary expression vector for production of human IL-10 in *Escherichia coli* and *Bifidobacterium longum*. *Biotechnology Letters*, 29(8) (2007) 1249–1253.
35. Mellman I., Coukos G., Dranoff G. Cancer immunotherapy comes of age. *Nature*, 480(7378) (2011) 480–489.

36. Alderton G K. Tumour immunology: Intestinal bacteria are in command. *Nature reviews*, 16(1) (2016) 4.
37. Sivan A., Corrales L., Hubert N., Williams J. B., Aquino-Michaels K., Earley Z. M., *et al.* Commensal *Bifidobacterium* promotes antitumor immunity and facilitates anti-PD-L1 efficacy. *Science*, 350(6264) (2015) 1084–1089.
38. Snyder A., Pamer E., Wolchok J. Could microbial therapy boost cancer immunotherapy? *Science*, 350(6264) (2015) 1031–1032.
39. Wu M. H., Pan T. M., Wu Y. J., Chang S. J., Chang M. S., Hu C. Y. Exopolysaccharide activities from probiotic *Bifidobacterium*: Immunomodulatory effects (on J774A.1 macrophages) and antimicrobial properties. *International Journal of Food Microbiology*, 144(1) (2010) 104–110.
40. Sekine K., Ohta J., Onishi M., Tatsuki T., Shimokawa Y., Toida T., *et al.* Analysis of antitumor properties of effector cells stimulated with a cell wall preparation (WPG) of *Bifidobacterium infantis*. *Biological & Pharmaceutical Bulletin*, 18(1) (1995) 148–153.
41. Iida N., Dzutsev A., Stewart C. A., Smith L., Bouladoux N., Weingarten R. A., *et al.* Commensal bacteria control cancer response to therapy by modulating the tumor microenvironment. *Science*, 342(6161) (2013) 967–970.
42. Sugahara H., Odamaki T., Fukuda S., Kato T., Xiao J. Z., Abe F., *et al.* Probiotic *Bifidobacterium longum* alters gut luminal metabolism through modification of the gut microbial community. *Scientific Reports*, 5(2015) 13548.
43. Yarden Y., Sliwkowski M. X. Untangling the ErbB signalling network. *Nature Reviews Molecular Cell Biology*, 2(2) (2001) 127–137.
44. Jiang H. Differentiation inducing effect of *Bifidobacterial* surface molecules on human colonic cancer cells. *Chinese Journal of Microbiology & Immunology*, 21(2) (2001) 186–190.
45. Kim S. W., Kim H. M., Yang K. M., Kim S. A., Kim S. K., An M. J., *et al.* *Bifidobacterium lactis* inhibits NF-κB in intestinal epithelial cells and prevents acute colitis and colitis-associated colon cancer in mice. *Inflammatory Bowel Diseases*, 16(9) (2010) 1514–1525.
46. Dachs G. U., Patterson A. V., Firth J. D., Ratcliffe P. J., Townsend K. M., Stratford I. J., *et al.* Targeting gene expression to hypoxic tumor cells. *Nature Medicine*, 3(5) (1997) 515–520.
47. Wei C., Xun A. Y., Wei X. X., Yao J., Wang J. Y., Shi R. Y., *et al.* *Bifidobacteria* expressing tumstatin protein for antitumor therapy in tumor-

bearing mice. *Technology in Cancer Research & Treatment*, 15(3) (2016) 498–508.

48. Li Z. J., Zhu H., Ma B. Y., Zhao F., Mao S. H., Liu T. G., *et al.* Inhibitory effect of *Bifidobacterium infantis*-mediated sKDR prokaryotic expression system on angiogenesis and growth of lewis lung cancer in mice. *BMC Cancer*, 12 (2012) 155–166.

49. Zhu H., Li Z., Mao S., Ma B., Zhou S., Deng L., *et al.* Antitumor effect of sFlt-1 gene therapy system mediated by *Bifidobacterium infantis* on Lewis lung cancer in mice. *Cancer Gene Therapy*, 18(12) (2011) 884–896.

50. Zhu L. P., Yin Y., Xing J., Li C., Kou L., Hu B., *et al.* Therapeutic efficacy of *Bifidobacterium longum*-mediated human granulocyte colony-stimulating factor and/or endostatin combined with cyclophosphamide in mouse-transplanted tumors. *Cancer Science*, 100(10) (2009) 1986–1990.

51. Hu B., Kou L., Li C., Zhu L. P., Fan Y. R., Wu Z. W., *et al. Bifidobacterium longum* as a delivery system of trail and endostatin cooperates with chemotherapeutic drugs to inhibit hypoxic tumor growth. *Cancer Gene Therapy*, 16(8) (2009) 655–663.

52. Li X., Fu G. F., Fan Y. R., Liu W. H., Liu X. J., Wang J. J., *et al. Bifidobacterium adolescentis* as a delivery system of endostatin for cancer gene therapy: selective inhibitor of angiogenesis and hypoxic tumor growth. *Cancer Gene Therapy*, 10(2) (2003) 105–111.

53. Yin Y., Kou L., Wang J. J., Xu G. X. Therapeutic efficacy of *Bifidobacterium longum*-mediated human interleukin-2 with endostatin or trail in transplanted tumors in mice. *Experimental and Therapeutic Medicine*, 3(3) (2012) 481–486.

54. Dang L. H., Bettegowda C., Huso D. L., Kinzler K. W., Vogelstein B. Combination bacteriolytic therapy for the treatment of experimental tumors. *Proceedings of the National Academy of Sciences of the United States of America*, 98(26) (2001) 15155–15160.

55. Slavin R. E., Millan J. C., Mullins G. M. Pathology of high dose intermittent cyclophosphamide therapy. *Human Pathology*, 6(6) (1975) 693–709.

56. Schrezenmeir J., de Vrese M. Probiotics, prebiotics, and synbiotics–approaching a definition. *The American Journal of Clinical Nutrition*, 73(2 Suppl) (2001) 361S–364S.

57. Challa A., Rao D. R., Chawan C. B., Shackelford L. *Bifidobacterium longum* and lactulose suppress azoxymethane-induced colonic aberrant crypt foci in rats. *Carcinogenesis*, 18(3) (1997) 517–521.

58. Rowland I. R., Rumney C. J., Coutts J. T., Lievense L. C. Effect of *Bifidobacterium longum* and inulin on gut bacterial metabolism and carcinogen-induced aberrant crypt foci in rats. *Carcinogenesis*, 19(2) (1998) 281–285.

59. Le Leu R. K., Hu Y., Brown I. L., Woodman R. J., Young G. P. Synbiotic intervention of *Bifidobacteriumlactis* and resistant starch protects against colorectal cancer development in rats. *Carcinogenesis*, 31(2) (2010) 246–251.

60. Pool-Zobel B L. Inulin-type fructans and reduction in colon cancer risk: Review of experimental and human data. *The British Journal of Nutrition*, 93(Suppl 1)(2005) S73–S90.

61. Femia A. P., Luceri C., Dolara P., Giannini A., Biggeri A., Salvadori M., *et al.* Antitumorigenic activity of the prebiotic inulin enriched with oligofructose in combination with the probiotics *lactobacillus* rhamnosus and *Bifidobacterium lactis* on azoxymethane-induced colon carcinogenesis in rats. *Carcinogenesis*, 23(11) (2002) 1953–1960.

62. Dias M. C., Vieiralves N. F. L., Gomes M. I. F. V., Salvadori D. M. F., Rodrigues M. A. M., Barbisan L. F. Effects of lycopene, synbiotic and their association on early biomarkers of rat colon carcinogenesis. *Food and Chemical Toxicology*, 48(3) (2010) 772–780.

63. Zhang Y. J., Li S., Gan R. Y., Zhou T., Xu D. P., Li H. B. Impacts of gut bacteria on human health and diseases. *International Journal of Molecular Sciences*, 16(4) (2015) 7493–7519.

64. Talib W. H., Mahasneh A. M. Combination of ononis hirta and *Bifidobacterium longum* decreases syngeneic mouse mammary tumor burden and enhances immune response. *Journal of Cancer Research and Therapeutics*, 8(3) (2012) 417–423.

65. Menter D. G., Sabichi A. L., Lippman S. M. Selenium effects on prostate cell growth. *Cancer Epidemiology, Biomarkers & Prevention*, 9(11) (2000) 1171–1182.

66. Sanmartin C., Plano D., Sharma A. K., Palop J. A. Selenium compounds, apoptosis and other types of cell death: An overview for cancer therapy. *International Journal of Molecular Sciences*, 13(8) (2012) 9649–9672.

67. Pophaly S. D., Poonam Singh P., Kumar H., Tomar S. K., Singh R. Selenium enrichment of lactic acid bacteria and *Bifidobacteria*: A functional food perspective. *Trends Food Science Technology*, 39(2) (2014) 135–145.

68. Yin Y., Wang R. R., Wang Y., Wang J. J., Xu G. X. Preparation of selenium-enriched *Bifidobacterium longum* and its effect on tumor

growth and immune function of tumor-bearing mice. *Asian Pacific Journal of Cancer Prevention: APJCP*, 15(8) (2014) 3681–3686.

69. Yin Y., Wang Q. X., Chen X., Xing J., Fan Y. R., Wu Z. W., *et al.* Antitumor efficacy of *Bifidobacterium longum* carrying endostatin gene enriched with selenium and the distribution of selenium. *African Journal of Microbiology Research*, 5(31) (2011) 5615–5621.
70. O'Callaghan A., van Sinderen D. *Bifidobacteria* and their role as members of the human gut microbiota. *Front Microbiology*, 7 (2016) 925.
71. O'Connell Motherway M., Fitzgerald G. F., Neirynck S., Ryan S., Steidler L., van Sinderen D. Characterization of apub, an extracellular type ii amylopullulanase from *Bifidobacterium breve* UCC2003. *Applied and Environmental Microbiology*, 74(20) (2008) 6271–6279.
72. O'Connell Motherway M., Zomer A., Leahy S. C., Reunanen J., Bottacini F., Claesson M. J., *et al.* Functional genome analysis of *Bifidobacterium breve* UCC2003 reveals type IVb tight adherence (Tad) pili as an essential and conserved host-colonization factor. *Proceedings of the National Academy of Sciences of the United States of America*, 108(27) (2011) 11217–11222.
73. O'Connell Motherway M., O'Driscoll J., Fitzgerald G. F., Van Sinderen D. Overcoming the restriction barrier to plasmid transformation and targeted mutagenesis in *Bifidobacterium breve* UCC2003. *Microbial Biotechnology*, 2(3) (2009) 321–332.
74. O'Connell Motherway M., Kinsella M., Fitzgerald G. F., van Sinderen D. Transcriptional and functional characterization of genetic elements involved in galacto-oligosaccharide utilization by *Bifidobacterium breve* UCC2003. *Microbial Biotechnology*, 6(1) (2013) 67–79.
75. O'Connell K. J., Motherway M. O., Liedtke A., Fitzgerald G. F., Paul Ross R., Stanton C., *et al.* Transcription of two adjacent carbohydrate utilization gene clusters in *Bifidobacterium breve* UCC2003 is controlled by laci- and repressor open reading frame kinase (ROK)-type regulators. *Applied and Environmental Microbiology*, 80(12) (2014) 3604–3614.
76. Fouhy F., O'Connell Motherway M., Fitzgerald G. F., Ross R. P., Stanton C., van Sinderen D., *et al.* In silico assigned resistance genes confer *Bifidobacterium* with partial resistance to aminoglycosides but not to beta-lactams. *PLOS One*, 8(12) (2013) e82653.
77. Egan M., O'Connell Motherway M., Ventura M., van Sinderen D. Metabolism of sialic acid by *Bifidobacterium breve* UCC2003. *Applied and Environmental Microbiology*, 80(14) (2014) 4414–4426.

78. Egan M., O'Connell Motherway M., van Sinderen D. A GntR-type transcriptional repressor controls sialic acid utilization in *Bifidobacterium breve* UCC2003. *FEMS Microbiology Letters*,362(4) (2015): doi: 10.1093/femsle/fnu056.

79. Egan M., Motherway M. O., Kilcoyne M., Kane M., Joshi L., Ventura M., van Sinderen D. Cross-feeding by *Bifidobacterium breve* UCC2003 during co-cultivation with *Bifidobacterium bifidum* PRL2010 in a mucin-based medium. *BMC Microbiology*, 14 (2014) 282–295.

80. Christiaen S. E., O'Connell Motherway M., Bottacini F., Lanigan N., Casey P. G., Huys G., *et al.* Autoinducer-2 plays a crucial role in gut colonization and probiotic functionality of *Bifidobacterium breve* UCC2003. *PLOS One*, 9(5) (2014) e98111.

81. Fukuda S., Toh H., Hase K., Oshima K., Nakanishi Y., Yoshimura K., *et al.* *Bifidobacteria* can protect from enteropathogenic infection through production of acetate. *Nature*, 469(7331) (2011) 543–547.

82. Fukiya S., Hirayama Y., Sakanaka M., Kano Y., Yokota A. Technological advances in bifidobacterial molecular genetics: Application to functional genomics and medical treatments. *Biosci Microbiota Food Health*, 31(2) (2012) 15–25.

83. Hirayama Y., Sakanaka M., Fukuma H., Murayama H., Kano Y., Fukiya S., *et al.* Development of a double-crossover markerless gene deletion system in *Bifidobacterium longum*: Functional analysis of the alpha-galactosidase gene for raffinose assimilation. *Applied and Environmental Microbiology*, 78(14) (2012) 4984–4994.

84. Sakaguchi K., He J. L., Tani S., Kano Y., Suzuki T. A targeted gene knockout method using a newly constructed temperature-sensitive plasmid mediated homologous recombination in *Bifidobacterium longum*. *Applied Microbiology and Biotechnology*, 95(2) (2012) 499–509.

85. Wang Y., Zhang Z. T., Seo S. O., Lynn P., Lu T., Jin Y. S., *et al.* Bacterial genome editing with CRISPR-Cas9: Deletion, integration, single nucleotide modification, and desirable "clean" mutant selection in *clostridium beijerinckii* as an example. *ACS Synthetic Biology*, 5(7) (2016) 721–732.

86. Wang Y., Zhang Z. T., Seo S. O., Choi K. J., Lu T., Jin Y. S., *et al.* Markerless chromosomal gene deletion in *clostridium beijerinckii* using CRISPR/Cas9 system. *Journal of Biotechnology*, 200 (2015) 1–5.

87. Xu T., Li Y., Shi Z., Hemme C. L., Li Y., Zhu Y., *et al.* Efficient genome editing in *Clostridium cellulolyticum* via CRISPR-Cas9 nickase. *Applied and Environmental Microbiology*, 81(13) (2015) 4423–4431.

88. Oh J. H., van Pijkeren J P. CRISPR-Cas9-assisted recombineering in *Lactobacillus reuteri. Nucleic Acids Research,* 42(17) (2014) e131.

89. Zeng H., Wen S., Xu W., He Z., Zhai G., Liu Y., *et al.* Highly efficient editing of the actinorhodin polyketide chain length factor gene in *Streptomyces coelicolor* M145 using CRISPR/Cas9-codA(sm) combined system. *Applied Microbiology and Biotechnology,* 99(24) (2015) 10575–10585.

90. Cobb R. E., Wang Y., Zhao H. High-efficiency multiplex genome editing of streptomyces species using an engineered CRISPR/Cas9 system. *ACS Synthetic Biology,* 4(6) (2015) 723–728.

91. Huang H., Zheng G., Jiang W., Hu H., Lu Y. One-step high-efficiency CRISPR/Cas9–mediated genome editing in streptomyces. *Acta Biochim Biophys Sin (Shanghai),* 47(4) (2015) 231–243.

92. Wei M. Q., Mengesha A., Good D., Anne J. Bacterial targeted tumour therapy-dawn of a new era. *Cancer Letters,* 259(1) (2008) 16–27.

Chapter 2

Therapy with Oncolytic *Clostridium novyi*-NT: From Mice to Men

Shibin Zhou

Ludwig Center for Cancer Genetics and Therapeutics, Sidney Kimmel Comprehensive Cancer Center, John Hopkins University School of Medicine, Baltimore, MD 21287, USA

sbzhou@jhmi.edu

Eradicating cancer cells without inflicting collateral damage is a major challenge in cancer therapy, which has prompted the recent development of a variety of targeted therapeutic approaches. Many of these approaches are aimed at proteins altered specifically in cancer cells. Several therapeutic agents have been used clinically to target oncogenes such as *ERBB2*, *EGFR*, and *BRAF* with genetic or epigenetic changes, and many more are in the pipeline [1–6]. Alternatively, unique physiological alterations at the tissue level can be exploited for targeted therapy.

2.1 Targeted Therapies at the Tissue Level

Healthy tissues maintain a blood supply through a regulated, highly efficient network of vessels that are organized hierarchically and distributed evenly to provide sufficient perfusion of oxygen and nutrients to and remove metabolic wastes from all cells in order to keep the tissues functional. In contrast, tumor vasculature

Microbial Infections and Cancer Therapy: Recent Advances
Edited by Ananda M. Chakrabarty and Arsénio M. Fialho

ISBN 978-981-4774-86-4 (Hardcover), 978-1-351-04190-4 (eBook)
www.panstanford.com

is leaky, disorganized, and preferentially localized in the periphery of an advanced solid tumor [7]. The uneven distribution of blood vessels and inefficient blood supply through the architecturally defective vessels lead to hypoxia and necrosis in the tumor [8, 9]. At the same time, the heterogenic perfusion makes a fraction of cancer cells inaccessible and/or insensitive to the chemo- and radiation therapies, thus leaving the "seeds" for future relapse [10]. Nevertheless, the aberrant tumor vasculature provides an opportunity for the development tumor tissue-selective therapeutic approaches.

One such approach exploits the so-called enhanced permeability and retention (EPR) effect, a biological phenomenon associated with the aberrant tumor vasculature [11, 12]. The histological basis for the EPR effect includes fenestrations on the vessel wall, defects generated during the development of tumor vessels, and the lack of a functional lymphatic system. These defects in the tumor vascular system allow increased permeation and retention of the macromolecular drugs or nanoparticles within an appropriate size range in the tumor parenchyma [13–16]. In contrast, the macromolecular and nanosized drug formulations are less likely to accumulate in normal tissues with a well-developed vascular system. The development of Doxil® exemplifies a successful clinical application of the EPR concept. Doxil is a PEGylated liposomal formulation of doxorubicin that has been approved by the US Food and Drug Administration (FDA) and the European Medicines Agency (EMA) for the treatment of AIDS-related Kaposi's sarcoma, recurrent ovarian cancer, metastatic breast cancer, and multiple myeloma [17]. However, the EPR effect can be highly variable among individual tumors because of the heterogeneity associated with the tumor vasculature [18], limiting the application of the macromolecular and nanosized drug formulations to a relatively small patient population.

Another approach capitalizes on the ability of certain bacterial species to colonize and proliferate in tumors with necrosis or hypoxia, conditions not found in healthy metabolically active tissues. Using bacteria to fight cancer is not a modern concept. The history goes back to the late 1800s, when Dr. William B. Coley, a surgeon at the then New York Cancer Hospital, inoculated his patients in a systematic way with cultures of the erysipelas-causing streptococcal bacteria [19, 20]. Coley hypothesized that the bacterial infection would elicit a robust anticancer immune response. This practice has earned him the reputation as a pioneer in cancer immunotherapy. The initial streptococcal inoculation and subsequent use of the famous Coley's toxins, a mixture consisting of heat-inactivated *Streptococci* and *Serratia marcescens*, generated mixed results with sporadic success and significant toxicity. The idea revived years later when a better understanding about the tumor microenvironment was achieved and recombinant DNA technology became available to generate more potent and less toxic bacterial strains by genetic engineering. Many bacterial strains (mostly anaerobic) have since shown preferential targeting of solid tumors [21–28]. Among the most investigated are various strains of *Salmonella*, *Clostridium*, and *Listeria*, some of which have been tested in clinical trials [27, 29–33]. The clinical development of live bacteria as therapeutic agents for cancer has been challenging because of potential severe toxicities associated with infection from live bacteria. One remarkable clinical success is the use of bacillus Calmette-Guérin (BCG) in the treatment of bladder cancer [34]. BCG is an attenuated live strain of *Mycobacterium bovis* originally generated as a vaccine for tuberculosis. BCG therapy by intravesical administration was first documented in the 1970s and has since become an important treatment option for transitional-cell carcinoma *in situ* of the bladder [35–37]. It is believed that BCG's therapeutic effect is mainly due to its immunomodulatory activity [38–40].

2.2 Clostridia as Live Therapeutic Agents for Cancer Therapy

Clostridia are rod-shaped anaerobic bacteria that can form endospores in an unfavorable environment [41]. They are found commonly in the soil and less frequently in intestinal and female lower reproductive tracks of humans [42–44]. The genus of *Clostridium* consists of several clinically important human pathogens, including *Clostridium difficile*, *C. botulinum*, *C. tetani*, and *C. perfringens*, which cause *Clostridium difficile* infection (CDI), botulism, tetanus, and gas gangrene, respectively.

As anaerobic bacteria, clostridia have been tested for the treatment of solid tumors since the early 20th century [45]. Parker *et al.* treated transplantable mouse fibrosarcoma and adenocarcinoma with *C. histolyticum* [46]. They hypothesized that bacterial toxins produced during the local infection established following intratumoral (IT) spore injection would lyse the tumor cells, while systemic administration of antitoxin and penicillin would help control the resulting toxemia and spreading of the infection into the surrounding healthy tissue, respectively. All of the sarcomas treated with the spores alone showed tumor lysis, but the mice died within a few days of spore administration, apparently because of infection-related toxicity. Antitoxin and penicillin somewhat protected the mice without substantially reducing the efficacy. Nevertheless, all the mice that survived infection-related toxicity eventually succumbed to tumor regrowth. The adenocarcinomas did not show regression following spore treatment, likely due to a lack of robust germination. Malmgren and Flanigan later showed that *C. tetani* spores administered intravenously germinated in both spontaneous and transplanted mouse tumors [47]. Importantly, the vegetative bacteria were confined within the tumors and germination did not take place in normal tissues.

Möse and Carey were among the first to treat human patients with clostridia [29, 48–50]. Möse and Möse of the Institute for Hygiene, University of Graz, Austria, used a *C. butyricum* strain called M55 that was later on reclassified as *C. sporogenes* ATCC 13732. In a heroic effort, they first injected themselves with the M55 spores to demonstrate the safety of systemic injection, before treating cancer patients [51]. Patients with several different tumor types, including glioblastoma, were then treated with billions of the M55 spores by injection through the internal carotid artery or a vein. Signs of germination and tumor lysis, but not complete tumor regression, were observed following spore administration. The majority of the patients seemed to tolerate the treatment well, but many patients with glioblastoma required surgical interventions to manage the brain abscess formed following clostridial infection, and occasional fatal toxic response also took place.

These and other earlier attempts demonstrated that clostridial spores can selectively germinate inside solid tumors and induce a significant therapeutic response. However, highly variable therapeutic responses among patients and substantial treatment-related toxicity hindered further clinical development. To overcome these challenges, genetic engineering approaches were employed to generate more efficacious and less toxic strains. Several engineered clostridial strains have been published, including those engineered to express prodrug-converting enzymes [52–58], tumor necrosis factor alpha (TNF-α) [59, 60], interleukin-2 (IL-2) [61], and an antibody against the hypoxia-inducible factor 1 alpha subunit (HIF1α) [62].

2.3 *C. novyi*-NT as a Live Therapeutic Agent for Cancer Therapy

2.3.1 *C. novyi*

C. novyi was first isolated in the late 19th century by Dr. Frederick G. Novy [63], a bacteriologist at the University of Michigan, and has been named *Bacillus oedematismaligni*, *B. novyi*, and *C. oedematiens* in the past. *C. novyi* is generally classified into four types on the basis of the toxins produced [64]. The type A *C. novyi* produces α-toxin [65, 66], a lethal toxin that exerts its toxic effect by inactivating GTPases of Rho family by catalyzing the covalent attachment of an *N*-acetylglucosamine moiety, leading to disruption of the actin cytoskeleton and intercellular junctions [67–70]. *In vivo*, α-toxin shows lethal and edematizing activities and is a major virulence factor for the toxic shock and gas gangrene syndromes associated with *C. novyi* infection.

Type A is the most common human pathogen among the three types of *C. novyi* [42]. In contrast, type B only occasionally causes opportunistic infection in humans [71, 72]. Type C does not produce the major toxins and is considered nonpathogenic. *C. novyi* was associated with approximately 30% of the wound-related gas gangrene cases in World War I [42]. More recently, type A *C. novyi* was identified in a major outbreak of lethal infections among injection heroin users [73–76]. Patients developed injection site infection with severe local inflammation manifested as edema, erythema, pain, and abscess formation without obvious pus. In many cases, rapid systemic deterioration leading to hypotension and cardiogenic shock followed. Notably, the purity of the heroin involved in many of the cases was high and thus the heroin required more than the usual amount of citric acid to dissolve [76, 77]. Essentially all the patients injected the drug into the skin or muscle at the site of infection, rather than into the vein. These facts led to the hypothesis that the high concentrations of citric acid had damaged the soft tissue, resulting in necrosis around the injection site, which served as a niche for *C. novyi* spores contaminating the heroin supply to germinate and start the infection.

Even though not a significant pathogen in human diseases, the type B *C. novyi* is an etiologic agent for infectious necrotic hepatitis, commonly known as "black disease," in sheep and cattle [78]. The *C. novyi* outbreaks are often associated with liver fluke endemic. The necrotic lesions caused by migration of the young flukes inside the liver provide a favorable environment for the germination of *C. novyi* spores. Thus, in both humans and animals, *C. novyi* infection seems to take place only when pre-existing hypoxic lesions are present.

2.3.2 *C. novyi*-NT

In an effort to identify additional bacterial strains with robust antitumor activities, an *in vivo* screen was carried out with 26 anaerobic bacterial strains belonging to the genera of *Bifidobacterium*, *Lactobacillus*, and *Clostridium* [79]. Individual bacterial strains were injected into mice bearing subcutaneous B16 tumors, which were later dissected for the assessment of bacterial colonization. A type A *C. novyi* strain (ATCC19402) and a *C. sordellii* strain stood out in this screen because of their ability to not only germinate robustly but also spread throughout the poorly vascularized regions of the tumor. Although no clinical side effects were observed in healthy mice injected with a large number of the *C. novyi* and *C. sordellii* spores, all tumor-bearing mice died soon after the treatment, presumably due to the lethal toxins released from the vegetative bacteria proliferating inside the tumors [80, 81]. The *C. novyi* strain was selected for further development because it carries only a single lethal toxin (α-toxin) gene located on a phage episome [66, 82, 83].

As an extrachromosomal element, the *C. novyi* phage episome can be lost randomly from the bacterial cell, which allows relatively easy isolation of *C. novyi* clones devoid of the phage. To achieve this, the *C. novyi* ATCC19402 spores were heated to 70°C for 15 min., after which the heated spores were plated on agar plates for cloning. Heating serves to inactivate any exogenous phage in the spore preparation, thus preventing the phage-free clones from being transduced again during vegetative growth on solid agar [83]. A polymerase chain reaction (PCR) was then performed on individual colonies to identify *C. novyi* clones free of the *α-toxin* gene. One such clone was named *C. novyi*-NT and chosen for subsequent characterization and development [79].

Like other type A *C. novyi* strains, *C. novyi*-NT is a gram-positive spore-forming anaerobe (Fig. 2.1). The vegetative form of *C. novyi*-NT displays multiple long flagella, likely responsible for its ability to disperse within the infected tumor. The vegetative bacteria are exquisitely sensitive to oxygen, and the spores can only germinate at an oxygen level of 0.3% or below [84]. Their extraordinary sensitivity to oxygen makes it technically challenging to deliver viable vegetative form of clostridia to solid tumors, especially when delivered through a systemic route. Therefore, suspension of bacterial spores is the preferred formulation in practice [29, 32].

The *C. novyi*-NT spore is approximately 1–1.5 μm in diameter, with a multilayered spore coat to ensure its resilience in a potentially hostile environment. Ultrastructural studies suggest that formation of the spore coat layers follows a self-assembly process similar to crystallization, which could be influenced by pH, salt concentrations, and impurities in the sporulation culture [85]. Thus, the protocol for spore manufacture should be standardized to minimize variation in the quality of spores. Mature *C. novyi*-NT spores contain mRNA enriched in those encoding proteins for biosynthesis and degradation of the spores [86]. The mRNA molecules are quite stable despite incubation of the spores at 37°C for 14 days followed by storage at 4°C for a year. The mRNA stored in spores could allow rapid synthesis of proteins that are required in the initial stage of germination. The spore-specific mRNA also includes those predicted to code for proteins with redox activity, such as glutathione peroxidase, NADPH thioredoxin reductase, and glutaredoxin. Interestingly, the genes for these proteins are organized into a single operon. Furthermore, glutathione peroxidases have been implicated as major scavengers for hydrogen peroxide and several organic hydroperoxides in other organisms [86–88]. Thus, it is tempting to speculate that the pre-existing mRNA would allow rapid reconstitution of a redox chain during germination to ensure the reduced microenvironment necessary for the survival of a nascent oxygen-sensitive vegetative bacterium.

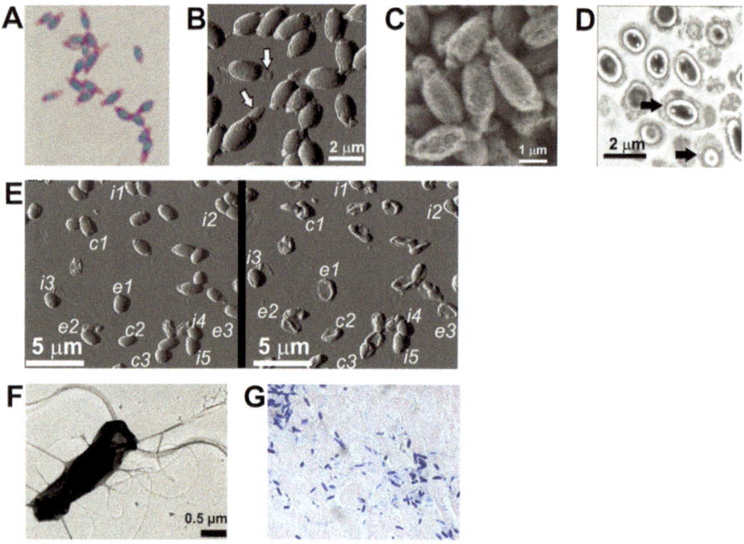

Figure 2.1 Micrographs of *C. novyi*-NT. (A) Malachite green/eosin-stained spores. (B) Atomic force micrograph (AFM) of air-dried spores. White arrows point to the "tails" also seen in (A). (C) Environmental scanning electron micrograph of wet spores. (D) Transmission election micrograph of spores. Spores are shown with a dark core and a white cortex, surrounded by amorphous shells. Black arrows indicate spores with large shells. (E) AFM amplitude images showing the same spores before (left) and 24 h after (right) exposure to the germination medium. Spores that remained intact (i1–i5) collapsed after germination (c1–c3) and had fully outgrown with only an empty spore coat left behind (e1–e3) are indicated. (F) Transmission electron micrograph of a vegetative bacterium highlighting numerous long flagella. (G) Gram-stained vegetative bacteria (1000X) in a section of an infected mouse tumor. (B–E) are reprinted from Ref. [85], Copyright 2007, American Society for Microbiology; (F) is reprinted from Ref. [127], Copyright 2003, *National Academy of Sciences*, USA; (G) is reprinted from Ref. [111], Copyright 2004, *National Academy of Sciences*, USA.

C. novyi-NT spores germinate in response to special environmental cues, such as germinants and low oxygen concentrations [89, 90]. Interestingly, heating to 70°C–80°C for 30 min. can dramatically accelerate and maximize spore germination [85]. Thermal ablative approaches, such as radiofrequency ablation (RFA), microwave ablation (MWA), and high-intensity focused ultrasound (HIFU), can create extensive necrotic lesions by inducing local hyperthermia [91–95], potentially providing an optimal condition for *C. novyi* spores to germinate. Therefore, a combination therapy with spores administered first, followed by a thermal ablative treatment could prove beneficial clinically, especially for the tumors without significant pre-existing necrosis.

C. novyi-NT has a single circular genome of 2,547,720 base pairs (bp), which is highly A+T rich, with an overall A+T content of 71.1% [86]. No extrachromosomal sequences were identified in the *C. novyi*-NT DNA, consistent with loss of the phage episome harboring the α-*toxin* gene. Among 23 published clostridial genomes, the *C. novyi*-NT genome was found most closely related to the *C. botulinum* C-Eklund genome [96]. A total of 2325 coding sequences were predicted from the *C. novyi*-NT genome, many of which are transcriptionally regulated in growth phase–specific patterns. The majority of the genes involved in basic cellular metabolism functions, such as protein and nucleic acid synthesis, are shared by other clostridial genomes [86]. Conversely, many genes for cell surface or secreted proteins, such as transporters, degrading enzymes, and sensor proteins, appear to be *C. novyi*-NT specific, implying a unique way in which *C. novyi*-NT interacts with its environment.

Among the 153 predicted cell surface–associated or secreted proteins, several are potentially cytolytic because of their ability to degrade lipids or proteins (Table 2.1) [86]. The genes for these proteins were expressed not only by vegetative *C. novyi*-NT growing *in vitro* but also by the bacteria infecting the experimental tumors. Particularly interesting are those involved in lipid degradation. Phospholipase C (PLC, γ-toxin in *C. novyi*) was expressed at very high levels in two infected experimental tumors and was found to share 61% of the amino acid identity with its homolog in *C. perfringens* (called α-toxin in *C. perfringens*), consistent with prior biochemical studies showing that the two have similar activities [97]. A *C. novyi*-NT strain with the *plc* gene inactivated by targeted insertional mutagenesis has been generated. This *plc* mutant strain has lost the ability of *β*-hemolysis (unpublished data). As the *plc* gene in *C. perfringens* encodes a major lethal toxin and is required for the virulence of this bacterium [98, 99], it will be interesting to see whether the *C. novyi*-NT *plc* mutant strain is even safer than the parental *C. novyi*-NT in the mouse tumor models. Notably, the *plc* gene and two lipase genes were among the most highly expressed in the infected tumors as per genome-wide transcriptome analysis. One of the lipases (NT01CX2047) was later shown to be able to affect the structure of the lipid bilayer and alter its permeability, making the enzyme potentially cytotoxic [100]. It is conceivable that these lipid-disrupting enzymes are largely responsible for tumor destruction by the oncolytic bacteria. This hypothesis can be tested using bacterial strains with these genes deleted.

In addition to the lipid-disrupting enzymes, a number of genes involved in fatty acid and lipid metabolism were highly expressed by *C. novyi*-NT infecting the experimental tumors [86]. As degraded biological membranes and plasma exudates can be quite abundant in the infected tissues, the metabolic pathways in *C. novyi*-NT may be shifted accordingly to adapt to a new carbon/energy source. It has been shown *in vitro* that relevant enzymes can be induced to allow bacteria to use fatty acids and glycerol as carbon/energy sources when these substrates are present in the culture medium [101, 102].

Several spore-related genes were also expressed at very high levels in the infected tumors [86]. As the spores were not injected directly into the tumors, this observation suggested that massive sporulation was taking place in the tumors. This is consistent with the result from a microbiological study that showed a 30-fold increase in the number of viable spores inside the tumor within 24 h of systemic spore administration [84]. Therefore, there appears to be a dynamic process of germination and sporulation, indicating a continued struggle of the anaerobic bacteria with their hostile environment.

Table 2.1 Extracellular degradative enzymes

Gene ID	Gene name	mRNA Abundance*						
		Early log	**Mid log**	**Late log**	**HCT116 (infected)**	**CT26 (infected)**	**HCT116 (uninfected)**	**CT26 (uninfected)**
NT01CX0021	serine protease, subtilase family	10497	16727	16861	161	154	74	47
NT01CX0560	thermolysin metallopeptidase	318	373	276	228	271	128	63
NT01CX0630	lipase	4212	7759	14830	3187	848	130	101
NT01CX0944	serine protease, subtilase family	786	527	659	272	303	121	125
NT01CX0979	phospholipase C	7419	28960	29177	5793	2191	114	155
NT01CX1195	clostridiopeptidase B	2659	13541	12452	451	236	58	92
NT01CX1544	protease/ transglutaminase	2784	12774	14905	844	271	93	140
NT01CX2047	lipase	4939	18684	20366	8047	3040	59	81

Source: Assembled with data published in Ref. [86].

*Determined by microarray analysis; values normalized across arrays.

2.4 Preclinical Studies: Toxicity Associated with *C. novyi*-NT Treatment

C. novyi-NT is substantially less toxic than its parental strain, *C. novyi* ATCC19402, in experimental tumor models. In contrast to the parental strain, which kills 100% of tumor-bearing mice within 16 h of spore administration, the vast majority of tumor-bearing mice can survive IT *C. novyi*-NT infection unless the tumors are extraordinarily large (>2000 mm^3) [84]. Nevertheless, toxicity associated with *C. novyi*-NT treatment has been routinely observed.

There are two types of toxicity, one caused by vegetative bacteria germinated inside the tumor and the other by spores themselves, which can be observed even in tumor-free animals where spores do not germinate. Even though no clinical signs of toxicity were observed when tumor-free healthy mice were injected intravenously with *C. novyi*-NT spores, histological examination revealed transient multifocal subacute hepatitis and reactive splenic hyperplasia at doses above 500 million spores/kg [84]. A biodistribution study showed that the majority of the viable spores were localized in the liver and spleen following intravenous (IV) administration. Thus, the histologic abnormalities likely signify a response of the mononuclear phagocytic system (MPS) in the liver and spleen to a large load of spores that are in the size range particularly well suited for phagocytosis [103]. Similar pathological changes were observed in tumor-free rabbits as well. These changes resolved spontaneously over time.

Clinical signs of toxicity are often seen when mice bearing large tumors are treated with spores through the IV or IT route, and the toxicity is always associated with robust germination. Both the efficacy and severity of the toxicity seem to be correlated with the tumor size: a significant therapeutic effect was observed more often in mice with larger tumors, but these animals would be more likely to die due to acute toxicity [84, 104]. The common signs of toxicity are fever, lethargy, poor grooming, loss of weight, and death (usually within five days), which are expected in a serious infection, such as a large abscess. However, it is not clear precisely what pathophysiological events lead to death in a fraction of animals with large *C. novyi*-NT-infected tumors. Regardless, toxicity can be prevented or minimized by aggressive fluid resuscitation as supportive care and administration of antibiotics, two measures often required for treating serious bacterial infections in human patients. *C. novyi*-NT is highly sensitive to a number of commonly used antibiotics, making its infection relatively easy to control. Toxicity can be minimized even when antibiotics are administered as late as 24 h after spore injection, when robust germination is already evident. However, antibiotics protect animals at the expanse of efficacy because antibiotic treatment will effectively terminate the infection before it has a chance to run its course for a complete oncolysis.

Hypoxic lesions unrelated to neoplasia, such as those found in ischemic heart and brain diseases, are naturally a safety concern for therapies using anaerobic bacteria. Atheromatous plaques and myocardial infarcts were generated in different mouse models to address this issue [84]. Mice harboring these lesions did not show any clinical toxicity after IV injection of billions of *C. novyi*-NT spores. Gram staining did not reveal any sign of bacterial colonization or germination within or around the lesions either. Interestingly, Möse and his colleagues also observed in the autopsy of a patient treated with the *C. butyricum* strain M55 that massive germination had taken place in the tumor, a bronchial carcinoma, but not in embolic kidney infarct or embolic cerebromalacia [105], providing anecdotal evidence that nonmalignant necrotic lesions may not support germination of clostridia in humans either. It is unclear why *C. novyi*-NT spores are able to germinate within the necrotic and hypoxic regions of tumors but not in the necrotic lesions not associated with a tumor. One possibility is that the oxygen levels in the atheromatous/infarcted tissues are slightly higher than in tumors, making these tissues less supportive of germination of *C. novyi*-NT, a bacterium known for its exquisite sensitivity to oxygen. In addition, unknown tumor-specific factors could make *C. novyi*-NT tolerate higher concentrations of oxygen. Vegetative bacteria have been observed not only within microinvasive lesions where necrosis was not evident but also around neoplastic vessels in glioma models [32, 106]. Alternatively, it is possible that the atheromatous and infarcted lesions are inaccessible to *C. novyi*-NT spores because the supplying vasculature around these lesions is not as chaotic and leaky as that inside a tumor.

2.5 Preclinical Studies: Therapeutic Effects

It remains unknown how systemically administered nonmotile spores are translocated into the tumor. Conceptually, spores can enter tumor parenchyma through the inherently leaky tumor endothelium, similar to circulating macromolecules and nanoparticles [107–109]. Alternatively, systemically administered spores could be phagocytosed by the phagocytic cells, which then carry them through the endothelial barrier [110]. Biodistribution studies show that only a tiny fraction of the intravenously injected spores were localized within the tumor [84], and yet, they can induce profound tumor destruction, owing to the proliferative capacity of live bacteria. A dosing study demonstrated that extensive tumor necrosis could result from an estimated 10 spores within a tumor, achieved by IV injection of ~1000 spores (unpublished data). However, at such low doses, spore germination becomes more stochastic and consequently less predictable.

Germination is a prerequisite for the therapeutic effect of *C. novyi*-NT spores. Germination usually peaks in most tumor-bearing mice within 48 h of spore administration, as evidenced by hemorrhagic necrosis in the tumor (Fig. 2.2). It often takes longer to germinate for spores directly injected into a tumor than those delivered by IV injection, perhaps because of the time needed for the oxygen dissolved in the spore solution to dissipate. In both CT26 (syngeneic mouse colorectal cancer, Fig. 2.2A) and HCT116 (human colorectal cancer xenograft, Fig. 2.2B) subcutaneous models, the tumors turn black quickly following germination as hemorrhagic necrosis progresses. The necrosis generally stops around the tumor perimeter. Histological assessment revealed swarming vegetative bacteria within the hypoxic core and a band of inflammatory cells around the tumor rim to prevent the bacteria from spreading into the surrounding normal tissue [106, 111]. Thus, the infection is essentially confined within the tumor by both normoxia and a potent local inflammatory response. Over a period of five to seven days, the black lesion would "dry out," forming a scab. Tumor is usually eradicated if the entire tumor turns black, with no viable tumor rim visible (Fig. 2.2A, top panel), which happens in approximately 30% of the treated CT26 tumors but not HCT116 xenografts. Those with a viable tumor rim or even a small nodule remaining would eventually relapse. Thus far, a robust tumor response to *C. novyi*-NT treatment resulting in cures has been observed in several tumor models, including CT26, RENCA, Panc02, VX2, and 060919 (Table 2.2). The first four syngeneic tumor models

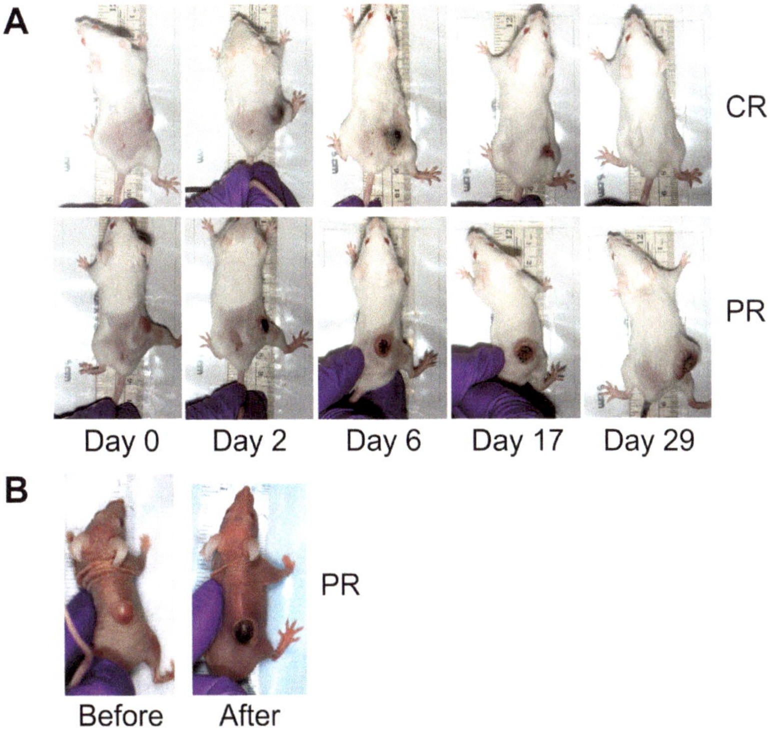

Figure 2.2 Tumor responses to *C. novyi*-NT spore treatment. (A) BALB/c mice bearing CT26 tumors. Representative mice with complete tumor response (CR, top panel) and limited response (bottom panel) are shown. Note that the tumor showing complete response turned black entirely without leaving any viable tumor rim on day 2. (B) An athymic nu/nu mouse with an HCT116 xenograft tumor that showed a partial response (PR) to the spore treatment. Before *C. novyi*-NT spore treatment; after *C. novyi*-NT spore treatment.

Table 2.2 Responses of different tumor models to *C. novyi*-NT monotherapy

Tumor model	Origin	Host	Tumor type	Transplant location	Chemically induced	Best cure rate observed	Reference
CT26	Mouse	BALB/c mouse	Colorectal	Subcutaneous	Y	~30%	[111]
RENCA	Mouse	BALB/c mouse	Renal	Subcutaneous	N	~30%	[111]
Panc02	Mouse	C57Bl/6N mouse	Pancreatic	Subcutaneous	Y	>50%	[104]
4T1	Mouse	BALB/c mouse	Breast	Subcutaneous	N	0%	Unpublished
HCT116	Human	Athymic nu/nu mouse	Colorectal	Subcutaneous	N/A	0%	[79, 122]
HT29	Human	Athymic nu/nu mouse	Colorectal	Subcutaneous	N/A	0%	[122, 127]
LS174T	Human	Athymic nu/nu mouse	Colorectal	Subcutaneous	N/A	0%	[127]
CaPan-1	Human	Athymic nu/nu mouse	Pancreatic	Subcutaneous	N/A	0%	[122]
HuCC-T1	Human	Athymic nu/nu mouse	Cholangiocarcinoma	Subcutaneous	N/A	0%	[122, 127]
F98	Rat	F344 Fisher rat	Glioblastoma	Orthotopic	Y	0%	[106]
60919	Human	Athymic nu/nu rat	Glioblastoma	Orthotopic	N	~10%	[106]
VX2	Rabbit	New Zealand white rabbit	Squamous cell carcinoma	Liver	N	~30%	[111]

showed 30%–50% cure rate. The intrahepatic transplant of VX2 is a very aggressive tumor model, often killing the rabbits within two months. A single IV injection of *C. novyi*-NT spores was able to cure 7 out of 23 tumor-bearing rabbits [111]. In contrast, some tumor models, such as the 4T1 mouse breast cancer and the HT29 human colorectal cancer xenograft, do not show extensive necrosis and consequently *C. novyi*-NT treatment has never resulted in a complete response (CR) in these models. It is worth noting that CT26 and Panc02 were both derived from tumors induced by chemical mutagenesis, thus likely harboring a large number of mutations in their genomes and being more immunogenic, whereas 4T1 was generated from a spontaneous tumor with a limited number of somatic mutations in its genome [112–115].

Different mechanisms are involved in tumor destruction by *C. novyi*-NT infection. In addition to the toxins (hemolysins, lipases, etc.) secreted by *C. novyi*-NT, the host immune system is likely to play an important role in tumor destruction as well. Immunothrombosis, a pathophysiological process in response to bacterial infection, is a mechanism employed by the infected host to compartmentalize pathogens for their containment and localized inactivation but will inevitably damage tissues nourished by the affected vessels as well [116]. This "side effect," in conjunction with the effects of proinflammatory cytokines, such as TNF-α [117, 118], may be the underlying mechanism for the hemorrhagic necrosis developed in the *C. novyi*-NT–sensitive tumors following germination. In turn, the release of large amounts of pathogen-associated molecular patterns (PAMPs), damage-associated molecular patterns (DAMPs), and tumor-associated antigens (TAAs) resulting from tumor tissue destruction provides adjuvanticity and antigenicity, two critical factors for the induction of an adaptive antitumor immune response [119, 120]. Consistent with the hypothesis that adaptive immunity plays a role in tumor eradication, cures have been rarely achieved in athymic nu/nu mice defective in T cell–mediated immune response [79, 104, 111]. In the immunocompetent mouse models, one-third of the mice bearing CT26 and RENCA tumors were cured and rejected a rechallenge with the same tumor cell lines [111]. Furthermore, mice cured of RENCA tumors were resistant to any rechallenge with RENCA cells, but not

CT26 cells, suggesting a tumor-specific immune response. In comparison, the vast majority of the surgically cured animals were not able to reject the same rechallenge. Adoptive transfer experiments revealed that $CD8^+$ T cells, rather than $CD4^+$ T cells, mediated the antitumor immunity. This T cell–mediated immune response could potentially be effective against micrometastases not colonized by *C. novyi*-NT and help prevent recurrence after the target tumor has been eradicated. Apparently, the antitumor activity of *C. novyi*-NT involves both *C. novyi*-NT-derived factors and the host immune system.

2.6 Preclinical Studies: Combination Approaches for Optimized Efficacy

Despite 30%–50% cure rates with some of the syngeneic tumor models, *C. novyi*-NT alone was unable to eradicate the xenograft tumors and the other syngeneic ones, such as the 4T1 tumor, due to its inability to destroy the tumor rim. The reason is currently unclear but is thought to be either limited IT necrosis/hypoxia or massive inflammatory infiltrates pre-existing in those tumors. Contrary to tumor cells in the hypoxic core, those in the well-perfused, highly proliferative tumor rim are sensitive to the conventional cytotoxic therapies. Thus, combining *C. novyi*-NT treatment with chemo- or radiation therapy could prove effective in eradicating the entire tumor. The chemotherapeutic agents that have been tested in combination with clostridial spores include those classified as DNA damaging agents and microtubule inhibitors [79, 121, 122]. In one study, 20 drugs, mostly experimental, were tested either alone or in conjunction with *C. novyi*-NT spores [122]. Four microtubule inhibitors showed substantially improved antitumor activity in the combination setting. The combination treatment with *C. novyi*-NT spores and HTI-286, an experimental microtubule destabilizer, cured ~40% of the mice bearing subcutaneous HCT116 or HuCC-T1 xenograft tumors, whereas no cure was obtained with either agent alone. Consistent with prior observations that microtubule networks in tumor endothelial cells or perivascular smooth muscle cells were particularly sensitive to microtubule-destabilizing agents [123], histological assessment revealed that HTI-286 effectively shut down the tumor blood flow in a tumor-specific fashion, resulting in enhanced tumor hypoxia. Accordingly, the number of bacteria in the HCT116 tumors increased almost sevenfold when *C. novyi*-NT spores were combined with HTI-286. Apparently, the microtubule-destabilizing agents had disrupted the blood flow in the tumor rim and subsequently created an enlarged hypoxic niche for *C. novyi*-NT to invade and colonize. It is anticipated that the combination with microtubule destabilizers would be particularly beneficial in the treatment of tumors with minimal hypoxia. In contrast, the microtubule stabilizers, such as MAC-321 and docetaxel, appeared to eradicate the tumor rim by activities directly against the tumor cells, without obvious effect on the tumor vasculature [122]. Both MAC-321 and docetaxel have substantial antitumor activities themselves, but treatment with these drugs rarely leads to cures. Combination with *C. novyi*-NT spores increased the cure rate considerably. It is noteworthy that the efficacy described above was achieved with a single dose of both *C. novyi*-NT spores and the chemotherapeutic agents.

Due to their poor specificity, nontargeted chemotherapeutic agents inevitably have substantial toxicity. One way to reduce their toxicity is to encapsulate the cytotoxic drugs in liposomes. Liposomes are phospholipid-based spherical vesicles ~100 nm in diameter and can preferentially accumulate in tumor tissue through the EPR effect as discussed earlier. Once inside the tumor tissue, they slowly release their payload, raising local drug concentrations. *C. novyi*-NT can augment the efficacy of liposomal drugs through two distinct mechanisms. First, the local inflammation in response to *C. novyi*-NT infection has been shown to increase vascular permeability, further enhancing the accumulation of liposomes in the infected tumor and resulting in a remarkable increase in the tumor-to-blood ratio of systemically administered liposomes [118]. Second, the hemolysins and a lipase (NT01CX2047) named liposomase are able to disrupt the lipid bilayer of the liposomes, leading to accelerated release of the drug content [100]. Through these mechanisms, *C. novyi*-NT was able to increase drug exposure of the tumor cells approximately sixfold without increasing drug concentrations in normal tissues. Consequently, approximately 65% of mice carrying CT26 or HCT116 tumors were cured by the combination treatment with *C. novyi*-NT spores and Doxil, compared to 0% by Doxil alone. Notably, combination with heat-inactivated *C. novyi*-NT spores did not show enhanced tumor regression. Similar therapeutic results were also obtained with liposomal CPT-11 (irinotecan), which is a topoisomerase inhibitor widely used in cancer therapy. Thus, this approach is in principle applicable to a variety of chemotherapeutic agents that can be encapsulated in a liposome.

Ionizing radiation is another form of cytotoxic therapy that is often used effectively in an adjuvant setting. It is well known that the efficacy of radiation therapy is dependent on oxygen and hypoxic cells are more resistant to ionizing radiation than normoxic cells [124–126]. Therefore, like chemotherapeutic agents, ionizing radiation should complement *C. novyi*-NT spores well in the treatment of solid tumors. This notion has been tested in mouse tumor models with three major modes of radiation therapy: external beam, brachytherapy, and radioimmunotherapy (RAIT) [127]. *C. novyi*-NT spores substantially enhanced the efficacy of fractionated external beam radiation (2 Gy × 5 daily doses) in several tumor models. However, cures were rarely achieved. Higher doses of external beam radiation were not possible because of significant morbidity. Localized radiation with brachytherapy allowed the delivery of higher doses without causing increased morbidity. In conjunction with *C. novyi*-NT spores, brachytherapy using plaques implanted with I-125 seeds delivering a dose as high as 50 Gy achieved a remarkable 100% cure rate in two xenograft tumor models. In comparison, brachytherapy alone was able to eradicate about 30% of the tumors in either model.

RAIT is a promising therapeutic approach for the treatment of widespread metastatic disease, because it is delivered systemically. However, its use is often limited for tumors with significant hypoxia due to its dependence on oxygen and the inability of radiolabeled therapeutic agents to access poorly vascularized tumor regions [128]. Again, *C. novyi*-NT can be the answer for both issues. As noted above, *C. novyi*-NT can destroy the hypoxic portion of a solid tumor and its infection augments the EPR effect, which would result in enhanced selective enrichment in solid tumors of the macromolecular drug formulations, such as antibodies. Treatment with *C. novyi*-NT spores was shown to enhance the IT accumulation of radioactively labeled IgG nearly threefold without affecting its concentrations in normal tissues [118]. Thus, *C. novyi*-NT treatment is expected to enhance the therapeutic effect of RAIT as well. Carcinoembryonic antigen (CEA) is a tumor antigen overexpressed on the surface of many colorectal cancer cells. RAIT using a humanized anti-CEA antibody has shown some clinical benefit for small-volume metastatic disease of colorectal cancer [129]. In a study with mice harboring a human colorectal cancer xenograft that expresses CEA, combination therapy with an anti-CEA antibody and *C. novyi*-NT spores showed significantly enhanced tumor regression compared to monotherapy with the antibody alone [127].

The results described above support the notion that by virtue of their distinct mechanisms of action, bacterial and cytotoxic therapies synergize to eradicate solid tumors. In addition, cytotoxic agents are able to create or enlarge necrotic/hypoxic areas in solid tumors, providing an optimal niche for bacteria to colonize in otherwise uninhabitable tumors.

2.7 From Bench to Bedside

Results from the vast majority of studies performed with laboratory animals cannot be reproduced in clinical trials. The reasons are many, but particularly worth mentioning are the following. Model organisms from yeast to mice share many genetic elements and biological pathways with humans, and yet there are fundamental differences that make them far from perfect models for human diseases. Moreover, disease models lack the heterogeneity always encountered in the real-world patient population. In a transplantable tumor model, all animals inoculated with the same cancer cell line are identical siblings carrying the same tumor. To the contrary, no two patients or their tumors are the same genetically. Therefore, all experimental therapeutic approaches, no matter how efficacious they are in laboratory animal models, have to pass the test in a real-world patient population.

Translation of any novel therapeutic agent from a laboratory bench to the bedside would be a tremendous effort but is especially challenging for live biologics, such as a replication-competent virus or bacterium. Safety is of paramount importance for these agents. Despite the fact that attenuated live vaccines have been used for more than two centuries, clinical use of replication-competent bacteria for cancer treatment still poses a major challenge to both clinicians and the regulatory authorities. Many issues have to be considered before live, replication-competent bacteria can be applied to humans, even in an experimental setting. A few are worth our special attention herein:

- Live genetically modified bacteria that carry antibiotic-resistant genes or mobile genetic elements (plasmids, transposons, bacteriophage, etc.) are generally not permitted for clinical studies. *C. novyi*-NT is simply a clone that has spontaneously lost its phage episome harboring the *α-toxin* gene, and thus it is not considered a genetically modified bacterium.
- Unlike most small molecules or other nonviable clinical agents, live bacteria or bacterial spores cannot be sterilized either by heating or by filtering, which presents a major challenge for making good manufacturing practices (GMP)-grade test articles. Thus, production and purification in dedicated clean rooms following strict aseptic protocols with frequent in-process monitoring is the only practical way to ensure "sterility" (meaning no contamination from other live microorganisms).
- Live bacteria are proliferative in the target tissue, and therefore, the effective (whether therapeutic or toxic) dose is not necessarily correlated with the administered dose. The effective dose depends more on the "quality" of the target tissue, which is defined by the accessibility, the extent of tumor necrosis/hypoxia, and the abundance of pre-existing tumor-infiltrating inflammatory cells. These factors determine how easily the systemically administered bacteria can enter their target tissue and whether the target tissue can support robust proliferation and spreading of the infection. Companion diagnostic approaches, such as those based on angiography and hypoxia/necrosis imaging, may help define the patient population that would benefit the most from bacterial therapy [130–132]. Additionally, germination and spreading of the bacteria may be monitored directly by

imaging the replicating bacteria [133–135]. It should also be noted that when low doses of spores are given, especially when administered systemically, germination is less predictable and may take much longer to occur. This could pose a greater risk to the patients, because they are likely to become less vigilant over time.

- Oncolytic bacterial therapy is a deliberate attempt to convert a tumor into a localized infection, which may have serious consequences if not managed properly. The severity of the infection-associated toxicity generally correlates positively with the tumor size and the extent of necrosis/hypoxia inside the tumor. As both therapeutic and toxic effects result from a robust infection, carefully calculated balance is critical. Practically, this is difficult to achieve because an antibiotic intervention too early would effectively eliminate the infection before an antitumor effect has been achieved, whereas a late intervention bears the risk of an unpredictable systemic inflammatory response. Effective management of the therapeutic infection requires experts from across disciplines, including oncologists, infectious disease specialists, and interventional radiologists or surgeons, for managing abscess or non-abscess-forming infections. Therefore, when and how to intervene after an IT infection has been established should be a team decision.
- When a live biological agent is used in a clinical setting, its potential impact on public health and environment is always a concern. The concern is somewhat lessened for bacteria like *C. novyi*-NT that are naturally present in the environment and have been attenuated [42, 43]. Bacterial spores are highly resistant to a variety of environmental insults [136]. It is worth noting that *C. novyi*-NT spores can be effectively inactivated by chlorine-based disinfectants.

2.8 Clinical Studies: Canine Trial

In addition to laboratory tumor models, tumors developed spontaneously in companion dogs provide an attractive model that shares several important biological features with human tumors [137, 138]. These tumors originate from cells with naturally occurring rather than engineered mutations, are of host origin, and are developed in hosts with heterogeneous genetic backgrounds.

In principle, systemic administration of *C. novyi*-NT spores is a preferred route for metastatic disease. In practice, direct target lesion injection ensures consistent amounts of spores being delivered into individual tumors, which is beneficial, especially in the early phase of dose-escalating clinical studies, because it would allow interpretation of the clinical results with less ambiguity. Canine soft tissue sarcomas serve as an excellent model because they represent one of the most common canine cancer types; share similar clinical, histopathological, and genomic features with human soft tissue sarcomas [32, 137, 138]; and are often located superficially. The superficially localized lesions provide easy access for spore administration, response assessment, and management of local toxicity. A clinical trial involving 16 companion dogs, most with spontaneous soft tissue sarcomas, was carried out [32]. Each dog received at least one cycle of treatment with 100 million *C. novyi*-NT spores injected directly into the target tumor. Fourteen of the dogs were evaluated and showed a 37.5% objective response rate. Interestingly, a CR and a partial response (PR) were observed in four out of seven (57%) evaluable cases of peripheral nerve sheath tumors. The numbers were too small to achieve statistical significance but encourage further studies to investigate whether this type of cancer is particularly sensitive to bacterial therapy. The observed therapeutic response often, but not always, involved abscess formation, which required surgical management such as debridement. The debrided tissue available for histopathological assessment revealed a large number of gram-positive bacilli morphologically consistent with *Clostridium* spp., accompanied by extensive necrosis and inflammation. Adverse events included fever, lethargy, anorexia, tumor inflammation, tumor pain, and tumor discharge, all expected for a typical soft tissue infection. The therapeutic response, the toxicity, and the process of wound healing were remarkably similar to those observed in preclinical models, which confirmed the relevance of the experimental tumors in modeling the response of naturally occurring cancers to *C. novyi*-NT therapy.

2.9 Clinical Studies: Phase I Human Trial

Encouraged by the promising results from the canine trial, a Phase I clinical trial has been initiated in human patients with solid tumors unresponsive to standard therapies (ClinicalTrials.gov, Identifier: NCT01924689) [32]. The first patient enrolled in the trial had a retroperitoneal leiomyosarcoma. Despite multiple surgical resections followed by chemo- and radiation therapies, the disease progressed, and metastases were found in the liver, lungs, peritoneum, and soft tissue in the right shoulder and adjacent right humerus. The patient was treated with 10,000 *C. novyi*-NT spores injected directly into the metastasis in the right shoulder. An 18-gauge multipronged needle was used for spore injection to maximize the chances of delivery of the spores into a necrotic or hypoxic region. Signs of germination showed up within two days. In addition to fever, with a peak temperature at 39.2° C, and an increased leukocyte count (of 18,300/mL), both indicative of germination and an established infection, the major adverse event was an intense pain in the right shoulder and scapula that required IV patient-controlled analgesia with hydromorphone. Extensive destruction with gas pockets in the tumor was shown on a computed tomography (CT) scan of the right upper extremity that was taken on day three of the treatment. *C. novyi*-NT was identified from a CT-guided tumor aspirate after growth under anaerobic culture conditions. Antibiotics, including piperacillin/tazobactam, metronidazole, and vancomycin, were started on day three and the patient's fever soon diminished, confirming the sensitivity of *C. novyi*-NT to antibiotic treatment. Magnetic resonance imaging (MRI) of the right upper extremity on day four revealed markedly reduced enhancement in the tumor mass compared to baseline, again suggesting massive tumor destruction. Tumor biopsies showed numerous gram-positive bacteria and an absence of viable tumor cells. The patient was discharged on oral antibiotics metronidazole and doxycycline per protocol. On day 55, the patient presented with localized pain resulting from an effort-induced pathological fracture of the necrotic right proximal humerus and was managed surgically. Histopathology with samples collected at the surgery revealed extensive necrosis with small foci of residual tumor cells. Once again, the therapeutic response of a human spontaneous tumor to *C. novyi*-NT spore treatment has closely resembled that observed in laboratory models.

2.10 Summary and Future Perspectives

Valuable lessons have been learned from both preclinical and clinical studies with *C. novyi*-NT. Firstly, efficacy and toxicity observed in preclinical studies have been faithfully recapitulated in canine and human clinical trials. Thus, experimental tumors modeled the real-world malignancy well for the effects of *C. novyi*-NT. Secondly, *C. novyi*-NT spores can robustly germinate and eradicate spontaneous tumors. However, many tumors are still resistant to *C. novyi*-NT treatment, which suggests that other approaches, such as cytotoxic therapies, are needed to boost germination or to help eradicate the normoxic tumor component. Thirdly, an effective immune response against nontarget metastatic lesions was not observed in preclinical models (unpublished data) or in the human patient even though *C. novyi*-NT spores germinated robustly in the target lesion and resulted in a robust inflammatory response. It is well known that cancer can hijack the regulatory mechanisms, such as checkpoints, regulatory T cells, and myeloid-derived suppressor cells (MDSCs), in the immune system to their advantage [139–141]. *C. novyi*-NT-induced tumor destruction and inflammation can provide a strong positive signal for an antitumor immune response, but the negative regulatory mechanisms have to be dismantled as well to fully realize *C. novyi*-NT's immune-stimulatory effect. Thus, combination therapy with approaches that can overcome the negative regulatory mechanisms (e.g., checkpoint blockade) is particularly attractive to explore. Fourthly, a robust IT infection poses the risk of causing a serious systemic inflammatory response. At present, oncolytic bacteria like *C. novyi*-NT are intended to treat patients with advanced diseases that are unresponsive to standard therapies only and the risk may be worth taking if clear therapeutic benefit is demonstrated. For other patients, a safer version of the therapy is required.

Further improvement in both safety profile and efficacy is clearly needed for a successful clinical translation of the therapy. As discussed earlier, the improvement can be made by combination with other therapeutic agents. Alternatively, improvement can be made by generating *C. novyi*-NT clones with additional desired properties. Targeted knockout, knock-in, or knockdown approaches can be employed to obtain such clones. Bacteria harboring antibiotic resistance genes or mobile genetic elements cannot be used in clinical studies. To address this issue, new technologies have been developed to enable targeted genomic manipulation without introducing those elements [58, 142–145]. Using these technologies, the genes encoding putative toxins can be knocked out individually or in combination. The resulting clones can then be tested for reduced toxicity *in vivo* using mouse tumor models. Clones with enhanced efficacy can be obtained by genetic engineering, with heterologous genes encoding a variety of therapeutic proteins.

C. novyi-NT is but one bacterial anticancer agent being developed. Many others are under preclinical development and equally promising. The lessons learned from the preclinical and translational works with *C. novyi*-NT will hopefully help to accelerate clinical translation of the others as well.

Acknowledgment

This work was supported by BioMed Valley Discoveries, Inc., Virginia and D. K. Ludwig Fund for Cancer Research, and NIH CA062924.

Competing Interests

Under a licensing agreement between BioMed Valley Discoveries, Inc., and the Johns Hopkins University, Shibin Zhou is entitled to a share of royalties received by the university on sales of products described in this article. The terms of the arrangement are under ongoing management by the Johns Hopkins University in accordance with its conflict-of-interest policies.

References

1. Piccart-Gebhart M. J., Procter M., Leyland-Jones B., Goldhirsch A., Untch M., Smith I., *et al.* Trastuzumab after adjuvant chemotherapy in HER2-positive breast cancer. *New England Journal of Medicine,* 353 (2005) 1659–1672.
2. Romond E. H., Perez E. A., Bryant J., Suman V. J., Geyer C. E. Jr., Davidson N. E., *et al.* Trastuzumab plus adjuvant chemotherapy for operable HER2-positive breast cancer. *New England Journal of Medicine,* 353 (2005) 1673–1684.
3. Lynch T. J., Bell D. W., Sordella R., Gurubhagavatula S., Okimoto R. A., Brannigan B. W., *et al.* Activating mutations in the epidermal growth factor receptor underlying responsiveness of non-small-cell lung cancer to Gefitinib. *New England Journal of Medicine,* 350 (2004) 2129–2139 .
4. Messersmith W. A., Ahnen D. J. Targeting EGFR in colorectal cancer. *New England Journal of Medicine,* 359 (2008) 1834–1836.
5. Bollag G., Hirth P., Tsai J., Zhang J., Ibrahim P. N., Cho H., *et al.* Clinical efficacy of a RAF inhibitor needs broad target blockade in BRAF-mutant melanoma. *Nature,* 467 (2010) 596–599.
6. Flaherty K. T., Infante J. R., Daud A., Gonzalez R., Kefford R. F., Sosman J., *et al.* Combined BRAF and MEK inhibition in melanoma with BRAF V600 mutations. *New England Journal of Medicine,* 367 (2012) 1694–1703.
7. Carmeliet P., Jain R. K. Angiogenesis in cancer and other diseases. *Nature,* 407 (2000) 249–257.
8. Cerar A., Zidar N., Vodopivec B. Colorectal carcinoma in endoscopic biopsies; additional histologic criteria for the diagnosis. *Pathology-Research and Practice,* 200 (2004) 657–662.
9. Wilson W. R., Hay M. P. Targeting hypoxia in cancer therapy. *Nature Reviews Cancer,* 11 (2011) 393–410.
10. Brown J. M. Tumor hypoxia in cancer therapy. *Methods in Enzymology,* 435 (2007) 297–321.
11. Matsumura Y., Maeda H. A new concept for macromolecular therapeutics in cancer chemotherapy: Mechanism of tumoritropic accumulation of proteins and the antitumor agent smancs. *Cancer Research,* 46 (1986) 6387–6392.
12. Fang J., Sawa T., Maeda H. Factors and mechanism of "EPR" effect and the enhanced antitumor effects of macromolecular drugs

including SMANCS. *Advances in Experimental Medicine and Biology*, 519 (2003) 29–49.

13. Maeda H., Fang J., Inutsuka T., Kitamoto Y. Vascular permeability enhancement in solid tumor: Various factors, mechanisms involved and its implications. *International Immunopharmacology*, 3 (2003) 319–328.
14. Drummond D. C., Meyer O., Hong K., Kirpotin D. B., Papahadjopoulos D. Optimizing liposomes for delivery of chemotherapeutic agents to solid tumors. *Pharmacological Reviews*, 51 (1999) 691–743.
15. Torchilin V. P. Micellar nanocarriers: Pharmaceutical perspectives. *Pharmaceutical Research*, 24 (2007) 1–16.
16. Maeda H., Bharate G. Y., Daruwalla J. Polymeric drugs for efficient tumor-targeted drug delivery based on EPR-effect. *European Journal of Pharmaceutics and Biopharmaceutics*, 71 (2009) 409–419.
17. Barenholz Y. Doxil®—the first FDA-approved nano-drug: Lessons learned. *Journal of Controlled Release*, 160 (2012) 117–134 .
18. Maeda H. Toward a full understanding of the EPR effect in primary and metastatic tumors as well as issues related to its heterogeneity. *Advanced Drug Delivery Reviews*, 91 (2015) 3–6.
19. Coley W. B. The treatment of malignant tumors by repeated inoculations of erysipelas. With a report of ten original cases. 1893. *Clinical Orthopaedics and Related Research*, 262 (1991) 3–11.
20. McCarthy E. F. The toxins of William B. Coley and the treatment of bone and soft-tissue sarcomas. *Iowa Orthopaedic Journal*, 26 (2006) 154–158.
21. Bermudes D., Zheng L. M., King I. C. Live bacteria as anticancer agents and tumor-selective protein delivery vectors. *Current Opinion in Drug Discovery & Development*, 5 (2002) 194–199.
22. Theys J., Barbe S., Landuyt W., Nuyts S., Van Mellaert L., Wouters B., *et al.* Tumor-specific gene delivery using genetically engineered bacteria. *Current Gene Therapy*, 3 (2003) 207–221.
23. Chakrabarty A. M. Microorganisms and cancer: Quest for a therapy. *Journal of Bacteriology*, 185 (2003) 2683–2686.
24. Minton N. P. Clostridia in cancer therapy. *Nature Reviews Microbiology*, 1 (2003) 237–242.
25. Van Mellaert L., Barbe S., Anne J. *Clostridium* spores as anti-tumour agents. *Trends in Microbiology*, 14 (2006) 190–196.
26. Forbes N. S. Engineering the perfect (bacterial) cancer therapy. *Nature Reviews Cancer*, 10 (2010) 785–794.

27. Gravekamp C., Paterson Y. Harnessing *Listeria monocytogenes* to target tumors. *Cancer Biology & Therapy*, 9 (2010) 257–265.

28. Hoffman R. M. Tumor-seeking *Salmonella* amino acid auxotrophs. *Current Opinion in Biotechnology*, 22 (2011) 917–923.

29. Heppner F., Möse J. R. The liquefaction (oncolysis) of malignant gliomas by a non pathogenic *Clostridium*. *Acta Neurochirurgica* (Wien), 42 (1978) 123–125.

30. Toso J. F., Gill V. J., Hwu P., Marincola F. M., Restifo N. P., Schwartzentruber D. J., *et al.* Phase I study of the intravenous administration of attenuated *Salmonella typhimurium* to patients with metastatic melanoma. *Journal of Clinical Oncology*, 20 (2002) 142–152.

31. Nemunaitis J., Cunningham C., Senzer N., Kuhn J., Cramm J., Litz C., *et al.* Pilot trial of genetically modified, attenuated *Salmonella* expressing the *E. coli* cytosine deaminase gene in refractory cancer patients. *Cancer Gene Therapy*, 10 (2003) 737–744.

32. Roberts N. J., Zhang L., Janku F., Collins A., Bai R. Y., Staedtke V., *et al.* Intratumoral injection of *Clostridium novyi*-NT spores induces antitumor responses. *Science Translational Medicine*, 6 (2014) 249ra111.

33. Le D. T., Wang-Gillam A., Picozzi V., Greten T. F., Crocenzi T., Springett G., *et al.* Safety and survival with GVAX pancreas prime and *Listeria monocytogenes*-expressing mesothelin (CRS-207) boost vaccines for metastatic pancreatic cancer. *Journal of Clinical Oncology*, 33 (2015) 1325–1333.

34. Lamm D. L. BCG immunotherapy for transitional-cell carcinoma in situ of the bladder. *Oncology* (Williston Park), 9 (1995) 947–952, 955, discussion 955–965.

35. Morales A., Eidinger D., Bruce A. W. Intracavitary bacillus Calmette-Guerin in the treatment of superficial bladder tumors. *The Journal of Urology*, 116 (1976) 180–183.

36. De Jager R., Guinan P., Lamm D., Khanna O., Brosman S., De Kernion J., *et al.* Long-term complete remission in bladder carcinoma in situ with intravesical TICE bacillus Calmette Guerin. Overview analysis of six phase II clinical trials. *Urology*, 38 (1991) 507–513.

37. Herr H. W., Schwalb D. M., Zhang Z. F., Sogani P. C., Fair W. R., Whitmore W. F. Jr., *et al.* Intravesical bacillus Calmette-Guerin therapy prevents tumor progression and death from superficial bladder cancer: Ten-year follow-up of a prospective randomized trial. *Journal of Clinical Oncology*, 13 (1995) 1404–1408.

38. Bohle A., Gerdes J., Ulmer A. J., Hofstetter A. G., Flad H. D. Effects of local bacillus Calmette-Guerin therapy in patients with bladder carcinoma on immunocompetent cells of the bladder wall. *The Journal of Urology*, 144 (1990) 53–58.

39. Thalmann G. N., Sermier A., Rentsch C., Mohrle K., Cecchini M. G., Studer U. E. Urinary interleukin-8 and 18 predict the response of superficial bladder cancer to intravesical therapy with bacillus Calmette-Guerin. *The Journal of Urology*, 164 (2000) 2129–2133.

40. Sharma P., Old L. J., Allison J. P. Immunotherapeutic strategies for high-risk bladder cancer. *Seminars in Oncology*, 34 (2007) 165–172.

41. Wells C. L., Wilkins T. D. Clostridia: Sporeforming Anaerobic Bacilli. *Medical Microbiology*, Baron S. (ed.), 4th edn, (1996), University of Texas Medical Branch at Galveston, Galveston (TX).

42. Maclennan J. D. The histotoxic clostridial infections of man. *Bacteriological Reviews*, 26 (1962) 177–276.

43. Nishida S., Nakagawara G. Isolation of toxigenic strains of *Clostridium novyi* from soil. *Journal of Bacteriology*, 88 (1964) 1636–1640.

44. Chong E., Winikoff B., Charles D., Agnew K., Prentice J. L., Limbago B. M., *et al.*; NCT01283828 Study Team. Vaginal and rectal *Clostridium sordellii* and *Clostridium perfringens* presence among women in the United States. *Obstetrics & Gynecology*, 127 (2016) 360–368.

45. Torrey J. C., Kahn M. C. The treatment of Flexner-Jobling rat carcinomas with bacterial proteolytic ferments. *Journal of Cancer Research*, 11 (1927) 334–376.

46. Parker R. C., Plummer H. C., Siebenmann C. O., Chapman M. G. Effect of histolyticus infection and toxin on transplantable mouse tumors. *Proceedings of the Society for Experimental Biology and Medicine*, 66 (1947) 461.

47. Malmgren R. A., Flanigan C. C. Localization of the Vegetative form of *Clostridium* tetani in mouse tumors following intravenous spore administration. *Cancer Research*, 15 (1955) 473–478.

48. Heppner F., Möse J. R. *Onkolyse maligner Gliome durch apathogene Clostridien. Zentralblatt Fur Neurochirurgie*, 27 (1966) 184–192.

49. Möse J. R., Möse G., Propst A., Heppner F. *Onkolyse maligner Tumoren durch den Clostridienstamm M55. Medizinische Klinik*, 62 (1967) 189–225.

50. Carey R. W., Holland J. F., Whang H. Y., Neter E., Bryant B. Clostridial oncolysis in man. *European Journal of Cancer*, 3 (1967) 37–46.

51. Schmidt W., Fabricius E. M., Schneeweiss U. The tumour-*Clostridium* phenomenon: 50 years of developmental research (Review). *International Journal of Oncology*, 29 (2006) 1479–1492.

52. Fox M. E., Lemmon M. J., Mauchline M. L., Davis T. O., Giaccia A. J., Minton N. P., *et al.* Anaerobic bacteria as a delivery system for cancer gene therapy: in vitro activation of 5-fluorocytosine by genetically engineered clostridia. *Gene Therapy*, 3 (1996) 173–178.

53. Lemmon M. J., van Zijl P., Fox M. E., Mauchline M. L., Giaccia A. J., Minton N. P., *et al.* Anaerobic bacteria as a gene delivery system that is controlled by the tumor microenvironment. *Gene Therapy*, 4 (1997) 791–796.

54. Theys J., Landuyt W., Nuyts S., Van Mellaert L., van Oosterom A., Lambin P., *et al.* Specific targeting of cytosine deaminase to solid tumors by engineered *Clostridium acetobutylicum*. *Cancer Gene Therapy*, 8 (2001) 294–297.

55. Liu S. C., Minton N. P., Giaccia A. J., Brown J. M. Anticancer efficacy of systemically delivered anaerobic bacteria as gene therapy vectors targeting tumor hypoxia/necrosis. *Gene Therapy*, 9 (2002) 291–296.

56. Theys J., Pennington O., Dubois L., Anlezark G., Vaughan T., Mengesha A., *et al.* Repeated cycles of *Clostridium*-directed enzyme prodrug therapy result in sustained antitumour effects in vivo. *British Journal of Radiology*, 95 (2006) 1212–1219.

57. Liu S. C., Ahn G. O., Kioi M., Dorie M. J., Patterson A. V., Brown J. M. Optimized *clostridium*-directed enzyme prodrug therapy improves the antitumor activity of the novel DNA cross-linking agent PR-104. *Cancer Research*, 68 (2008) 7995–8003.

58. Heap J. T., Theys J., Ehsaan M., Kubiak A. M., Dubois L., Paesmans K., *et al.* Spores of *Clostridium* engineered for clinical efficacy and safety cause regression and cure of tumors in vivo. *Oncotarget*, 5 (2014) 1761–1769.

59. Theys J., Nuyts S., Landuyt W., Van Mellaert L., Dillen C., Bohringer M., *et al.* Stable *Escherichia coli–Clostridium acetobutylicum* shuttle vector for secretion of murine tumor necrosis factor alpha. *Applied and Environmental Microbiology*, 65 (1999) 4295–4300.

60. Nuyts S., Van Mellaert L., Theys J., Landuyt W., Bosmans E., Anne J., *et al.* Radio-responsive recA promoter significantly increases TNF-α production in recombinant clostridia after 2 Gy irradiation. *Gene Therapy*, 8 (2001) 1197–1201.

61. Barbe S., Van Mellaert L., Theys J., Geukens N., Lammertyn E., Lambin P., *et al.* Secretory production of biologically active rat interleukin-2 by *Clostridium acetobutylicum* DSM792 as a tool for anti-tumor treatment. *FEMS Microbiology Letters*, 246 (2005) 67–73.

62. Groot A. J., Verheesen P., Westerlaken E. J., Gort E. H., van der Groep P., Bovenschen N., *et al.* Identification by phage display of single-domain antibody fragments specific for the ODD domain in hypoxia-inducible factor 1alpha. *Laboratory Investigation*, 86 (2006) 345–356.

63. Novy F. G. Ein neuer anaërober *bacillus* des malignen Oedems. *Zeitschrift für Hygiene und Infektionskrankheiten*, 17 (1894) 209–232.

64. Oakley C. L., Warrack G. H., Clarke P. H. The toxins of *Clostridium* oedematiens (Cl. *novyi*). *Journal of General Microbiology*, 1 (1947) 91–107.

65. Ball D. W., Van Tassell R. L., Roberts M. D., Hahn P. E., Lyerly D. M., Wilkins T. D. Purification and characterization of alpha-toxin produced by *Clostridium novyi* type A. *Infection and Immunity*, 61 (1993) 2912–2918.

66. Hofmann F., Herrmann A., Habermann E., von Eichel-Streiber C. Sequencing and analysis of the gene encoding the alpha-toxin of *Clostridium novyi* proves its homology to toxins A and B of *Clostridium difficile*. *Molecular Genetics and Genomics*, 247 (1995) 670–679.

67. Hatheway C. L. Toxigenic clostridia. *Clinical Microbiology Reviews*, 3 (1990) 66–98.

68. Selzer J., Hofmann F., Rex G., Wilm M., Mann M., Just I., *et al.* *Clostridium novyi* alpha-toxin-catalyzed incorporation of GlcNAc into Rho subfamily proteins. *Journal of Biological Chemistry*, 271 (1996) 25173–25177.

69. Busch C., Schomig K., Hofmann F., Aktories K. Characterization of the catalytic domain of *Clostridium novyi* alpha-toxin. *Infection and Immunity*, 68 (2000) 6378–6383.

70. Popoff M. R., Bouvet P. Clostridial toxins. *Future Microbiology*, 4 (2009) 1021–1064.

71. Ma M., Boyd J. T., Trinh H. T., Coombs J. W., Fermann G. J. Fatal myocarditis due to *Clostridium novyi* type B in a previously healthy woman: Case report and literature review. *Scandinavian Journal of Infectious Diseases*, 39 (2007) 77–80.

72. Abdel-Haq N. M., Chearskul P., Salimnia H., Asmar B. I. Clostridial liver abscess following blunt abdominal trauma: Case report and

review of the literature. *Scandinavian Journal of Infectious Diseases*, 39 (2007) 734–737.

73. McGuigan C. C., Penrice G. M., Gruer L., Ahmed S., Goldberg D., Black M., *et al.* Lethal outbreak of infection with *Clostridium novyi* type A and other spore-forming organisms in Scottish injecting drug users. *Journal of Medical Microbiology*, 51 (2002) 971–977.
74. Jones J. A., Salmon J. E., Djuretic T., Nichols G., George R. C., Gill O. N., *et al.* An outbreak of serious illness and death among injecting drug users in England during 2000. *Journal of Medical Microbiology*, 51 (2002) 978–984.
75. Finn S. P., Leen E., English L., O'Briain D. S. Autopsy findings in an outbreak of severe systemic illness in heroin users following injection site inflammation: An effect of *Clostridium novyi* exotoxin? *Archives of Pathology & Laboratory Medicine*, 127 (2003) 1465–1470.
76. Brett M. M., Hood J., Brazier J. S., Duerden B. I., Hahne S. J. Soft tissue infections caused by spore-forming bacteria in injecting drug users in the United Kingdom. *Epidemiology & Infection*, 133 (2005) 575–582.
77. Murray-Lillibridge K., Barry J., Reagan S., O'Flanagan D., Sayers G., Bergin C., *et al.* Epidemiological findings and medical, legal, and public health challenges of an investigation of severe soft tissue infections and deaths among injecting drug users—Ireland, 2000. *Epidemiology & Infection*, 134 (2006) 894–901.
78. Stämpfli H.R. Infectious necrotic hepatitis (*Clostridium novyi* infection, black disease) http://www.merckvetmanual.com/mvm/generalized_conditions/clostridial_diseases/infectious_necrotic_hepatitis.html.
79. Dang L. H., Bettegowda C., Huso D. L., Kinzler K. W., Vogelstein B. Combination bacteriolytic therapy for the treatment of experimental tumors. *Proceedings of the National Academy of Sciences of the United States of America*, 27 (2001) 27.
80. Boyd N. A., Walker P. D., Thomson R. O. The prevention of experimental *Clostridium novyi* gas gangrene in high-velocity missile wounds by passive immunisation. *Journal of Medical Microbiology*, 5 (1972) 459–465.
81. Bette P., Oksche A., Mauler F., von Eichel-Streiber C., Popoff M. R., Habermann E. A comparative biochemical, pharmacological and immunological study of *Clostridium novyi* alpha-toxin, C. *difficile* toxin B and C. *sordellii* lethal toxin. *Toxicon*, 29 (1991) 877–887.
82. Eklund M. W., Poysky F. T., Meyers J. A., Pelroy G. A. Interspecies conversion of *Clostridium botulinum* type C to *Clostridium novyi* type A by bacteriophage. *Science*, 186 (1974) 456–458.

83. Eklund M. W., Poysky F. T., Peterson M. E., Meyers J. A. Relationship of bacteriophages to alpha toxin production in *Clostridium novyi* types A and B. *Infection and Immunity*, 14 (1976) 793–803.

84. Diaz L. A. Jr., Cheong I., Foss C. A., Zhang X., Peters B. A., Agrawal N., *et al.* Pharmacologic and toxicologic evaluation of C. *novyi*-NT spores. *Toxicological Sciences*, 88 (2005) 562–575.

85. Plomp M., McCaffery J. M., Cheong I., Huang X., Bettegowda C., Kinzler K. W., *et al.* Spore coat architecture of *Clostridium novyi* NT spores. *Journal of Bacteriology*, 189 (2007) 6457–6468.

86. Bettegowda C., Huang X., Lin J., Cheong I., Kohli M., Szabo S. A., *et al.* The genome and transcriptomes of the anti-tumor agent *Clostridium novyi*-NT. *Nature Biotechnology*, 24 (2006) 1573–1580.

87. Arthur J. R. The glutathione peroxidases. *Cellular and Molecular Life Sciences*, 57 (2000) 1825–1835.

88. Moore T. D., Sparling P. F. Interruption of the gpxA gene increases the sensitivity of *Neisseria meningitidis* to paraquat. *Journal of Bacteriology*, 178 (1996) 4301–4305.

89. Setlow P. Spore germination. *Current Opinion in Microbiology*, 6 (2003) 550–556.

90. Paredes-Sabja D., Setlow P., Sarker M. R. Germination of spores of *Bacillales* and *Clostridiales* species: Mechanisms and proteins involved. *Trends in Microbiology*, 19 (2011) 85–94.

91. Friedman M., Mikityansky I., Kam A., Libutti S. K., Walther M. M., Neeman Z., *et al.* Radiofrequency ablation of cancer. *Cardiovascular and Interventional Radiology*, 27 (2004) 427–434.

92. Poggi G., Tosoratti N., Montagna B., Picchi C. Microwave ablation of hepatocellular carcinoma. *World Journal of Hepatology*, 7 (2015) 2578–2589.

93. Chan A. C., Cheung T. T., Fan S. T., Chok K. S., Chan S. C., Poon R. T., *et al.* Survival analysis of high-intensity focused ultrasound therapy versus radiofrequency ablation in the treatment of recurrent hepatocellular carcinoma. *Annals of Surgery*, 257 (2013) 686–692.

94. Facciorusso A., Di Maso M., Muscatiello N. Microwave ablation versus radiofrequency ablation for the treatment of hepatocellular carcinoma: A systematic review and meta-analysis. *International Journal of Hyperthermia*, 32 (2016) 339–344.

95. Facciorusso A., Serviddio G., Muscatiello N. Local ablative treatments for hepatocellular carcinoma: An updated review. *World Journal of Gastrointestinal Pharmacology and Therapeutics*, 7 (2016) 477–489.

96. Skarin H., Hafstrom T., Westerberg J., Segerman B. *Clostridium botulinum* group III: A group with dual identity shaped by plasmids, phages and mobile elements. *BMC Genomics*, 12 (2011) 185.

97. Songer J. G. Bacterial phospholipases and their role in virulence. *Trends in Microbiology*, 5 (1997) 156–161.

98. Stevens D. L., Troyer B. E., Merrick D. T., Mitten J. E., Olson R. D. Lethal effects and cardiovascular effects of purified alpha- and theta-toxins from *Clostridium perfringens*. *Journal of Infectious Diseases*, 157 (1988) 272–279.

99. Awad M. M., Bryant A. E., Stevens D. L., Rood J. I. Virulence studies on chromosomal alpha-toxin and theta-toxin mutants constructed by allelic exchange provide genetic evidence for the essential role of alpha-toxin in *Clostridium perfringens*-mediated gas gangrene. *Molecular Microbiology*, 15 (1995) 191–202.

100. Cheong I., Huang X., Bettegowda C., Diaz L. A. Jr., Kinzler K. W., Zhou S., *et al.* A bacterial protein enhances the release and efficacy of liposomal cancer drugs. *Science*, 314 (2006) 1308–1311.

101. Weeks G., Shapiro M., Burns R. O., Wakil S. J. Control of fatty acid metabolism. I. Induction of the enzymes of fatty acid oxidation in *Escherichia coli*. *Journal of Bacteriology*, 97 (1969) 827–836.

102. Kunau W. H., Dommes V., Schulz H. beta-oxidation of fatty acids in mitochondria, peroxisomes, and bacteria: A century of continued progress. *Progress in Lipid Research*, 34 (1995) 267–342.

103. Proffitt R. T., Williams L. E., Presant C. A., Tin G. W., Uliana J. A., Gamble R. C., *et al.* Liposomal blockade of the reticuloendothelial system: Improved tumor imaging with small unilamellar vesicles. *Science*, 220 (1983) 502–505.

104. Maletzki C., Gock M., Klier U., Klar E., Linnebacher M. Bacteriolytic therapy of experimental pancreatic carcinoma. *World Journal of Gastroenterology*, 16 (2010) 3546–3552.

105. Propst A. *Diskussion, abstr V Internationaler Kongress fur Chemotherapie*, Vien, (1967).

106. Staedtke V., Bai R. Y., Sun W., Huang J., Kibler K. K., Tyler B. M., *et al.* *Clostridium novyi*-NT can cause regression of orthotopically implanted glioblastomas in rats. *Oncotarget*, 6 (2015) 5536–5546.

107. Dvorak H. F., Nagy J. A., Dvorak J. T., Dvorak A. M. Identification and characterization of the blood vessels of solid tumors that are leaky to circulating macromolecules. *American Journal of Pathology*, 133 (1988) 95–109.

108. Dvorak H. F. Leaky tumor vessels: Consequences for tumor stroma generation and for solid tumor therapy. *Progress in Clinical and Biological Research*, 354A (1990) 317–330.

109. Hashizume H., Baluk P., Morikawa S., McLean J. W., Thurston G., Roberge S., *et al.* Openings between defective endothelial cells explain tumor vessel leakiness. *American Journal of Pathology*, 156 (2000) 1363–1380.

110. O'Brien D. K., Melville S. B. The anaerobic pathogen *Clostridium perfringens* can escape the phagosome of macrophages under aerobic conditions. *Cellular Microbiology*, 2 (2000) 505–519.

111. Agrawal N., Bettegowda C., Cheong I., Geschwind J. F., Drake C. G., Hipkiss E. L., *et al.* Bacteriolytic therapy can generate a potent immune response against experimental tumors. *Proceedings of the National Academy of Sciences of the United States of America*, 101 (2004) 15172–15177.

112. Brattain M. G., Strobel-Stevens J., Fine D., Webb M., Sarrif A. M. Establishment of mouse colonic carcinoma cell lines with different metastatic properties. *Cancer Research*, 40 (1980) 2142–2146.

113. Corbett T. H., Roberts B. J., Leopold W. R., Peckham J. C., Wilkoff L. J., Griswold D. P. Jr., *et al.* Induction and chemotherapeutic response of two transplantable ductal adenocarcinomas of the pancreas in C57BL/6 mice. *Cancer Research*, 44 (1984) 717–726.

114. Aslakson C. J., Miller F. R. Selective events in the metastatic process defined by analysis of the sequential dissemination of subpopulations of a mouse mammary tumor. *Cancer Research*, 52 (1992) 1399–1405.

115. Kim K., Skora A. D., Li Z., Liu Q., Tam A. J., Blosser R. L., *et al.* Eradication of metastatic mouse cancers resistant to immune checkpoint blockade by suppression of myeloid-derived cells. *Proceedings of the National Academy of Sciences of the United States of America*, 111 (2014) 11774–11779.

116. Engelmann B., Massberg S. Thrombosis as an intravascular effector of innate immunity. *Nature Reviews Immunology*, 13 (2013) 34–45.

117. Carswell E. A., Old L. J., Kassel R. L., Green S., Fiore N., Williamson B. An endotoxin-induced serum factor that causes necrosis of tumors. *Proceedings of the National Academy of Sciences of the United States of America*, 72 (1975) 3666–3670.

118. Qiao Y., Huang X., Nimmagadda S., Bai R., Staedtke V., Foss C. A., *et al.* A robust approach to enhance tumor-selective accumulation of nanoparticles. *Oncotarget*, 2 (2011) 59–68.

119. Galluzzi L., Buque A., Kepp O., Zitvogel L., Kroemer G. Immunogenic cell death in cancer and infectious disease. *Nature Reviews Immunology,* (2016) doi:10.1038/nri.2016.107.

120. Zitvogel L., Apetoh L., Ghiringhelli F., Kroemer G. Immunological aspects of cancer chemotherapy. *Nature Reviews Immunology,* 8 (2008) 59–73.

121. Theys J., Landuyt W., Nuyts S., Van Mellaert L., Bosmans E., Rijnders A., *et al.* Improvement of *Clostridium* tumour targeting vectors evaluated in rat rhabdomyosarcomas. *FEMS Immunology and Medical Microbiology,* 30 (2001) 37–41.

122. Dang L. H., Bettegowda C., Agrawal N., Cheong I., Huso D., Frost P., *et al.* Targeting vascular and avascular compartments of tumors with *C. novyi*-NT and anti-microtubule agents. *Cancer Biology & Therapy,* 3 (2004) 326–337.

123. Griggs J., Metcalfe J. C., Hesketh R. Targeting tumour vasculature: The development of combretastatin A4. *Lancet Oncology,* 2 (2001) 82–87.

124. Harrison L. B., Chadha M., Hill R. J., Hu K., Shasha D. Impact of tumor hypoxia and anemia on radiation therapy outcomes. *Oncologist,* 7 (2002) 492–508.

125. Wachsberger P., Burd R., Dicker A. P. Tumor response to ionizing radiation combined with antiangiogenesis or vascular targeting agents: Exploring mechanisms of interaction. *Clinical Cancer Research,* 9 (2003) 1957–1971.

126. Teicher B. A. Physiologic mechanisms of therapeutic resistance. Blood flow and hypoxia. *Hematology/Oncology Clinics of North America,* 9 (1995) 475–506.

127. Bettegowda C., Dang L. H., Abrams R., Huso D. L., Dillehay L., Cheong I., *et al.* Overcoming the hypoxic barrier to radiation therapy with anaerobic bacteria. *Proceedings of the National Academy of Sciences of the United States of America,* 100 (2003) 15083–15088.

128. Carter P. Improving the efficacy of antibody-based cancer therapies. *Nature Reviews Cancer,* 1 (2001) 118–129.

129. Behr T. M., Liersch T., Greiner-Bechert L., Griesinger F., Behe M., Markus P. M., *et al.* Radioimmunotherapy of small-volume disease of metastatic colorectal cancer. *Cancer,* 94 (2002) 1373–1381.

130. Kashiwagi N., Nakanishi K., Kozuka T., Sato Y., Tanaka K., Tsukaguchi I., *et al.* Vascular supply with angio-CT for superselective intra-arterial chemotherapy in advanced maxillary sinus cancer. *British Journal of Radiology,* 83 (2010) 171–178.

131. Fleming I. N., Manavaki R., Blower P. J., West C., Williams K. J., Harris A. L., *et al.* Imaging tumour hypoxia with positron emission tomography. *British Journal of Radiology*, 112 (2015) 238–250.

132. Egeland T. A., Gaustad J. V., Galappathi K., Rofstad E. K. Magnetic resonance imaging of tumor necrosis. *Acta Oncologica*, 50 (2011) 427–434.

133. Bettegowda C., Foss C. A., Cheong I., Wang Y., Diaz L., Agrawal N., *et al.* Imaging bacterial infections with radiolabeled 1-(2′-deoxy-2′-fluoro-beta-D-arabinofuranosyl)-5-iodouracil. *Proceedings of the National Academy of Sciences of the United States of America*, 102 (2005) 1145–1150.

134. Diaz L. A. Jr., Foss C. A., Thornton K., Nimmagadda S., Endres C. J., Uzuner O., *et al.* Imaging of musculoskeletal bacterial infections by [^{124}I]FIAU-PET/CT. *PLOS One*, 2 (2007) e1007.

135. Liu G., Bettegowda C., Qiao Y., Staedtke V., Chan K. W., Bai R., *et al.* Noninvasive imaging of infection after treatment with tumor-homing bacteria using Chemical Exchange Saturation Transfer (CEST) MRI. *Magnetic Resonance in Medicine*, 70 (2013) 1690–1698.

136. Nicholson W. L., Munakata N., Horneck G., Melosh H. J., Setlow P. Resistance of *Bacillus* endospores to extreme terrestrial and extraterrestrial environments. *Microbiology and Molecular Biology Reviews*, 64 (2000) 548–572.

137. Paoloni M., Khanna C. Translation of new cancer treatments from pet dogs to humans. *Nature Reviews Cancer*, 8 (2008) 147–156.

138. Vail D. M., MacEwen E. G. Spontaneously occurring tumors of companion animals as models for human cancer. *Cancer Investigation*, 18 (2000) 781–792.

139. Pardoll D. M. The blockade of immune checkpoints in cancer immunotherapy. *Nature Reviews Cancer*, 12 (2012) 252–264.

140. Josefowicz S. Z., Lu L. F., Rudensky A. Y. Regulatory T cells: Mechanisms of differentiation and function. *Annual Review of Immunology*, 30 (2012) 531–564.

141. Talmadge J. E., Gabrilovich D. I. History of myeloid-derived suppressor cells. *Nature Reviews Cancer*, 13 (2013) 739–752.

142. Cartman S. T., Kelly M. L., Heeg D., Heap J. T., Minton N. P. Precise manipulation of the *Clostridium difficile* chromosome reveals a lack of association between the tcdC genotype and toxin production. *Applied and Environmental Microbiology*, 78 (2012) 4683–4690.

143. Al-Hinai M. A., Fast A. G., Papoutsakis E. T. Novel system for efficient isolation of *Clostridium* double-crossover allelic exchange mutants

enabling markerless chromosomal gene deletions and DNA integration. *Applied and Environmental Microbiology,* 78 (2012) 8112–8121.

144. Heap J. T., Ehsaan M., Cooksley C. M., Ng Y. K., Cartman S. T., Winzer K., *et al.* Integration of DNA into bacterial chromosomes from plasmids without a counter-selection marker. *Nucleic Acids Research* 40 (2012) e59.

145. Huang H., Chai C., Li N., Rowe P., Minton N. P., Yang S., *et al.* CRISPR/Cas9-based efficient genome editing in *Clostridium ljungdahlii,* an autotrophic gas-fermenting bacterium. 5(12) (2016) 1355–1361, doi:10.1021/acssynbio.6b00044.

Chapter 3

Genetic Engineering of Clostridial Strains for Cancer Therapy

Maria Zygouropoulou,[a] Aleksandra Kubiak,[a] Adam V. Patterson,[b] and Nigel P. Minton[a]

[a]*Clostridia Research Group, BBSRC/EPSRC Synthetic Biology Research Centre (SBRC), School of Life Sciences, University of Nottingham, Nottingham, NG7 2RD, UK*
[b]*Auckland Cancer Society Research Centre and Maurice Wilkins Centre for Molecular Biodiscovery, School of Medical Sciences, University of Auckland, Auckland 1142, New Zealand*

nigel.minton@nottingham.ac.uk

Although tumor hypoxia hampers the efficacy of conventional cancer therapies, it can be exploited by anaerobic bacteria for the selective targeting of solid tumors. Certain *Clostridium* strains are well suited for this purpose, being nonpathogenic and spore-forming obligate anaerobes. Systemically delivered clostridial endospores are dispersed throughout the body and eventually cleared. Those spores that infiltrate a tumor, however, germinate as a consequence of the encountered hypoxic and/or necrotic environment. The predilection of clostridial endospores to colonize tumors is a totally natural phenomenon and exquisitely selective. As such, clostridia can fill an important gap in the repertoire of cancer therapies, being capable of using the presence of hypoxia to their advantage, unlike most other treatment modalities.

Microbial Infections and Cancer Therapy: Recent Advances
Edited by Ananda M. Chakrabarty and Arsénio M. Fialho

ISBN 978-981-4774-86-4 (Hardcover), 978-1-351-04190-4 (eBook)
www.panstanford.com

In the course of time, clostridia have been genetically modified and armed with a variety of anticancer functionalities, in an effort to fine-tune their oncolytic properties. Considerable research efforts have been invested into clostridial-directed enzyme prodrug therapy (CDEPT), whereby clostridia are equipped with prodrug-converting enzymes (PCEs) that can metabolize nontoxic prodrugs into toxic derivatives. Beyond CDEPT, clostridia have also been engineered to deliver desired antibodies and immunotherapeutic messengers. Moreover, to improve the utility of clostridial-based therapies, the incorporation of an imaging functionality has been explored. In the majority of cases, preclinical evaluations have been encouraging, thus gradually enabling the translation of clostridial delivery systems into clinical applications.

This chapter presents a complete synopsis of *all* clostridial genetic engineering activities that have been pursued to date in the context of cancer as well as an insight into the relevant genetic tools underpinning these efforts. It also discusses opportunities that could be pursued in the future, highlighting the great promise that clostridial delivery systems hold as a treatment for cancer.

3.1 Tumor Hypoxia and Necrosis: A Blessing in Disguise?

Solid tumors, defined as localized masses devoid of cysts or liquid areas, account for approximately 90% of annual cancer diagnoses [1]. A typical histological feature of this type of tumors is the presence of hypoxia (reduced oxygen) [2].

Hypoxia is the cumulative result of the uncontrolled growth of the cancer mass that outpaces the angiogenic processes required to support it. As a consequence, the blood vessel architecture of the tumor becomes seriously defective [3]. Angiogenesis is greatest at the interface between tumor and normal tissue but diminishes toward the inner layers, which gradually become hypoxic and/or anoxic [4]. Indicatively, approximately 50%–60% of advanced solid tumors may contain up to 75% of hypoxic or anoxic regions depending on their size [5], with oxygen concentrations below 1%, as opposed to 3%–15% in normal tissues [5, 6]. Limited oxygen (and nutrient) supply eventually leads to cell quiescence and/or necrosis [4].

These structural and functional defects create a number of protective shields for cancer, justifying the fact that tumor hypoxia is now widely accepted as a negative prognosis marker and is associated with aggressive and metastatic forms of cancer [7]. The resulting hypoxic tumor microenvironment not only undermines the effects of radiotherapy, for which a well-oxygenated environment is a prerequisite, but also exacerbates genetic instability and mutability and modulates a number of resistance pathways, including loss of apoptotic potential [8]. Furthermore, the diffusion of chemotherapeutic agents from the bloodstream into the site of the tumor is impeded, resulting in uneven drug distribution and regions of subtherapeutic exposure [5, 9]. Moreover, cell quiescence leads to attenuation of the cellular functions and consequently to the suppression of the drug targets for many chemotherapeutic agents. As a result, quiescent cells escape treatment while retaining their ability to regrow if oxygen and nutrient supply is restored [10].

Although the presence of tumor hypoxia, quiescence, and necrosis hampers traditional therapies, it surprisingly offers great opportunities for anaerobic *Clostridium* strains, which can exploit these conditions as a means of selectively targeting solid tumors [11, 12].

3.2 Clostridia as Cancer-Fighting Agents

The genus *Clostridium* comprises a heterogeneous group of gram-positive, obligate anaerobic, and spore-forming bacteria naturally found in soil, aquatic sediments, as well as the intestinal tract of animals and humans. The genus has gained considerable infamy owing to a few pathogenic strains and their associated diseases, such as *Clostridium perfringens* (gas gangrene), *C. difficile* (pseudomembranous colitis), *C. tetani* (tetanus), and *C. botulinum* (botulism). Nevertheless, it is at the same time the most intensely studied family of bacteria for application in cancer therapy, with references dating back to the beginnings of the 19th century. Different strains have been investigated throughout the years in pursuit of optimum efficacy and safety. A complete time line of the use of clostridia in cancer therapy can be found in Refs. [2, 13, 14].

The biggest advantage of employing clostridia in cancer therapy over other candidate bacteria (e.g., *Salmonella* and *Bifidobacteria* strains) is their spore-forming ability. Spores offer immense benefits in terms of handling, storage, stability, and formulation, as well as the fact that they are easier and cheaper to produce [5, 15]. From a clinical point of view, spores have further advantages, given that they are unlikely to be shed from human patients. Additionally, nongerminated spores, unlike living bacteria, are entirely devoid of immunogenicity and are rapidly cleared from circulation [11, 16].

3.2.1 Embodiment of Treatment

3.2.1.1 Administration route and form

In a clinical setting, a spore dose ranging from 10^6 to 10^{10} colony forming units (CFU) could be administered intravenously or intratumorally, usually with the former route being the one of choice [17]. The initial steps of the proposed pathway for tumor entry involve circulating spores entering tumors via the disrupted and leaky vasculature. Their entry may be reinforced by the enhanced permeability and retention (EPR) effect, according to which particles of certain sizes (typically in the nm–μm range, that is, the size of spores) accumulate in tumor tissue as opposed to normal tissue [18].

3.2.1.2 Tumor colonization

Tumor-selective bacterial colonization is guaranteed, given that the hypoxic and necrotic areas uniquely found in solid tumors are the only places in which spores can germinate and grow. Germinated spores can actively migrate and self-propel away from vasculature, penetrating deep into tumor tissue [9]; this is in contrast to drug molecules, which are transported passively, dependent on diffusion gradients. Following tumor colonization, an actively growing population of vegetative clostridial cells is established at the tumor site. As a result of their immunoevasive capabilities and the aberrant architecture of their vasculature, tumors are the ideal sanctuaries for clostridia to replicate in, unhindered by the immune and reticuloendothelial clearance mechanisms. Also, due to increased cell turnover, tumors have an abundance of nutrients that can be utilized by the replicating bacteria [9]. Clostridial growth is only halted by the well-oxygenated outer rim of the tumor; in this manner, potential spread to healthy tissues is prevented (an additional safety feature) while clostridial oncolysis acts with precision [19].

3.2.1.3 Mechanism of action

Even from the early days of clostridial therapies, it was hypothesized that the inherent oncolytic properties of the species stem from the expression of native cytolytic enzymes upon germination. In support of this, it has been shown that proteolytic strains have superior oncolytic properties and are now the preferred strains for cancer therapy. Whole genome sequencing of these strains has confirmed the expression of several secreted proteases, lipases, and other degradative enzymes, accounting for their cytolytic properties [13, 20]. Nevertheless, there is currently an increasing body of evidence suggesting that the immune system may also participate in the oncolytic process; host inflammatory responses may be elicited as a result of the presence of a localized bacterial infection, helping to induce antitumor immunity and subsequent tumor lysis [21, 22]. Moreover, lysis of cancer cells releases new tumor antigens, aiding the eventual recognition of still-surviving cancer cells as "foreign" [23]. Suppression of tumor growth may also be the result of bacteria competing with tumor cells for available nutrients. In all cases, it has been shown that bacterial-mediated oncolysis is independent of tumor heterogeneity and genetic background and is capable of eradicating even the stubborn hypoxic/quiescent cells, unlike conventional chemotherapeutics [9].

3.2.1.4 Termination of treatment

When termination of treatment is desired, vegetative clostridial cells can be easily eliminated with commonly available antibiotics, such as metronidazole [24].

3.2.2 Limitations of Clostridial Oncolysis

All studies to date have conclusively established that the use of clostridial spores for cancer treatment can be exquisitely selective, safe, and well tolerated. Any side effects that have been encountered were easily managed, resembling the common symptoms of bacterial infections, for example, fever [25].

However, it has been noted that the extent of tumor colonization is directly proportional to tumor volume. A threshold size of 3 cm^3 (2–4 g of tumor mass) is required in order for the bacteria to exert their native oncolytic effect [11, 26], probably because oxygen concentrations in larger tumors are lower and therefore would allow the germination of clostridial spores. Another important shortcoming is that clostridial-mediated tumor lysis spares the cancerous cells at the oxygenated periphery of the tumor. Presumably, once clostridia have destroyed the hypoxic core of a tumor (and with it its niche), the tumor perishes. This allows the tumor to regrow from the remaining cancerous cells, the so-called viable outer rim. This is perhaps why the majority of studies undertaken so far have failed to cure the cancers permanently, despite evident oncolysis [19].

Improvement of the colonization efficiency and elimination of the outer rim have been the focus of ongoing efforts in the development of clostridial cancer therapy. The administration of clostridial spores has been combined with conventional therapies and various strategies aiming to amplify the hypoxic conditions in the tumor. The expectation was that with the complementation and synergy of different approaches not only would the hypoxic core be lysed but also the viable outer rim ablated. On a preclinical level, clostridial spores have been combined with radiation [27, 28], cytotoxic chemotherapeutic drugs [5, 22] (e.g., mitomycin C, vinorelbine, and docetaxel), vascular targeting agents (dolastatin D-10 [5], combretastatin A-4 [12], and vadimezan [19]), as well as reduction of the oxygen levels in the respired air of animals [29] or induction of tumor hyperthermia [30].

For all the above combinations outcomes were encouraging, with improved tumor regression and even "cures" [14, 19, 26]. On some occasions, extreme and even fatal toxicity was observed, attributed to metabolic complications as a result of the rapid breakdown of tumors (the so-called tumor lysis syndrome) [5]. This is dependent on the size of the tumor as well as the dose of the administered therapy. Although the syndrome can, to a certain degree, be prevented and managed in humans, it is important that candidate therapies strike a balance between effectiveness and safety, as being "too effective" may prove lethal [31].

3.3 Genetic Engineering Approaches

In this light, genetic engineering of clostridial strains in an effort to further enhance, fine-tune, and optimize their oncolytic properties seemed a reasonable step in the direction of clinically advancing the genus for cancer therapy. Genetic engineering would allow the incorporation of different anticancer functionalities in the clostridial host, essentially turning it into a vector for gene therapy. With the strict definition of the term, gene therapy involves the delivery of corrective genetic material *into* target cells (i.e., tumor cells or "normal" cells of their microenvironment), with the aim of either modifying, deleting, and replacing abnormal genes or introducing new ones of a therapeutic value [32, 33]. In the case of clostridial species (which lack invasive capabilities), uptake *into* the target cells is not realized and the bacteria serve instead as "Trojan horses," carrying and themselves expressing the therapeutic genes in the tumor region [34]. Genetically engineered strains are often referred to as "armed" or "second-generation" clostridia.

The delivery and expression of therapeutic genes by the clostridial host in the tumor region offer important advantages, which in a clinical setting could translate into treatments with higher therapeutic ratios:

- The rapid bacterial replication can amplify the transgenes locally, without affecting healthy tissues (no systemic toxicity).
- *In situ* production of the therapeutic allows it to act for longer periods of time and at higher concentrations, especially if compared to the systemic administration of the same therapeutic as a drug molecule (higher effectiveness).

Table 3.1 A summary of all genetically engineered clostridial strains in the context of cancer therapy

Strain	Expressed protein	Promoter	Gene location	Gene transfer method	Secretion/ Signal peptide	Prodrug	Refs.
Clostridial-directed enzyme prodrug therapy							
***C. beijerinckii* NCIMB 8052**	CD	Pfdx	pMTL540FT	Electroporation	No secretion	5-FC	[37]
***C. acetobutylicum* DSM792** ***C. acetobutylicum* NI4082**	CD	Pclos	pKNT19	Electroporation	Secretion/clos	5-FC	[38]
***C. sporogenes* NCIMB 10696**	CD	Pfdx	pMTL540F	Electroporation	No secretion	5-FC	[11]
***C. beijerinckii* NCIMB 8052**	nfsB	Pfdx	pMTL500F/ pNTR500F	Electroporation	No secretion	CB1954	[39]
***C. sporogenes* NCIMB 10696** ***C. novyi*-NT**	HinNTR	Pfac2	pMTL555 (pOJP10/11)	Conjugation	No secretion	CB1954	[24]
***C. sporogenes* NCIMB 10696**	nfsB	Padc PglnA Pptb Pthl PabrB Pvgb Pfdx	pMTL540FT	Electroporation	No secretion	CB1954 and PR-104	[40]

Strain	Expressed protein	Promoter	Gene location	Gene transfer method	Secretion/ Signal peptide	Prodrug	Refs.
***C. sporogenes* NCIMB 10696**	NmeNTR nfsB	Pfdx	Chromosomal integration pyrE locus	Conjugation	No secretion	CB1954	[41]
***C. sporogenes* NCIMB 10696**	CPG2	Pfac2 Plac	pMTL5112 pMTL82251:YZ2	Conjugation	Secretion/eglA	N/A	[42, 43]
Clostridial-directed antibody therapy							
***C. sporogenes* NCIMB 10696** ***C. novyi*-NT**	Anti-HIF1a (VHH-AG2)	Pfac2	pMTL555	Conjugation	Secretion/eglA	N/A	[44]
***C. sporogenes* NCIMB 10696**	Anti-VEGFA	Pfdx	pMTL84153/ pMTL82251	Conjugation	Secretion/eglA	N/A	[42]
Immunotherapy							
***C. acetobutylicum* DSM792**	mTNFa	PeglA	pIMP1/ pKNT19	Electroporation	Secretion/eglA	N/A	[45]
***C. acetobutylicum* NI4082**	mTNFa	PeglA	pMTL500E	Electroporation	Secretion/eglA	N/A	[46]
***C. acetobutylicum* DSM792**	mTNFa	PrecA	pIMP1	Electroporation	Secretion/eglA	N/A	[47]

(*Continued*)

Table 3.1 (*Continued*)

Strain	Expressed protein	Promoter	Gene location	Gene transfer method	Secretion/ Signal peptide	Prodrug	Refs.
***C. acetobutylicum* DSM792**	mTNFa	PrecA + extra Cheo box	pIMP1	Electroporation	Secretion/eglA	N/A	[48]
C. acetobutylicum DSM792	mTNFa	PeglA	pIMP1	Electroporation	Secretion/eglA	N/A	[49]
***C. acetobutylicum* DSM793**	rIL2	PeglA	pIMP2	Electroporation	Secretion/eglA	N/A	[50]
***C. sporogenes* ATCC 3584**	mIL12	PeglA	pIMP1	Electroporation	Secretion/eglA	N/A	[51]
Additional functionalities							
***C. oncolyticum* M55**	colicin E3	PcolE3	pCoIE3-CA38	Phage V-mediated transfection	Secretion/colE3	N/A	[52]
***C. perfringens*-sod-ATCC 13124**	PVL	N/A	Chromosomal integration pfoR locus	Electroporation	Secretion/LukS-LukF	N/A	[53]

Most importantly, the use of clostridial hosts can circumvent limitations posed by other gene transfer systems, such as the limited specificity and efficiency of transduction, the high risk of insertional mutagenesis, and the restricted genetic flexibility with respect to the size of heterologous DNA that can be incorporated. The clostridial cell is an ideal environment for gene expression, given that any cofactors necessary for protein function would be provided intracellularly, without the need to rely on the unpredictable and heterogeneous tumor microenvironment [35, 36].

Table 3.1 provides a summary of all the studies carried out to date employing genetically engineered clostridial strains in the context of cancer therapy. These are discussed in more detail in Sections 3.3.2–3.3.5.

3.3.1 The Underpinning Science

3.3.1.1 Genetic tools

Historically, clostridial species have been notoriously difficult to genetically modify; conventional methods had proven ineffective in the genus while genus-specific genetic tools were not available. In recent years, however, genetic methods have advanced significantly, paving the way for the use of clostridial species in cancer and other fields. These include the formulation of standardized plasmid vector systems [54], procedures for creating directed [55–59] and random mutations [60, 61], methods for bringing about the rapid integration of DNA into the chromosome [62, 63], and most recently clustered regularly insterspaced short palindromic repeats (CRISPR)/Cas9-mediated genome editing [64–66]. The steps and developments needed to bring about desired genetic modifications in any *Clostridium* species have recently been reviewed [67].

Gene transfer technologies developed for clostridia involve either the transformation of vegetative cells with a plasmid by electric field permeabilization of the cell membrane (electroporation) or the conjugative transfer of "shuttle" plasmids from *Escherichia coli* into a clostridial host (conjugation).

In the very first clostridial systems that were constructed for cancer therapy using the aforementioned technologies, the genes of interest were expressed in the clostridial host from autonomous plasmids. Given that plasmids may be present in multiple copies in the cell at any one time plasmid-based systems enable the expression of large amounts of protein. Nevertheless, clinical exploitations of clostridial and more generally bacterial cancer therapies can only be realized if the genes of interest are integrated in the chromosome of the bacterial host. Strict regulations regarding the use of genetically engineered organisms as well as fears of growing antibiotic resistance would impede the use of plasmid-based DNA; the potential mobility of elements carried on plasmids and the associated risk of horizontal gene transfer would pose insurmountable safety concerns [68]. Additionally, plasmid DNA is segregationally unstable in the absence of the appropriate selective pressures, posing the risk that expression of the gene of interest would not be sustained in the bacterial host [69]. For the reasons outlined above, genomic integration is the only viable option, offering greater genetic stability as well as unlimited capacity regarding the size of the heterologous gene inserted [34].

In this context, a seminal moment in the development of genetic tools for clostridia was the recent implementation of an allele-coupled exchange (ACE) method, which allows the insertion of heterologous cargos into the host chromosome without the use of antibiotic resistance markers [62]. This method is based on the principle that the integration event yields a selectable phenotype by the means of *pyrE* inactivation. The *pyrE* gene is involved in pyrimidine biosynthesis, and its inactivation eliminates the ability of cells to metabolize 5-fluoroorotic acid (5-FOA) into the toxic metabolite 5-fluorouracil (5-FU). This serves primarily as a counterselection marker, rendering recombinant cells the ability to survive in the presence of 5-FOA, but it simultaneously confers uracil auxotrophy upon them. This is of particular value in cancer treatment, since it automatically provides an additional containment measure; uracil is abundant at the site of the tumor but not readily found in other environments [41]. An outline of the genetic events that take place during ACE can be found in Fig. 3.1.

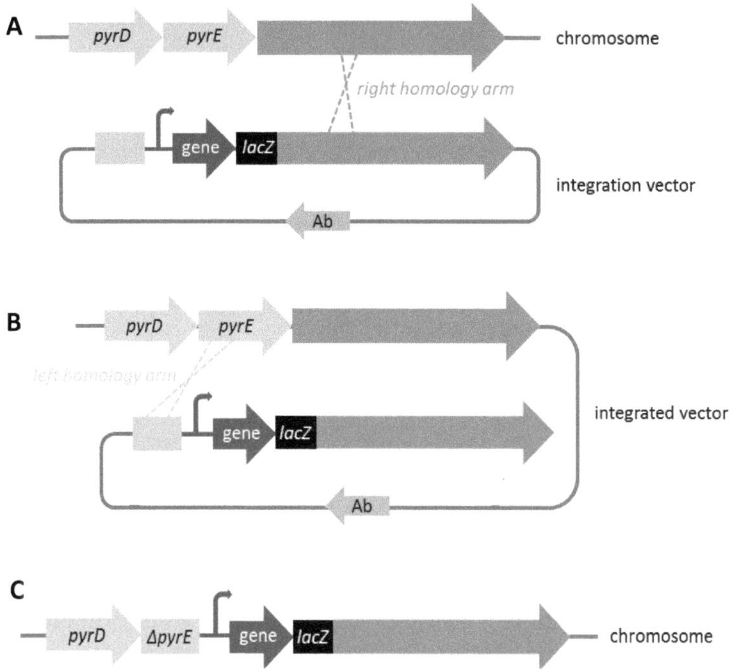

Figure 3.1 Allelic coupled exchange (ACE) for genomic integration in a clostridial host: (A) The gene of interest is integrated into the chromosome of the clostridial host using a segregationally unstable integration vector bearing a suitable antibiotic marker (Ab). This vector is designed so that the sequence to be integrated can be cloned immediately adjacent to a lacZ sequence, flanked by two arms homologous to genomic regions. Integration occurs in a two-step process consisting of two homologous recombination events. The two regions of homology are of very different lengths, in an attempt to direct the event order. The first recombination event (single-crossover) is mediated by a long region of homology between the vector and 1200 bp immediately downstream of the pyrE gene in the bacterial genome (right homology arm). (B) This results in the genomic integration of the entire plasmid. Given that the vector is segregationally unstable, single-crossover mutants have a growth advantage compared to non-single-crossover transconjugants and their colonies appear distinctly larger on media containing the antibiotic. The second recombination event (double-crossover) is mediated by a short region of homology between the vector and 300 bp of the pyrE gene (left homology arm); the complete gene is 576 bp. (C) A successful double-crossover event stably integrates the desired sequence in the chromosome while excising the plasmid and alongside the remaining 276 bp of the pyrE gene. This partial deletion leads to inactivation of the gene, yielding a selectable phenotype by the means of 5-FOA resistance.

However, chromosomal integration of the gene of interest implies that its expression will be carried out from a single gene copy, contrary to plasmid-based systems. Hence, overexpression strategies are of paramount importance in order to maximize the potential yield of the respective protein. Diverse overexpression strategies have now been implemented in a range of clostridial organisms; these include but are not limited to codon optimization [41, 40], mRNA stabilization strategies [70], and the provision of more effective transcription signals and ribosome binding sites (RBS) [71].

Depending on the intended action of the protein of interest, secretion in the extracellular space may be necessary. To that effect, a number of signal peptides functional in different clostridial hosts have been characterized and could be implemented accordingly. Another point to consider is whether constitutive or inducible expression of the genetic cargo is desired; in most cases, constitutive expression is preferred as it allows for a simpler genetic design. Occasionally though, gene expression may be placed under the control of external, tumor-specific stimuli, such as radio (*recA*, *recN*), hypoxia (HIP-1), SOS, or L-arabinose (Pbad) inducible promoters [19, 72, 73]. This could serve as an additional safety feature of the engineered vector, preventing activation in systemic circulation and healthy tissues. Nevertheless, in the case of clostridia such an approach is not essential, given that their administration in spore form guarantees that incorporated genetic cargos are kept inactive until spore germination occurs in tumors.

3.3.1.2 Strain selection

Initial genetic engineering efforts were undertaken using those strains for which there were gene transfer protocols available, including the saccharolytic *C. acetobutylicum* and *C. beijerinckii* [14, 43]. However, although these strains were more amenable to gene transfer, it was quickly established that they had far inferior colonizing and therefore oncolytic properties than most proteolytic strains. In fact, vegetative cell numbers in experimental tumors colonized by *C. beijerinckii* were 2 orders of magnitude lower than those in tumors colonized by *C. sporogenes* M55 (10^5–10^6 versus 1–2 × 10^8 bacteria/g of tumor, respectively) [11]. At the same time, in a direct comparison of 26 bifidobacteria, lactobacilli, and clostridial strains (including *C. acetobuyilicum*), it was found that two proteolytic strains, *C. novyi* and *C. sordelii*, were the only ones able to spread extensively in the poorly vascularized portions of tumors [5].

Fortunately, genetic tools have now progressed sufficiently enough that we can afford to select those strains that are better suited for cancer therapy based on their colonization and oncolytic properties. Nevertheless, it needs to be taken into account that in the context of genetic engineering, the use of proteolytic strains brings about an obvious trade-off; on one hand, the presence of proteolytic enzymes is instrumental for the colonization and oncolysis processes, but on the other hand it might compromise the yield of the recombinant protein as a consequence of enzymatic degradation. However, the relevance of this in *in vitro* and *in vivo* settings needs to be further investigated [74].

Most prominent among the proteolytic strains being investigated for cancer therapy is *C. sporogenes* (previously known as *C. butyricum* M55 or *C. oncolyticum* M55) and *C. novyi*-NT (nontoxic). The strain of *C. sporogenes* used in current studies (NCIMB 10696 or ATCC 3584) is different to *C. sporogenes* M55 (ATCC 13732) used in older experiments, substituted for its greater amenability to DNA transfer and genetic manipulation [43, 75]. While *C. sporogenes* is entirely nonpathogenic, *C. novyi*-NT is an attenuated form of the pathogenic strain *C. novyi* obtained after heat treatment and consequent removal of a lethal toxin carried on a bacteriophage.

In the context of genetic engineering, it seems that *C. sporogenes* is probably the preferred strain of the two, given that it has a bigger genome and coding capacity than *C. novyi*-NT (4.14 Mb and 2.55 Mb, respectively) [13, 20]. Furthermore, *C. sporogenes* has the advantage of being a truly nonpathogenic strain, hence posing fewer safety concerns; any retained virulence could be problematic for immunocompromised late-stage cancer patients while in the genetically unstable environment of the tumor as there is a theoretical risk of attenuated strains reverting to wild type or acquiring other toxic/virulent characteristics [15]. Most importantly, an optimized and refined codon optimization algorithm is now in place, developed exclusively for *C. sporogenes* by DNA 2.0. Implementation of this algorithm will contribute greatly to the maximization of expression of any heterologous gene in this strain [71].

3.3.2 Clostridial-Directed Enzyme Prodrug Therapy

Most efforts with genetically engineered clostridial spores have concentrated on the incorporation of genes for prodrug-converting enzymes (PCEs), thereby giving rise to clostridial-directed enzyme prodrug therapy (CDEPT) [75]. Prodrugs are inert precursors that can be activated by PCEs into potent (anticancer) drugs. Following selective spore germination in the tumor, expression of the PCE is highly localized. The prodrug is then systemically administered, but its activation and subsequent anticancer activity take place inside the tumor where it has encountered the PCE. Even more conveniently, as with all enzymatic reactions, one molecule of PCE can metabolize large quantities of the prodrug. CDEPT, which falls under the category of suicide gene therapies [76], is a promising and, most importantly, safe approach for overcoming the limitations associated with incomplete clostridial oncolysis [77]. An outline of CDEPT is shown in Fig. 3.2.

The success of CDEPT is reliant on various elements:

- **Suitable PCE:** An enzyme that is ideally absent or otherwise present in insignificant levels in humans or exclusively expressed in the tumor. If a human enzyme homolog of the PCE exists, it should have different structural requirements with respect to the substrate. It should also be sufficiently active at body temperature (37° C) and have access to any cofactors required for catalysis. The PCE can either be exported or exert its actions from the inside of the clostridial cell.
- **Suitable prodrug:** A prodrug should have optimal physicochemical properties (i.e., solubility and stability) and be able to diffuse into bacterial cells (if the enzyme is not secreted). The active metabolite should be able to diffuse out. A high differential toxicity between the prodrug and the active metabolite is also necessary.
- **Suitable PCE/Prodrug combination:** The combination should be kinetically favorable, allowing for a high reaction rate, catalytic efficiency, and product yield.
- **Sufficient PCE expression:** Although bacterial replication can amplify the transgene, strong constitutive expression of the PCE from the clostridial vegetative cells is highly

desired, such that a maximal level of enzyme is produced throughout the growth cycle of the bacterium and that enzyme concentration is not rate limiting in the conversion reaction.

- **Bystander effect:** It is essential for the toxic prodrug metabolite to be able to diffuse from the site of generation toward viable cancer cells, hence generating a localized cytotoxic effect and thus allowing the majority of tumor cells to be treated.

To date, a number of enzyme–prodrug combinations have been explored in the more general context of enzyme–prodrug strategies. Those that have been implemented in clostridial species are described below.

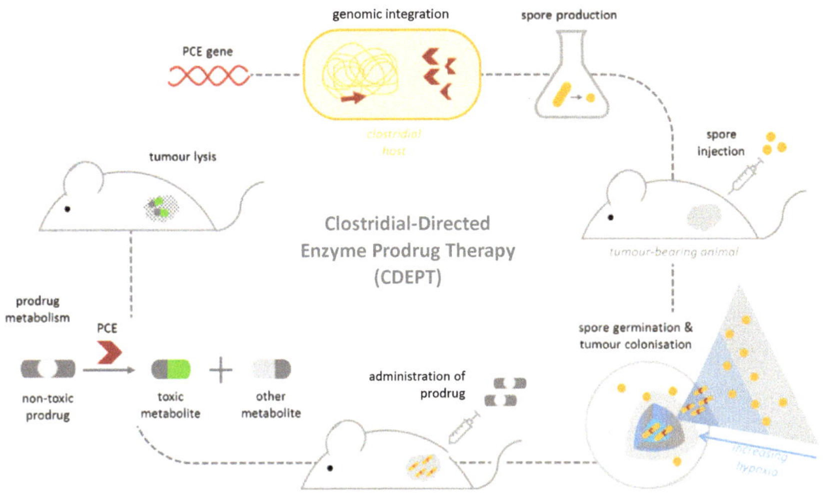

Figure 3.2 Clostridial-directed enzyme prodrug therapy (CDEPT): (From top-left corner, clockwise) A gene encoding a suitable prodrug-converting enzyme (PCE) is integrated into the bacterial chromosome. A spore stock of the recombinant cells is prepared, and an appropriate spore dose is administered intravenously into a tumor-bearing animal. The spores germinate only in the hypoxic environment of the tumor; the resulting vegetative cells replicate locally and colonize the tumor. A nontoxic prodrug is then administered systemically. Its conversion into an active drug occurs only within the tumor, whereby the PCE is being expressed by the vegetative clostridial cells. The active drug leads to cancer cell death and tumor regression.

3.3.2.1 Cytosine deaminase

Cytosine deaminase (CD) is an enzyme whose normal function is to catalyze the deamination of cytosine to uracil. It is part of the pyrimidine salvage pathway, whereby it allows the utilization of cytosine for pyrimidine nucleotide synthesis. In the context of CDEPT, CD is matched with 5-fluorocytosine (5-FC) as the prodrug of choice; CD catalyzes the conversion of 5-FC into 5-FU, which is then further metabolized into inhibitors of RNA and DNA biosynthesis. Employing CD in CDEPT was a rational choice, given the lack of a mammalian enzyme counterpart, the large differential in toxicity between the prodrug (5-FC) and the metabolite (5-FU), as well as the existing clinical experience with 5-FU as a chemotherapeutic and radiosensitizer agent [37]. In addition 5-FU has been associated with a number of unwanted side effects following systemic administration, which could in principle be circumvented with CDEPT.

So far, CD expression has been demonstrated in three different clostridial strains: *C. beijerinckii*, *C. acetobutylicum*, and *C. sporogenes*. In all cases the CD employed was that of *E. coli*, with the *codA* gene (UniProt P25524) carried on a shuttle plasmid. Fox and colleagues were the first to show that in clonogenic survival assays, culture supernatants of CD-expressing *C. beijerinckii* NCIMB 805 cells can increase the sensitivity of murine EMT6 carcinoma cell lines to 5-FC up to 500-fold. Although CD was not engineered to be secreted, activity in the culture supernatants is thought to have arisen as a result of bacterial cell death and subsequent release of the protein into the external milieu [37].

A few years later, Theys and colleagues engineered two different strains of *C. acetobutylicum* (DSM 792, NI4082) to express and secrete the same protein. The recombinant spores were delivered to WAG/Rij rats bearing subcutaneous rhabdomyosarcomas. CD activity could be detected in 10/18 tumors treated with strain DSM 792 and 4/6 tumors treated with strain NI4082, while no activity was detected in healthy tissues. When strain NI4082 was combined with Combretastatin A-4 phosphate (CombreAp), proven to promote vascular collapse and amplify hypoxia, the incidence of CD activity in tumors increased to 100% (6/6 tumors). Most importantly, it was shown that the efficiency of conversion of 5-FC to 5-FU achieved could enable clinically relevant sensitization of tumors to radiotherapy [38, 46].

Although these studies were useful as a proof of that concept that CD expression and secretion in clostridia was indeed feasible and worthwhile, it was not until *C. sporogenes* was employed that a clear antitumor effect was demonstrated. Once a DNA transfer methodology via electroporation was developed for the strain, *C. sporogenes* was engineered to express a nonsecreted form of CD. Following intravenous (IV) administration of recombinant spores in C3H/Km mice harboring SCCVII tumors, tumor growth delay was observed, greater than that achieved by a maximum tolerated dose of 5-FU. Additionally, the researchers were able to establish that the numbers of clostridial vegetative cells in tumors were unaffected by the treatment, allaying concerns around selective bacterial cell death. However, employing clostridia did not prove successful in preventing development of tumor resistance to 5-FU, a previously known shortcoming. In fact, after seven days of treatment, tumors became refractory to the toxic metabolite and tumor growth of treated mice (with 5-FU only or with recombinant spores and 5-FC) resembled that of control animals [11].

It seems that this inherent disadvantage of the CD/5-FC combination halted research efforts employing this particular system; to date no follow-up studies have been published. Instead, it appears that scientific interest was shifted to alterative CDEPT strategies and predominantly to systems that employ nitroreductases (NTRs) as the PCEs.

3.3.2.2 Nitroreductases

NTRs represent a large family of nicotinamide adenine dinucleotide (phosphate) [NAD(P)H]-dependent flavoenzymes that can catalyze the reduction of nitro groups. They have broad substrate specificity and can accommodate a great variety of polynitrated aromatic compounds, usually generating hydroxylamino or amino derivatives, as terminal reduction products [78]. In the context of directed enzyme prodrug therapy (DEPT) strategies employing NTRs, CB1954 has traditionally been the mainstay prodrug utilized. CB1954 (tetrazicar) is the prototype of the dinitrobenzamide family of prodrugs, and its activation by NTRs leads to the production of 2-hydroxylamine (2HX) and 4-hydroxylamine (4HX) derivatives. The 4HX derivative, a bifunctional alkylator, is 10,000-fold more toxic than CB1954 and is further metabolized to form interstrand crosslinks in DNA. The crosslinks are poorly repaired and lead to cell death independently of the cell cycle stage, also killing cells that are not rapidly proliferating [19, 78–80]. The 2HX product despite being less cytotoxic may also contribute to tumor cell killing as it diffuses more readily and displays a more pronounced bystander effect [81].

Although clostridial cells natively express a range of NTRs, it has been shown that the level of endogenous NTR activity is not sufficient to metabolize efficiently prodrugs of interest and generate significant anticancer effects [24, 41, 40]; as a result, engineering of the clostridial host in order to (over)express a specific NTR gene selected and matched with a given product is necessary. To date, clostridial strains engineered to express NTRs include *C. beijerinckii* and *C. sporogenes*. In all cases the enzymes have been introduced in a nonsecreted form, assuming that the prodrugs employed can diffuse in the bacterial cell while their metabolites can diffuse out.

E. coli nfsB, also known as EcoNTR (UniProt P38489), was the first bacterial NTR employed in CDEPT. *In vitro* treatment of EMT6 and SCCVII cancer cell lines with supernatants of nfsB-expressing *C. beijeirinckii* cell cultures and CB1954 resulted in a 22-fold higher killing than wild-type *C. beijeirinckii* cell culture supernatants combined with the same prodrug. *In vivo*, significant NTR activity was confirmed in 10/10 tumors after IV injection of recombinant spores in Balb/c female mice harboring EMT6 mammary carcinomas, while tumors of mice injected with nonrecombinant spores were devoid of NTR activity [39]. A few years later, a codon-optimized version of the same gene (sNTR) in combination with more efficient transcription signals than those employed previously was introduced in *C. sporogenes*, in an effort to eliminate codon bias and improve expression levels in the clostridial host. Indeed, expression of the gene was improved 20- to 30-fold and was critical in achieving statistically significant antitumor activity *in vivo*. When sNTR-recombinant spores were injected in immunodeficient nude mice with SiHa human cervical carcinomas, significant tumor growth delay was observed in combination with the CB1954 or PR-104 prodrugs. On the contrary, treatment with recombinant spores carrying the native version of the gene in combination with the same prodrugs failed to generate significant antitumor activity, presumably due to lower NTR expression [40]. This serves to highlight the importance of adequate PCE expression for clinical implementations of CDEPT.

Despite these encouraging results, the nfsB/CB1954 combination is far from ideal. CB1954 is not a natural substrate for nfsB. So the enzyme affinity, reaction rate, and product yield are suboptimal. Consequently, efforts have concentrated on finding more efficient combinations.

In this respect, HinNTR, an alternative nfsB-type NTR, was identified from *Haemophilus influenzae* (UniProt Q4QJZ7) with an improved CB1954 turnover rate. Additionally, HinNTR was found to exclusively metabolize CB1954 to the 4HX toxic metabolite, as opposed to nfsB, which generates an equimolar amount of the 4HX and 2HX derivatives. A plasmid carrying a codon-optimized version of the HinNTR gene was introduced for the first time in *C. sporogenes* by conjugation. When nu/nu mice xenografted with subcutaneous HCT116 tumors were treated with recombinant spores, followed by CB1954 administration, a significant antitumor activity was observed in tumor regrowth delay assays. Most importantly antitumor efficacy was maintained even after repeated cycles of treatment, analogous to many chemotherapeutic anticancer regimens [24].

Although the above studies generated a body of useful preclinical data, the clinical exploitation of CDEPT can only be realized if the PCE is integrated in the chromosome of the clostridial host. Thus, in the most comprehensive CDEPT study to date, a codon-optimized version of the NmeNTR gene was stably integrated into the chromosome of *C. sporogenes* using ACE. NmeNTR, an enzyme from *Neisseria meningitis* (UniProt Q9K022), is also an nfsB-type NTR with kinetics superior to that of nfsB. Metabolism of CB1954 by NmeNTR generates only the 4HX toxic derivative, while its affinity for the prodrug (K_M = 2.47 μM) is lower than the maximum concentration of CB1954, which can be safely tolerated in a patient's serum (6.3 μM), indicating that enzyme saturation and efficient prodrug activation would be feasible in a clinical setting. As expected, treatment of human colorectal HCT116 carcinoma in NMRI nu/nu mice with CB1954 and spores of the

NmeNTR-expressing strain delayed tumor growth significantly and to a greater extent than treatment with nfsB-recombinant spores; complete tumor regression was also seen in some cases (4/16 tumors) [41].

Despite the encouraging outcomes above, identifying a kinetically favorable NTR/prodrug combination has proven challenging. Some of the most noteworthy naturally occurring NTRs that have been characterized for their catalytic activity toward CB1954 are included in Table 3.2; however, only the ones mentioned above have been expressed in clostridial hosts. From Table 3.2 it becomes apparent that there is no single enzyme with ideal kinetics toward CB1954. As an example, although NmeNTR seems to satisfy the K_M requirement, it has a very low catalytic efficiency with respect to CB1954, which automatically renders it a less attractive choice. On the other hand, YfkO from *Bacillus licheniformis* (UniProt Q65MG6), which possesses by far the greatest published catalytic efficiency toward CB1954, has a lower-than-desired affinity for the prodrug (K_M > 6.3 μM). Consequently, researchers opted to engineer natural NTRs with the aim of improving their activity toward CB1954. This was largely achieved by random and/or site-directed mutagenesis as well as directed evolution of the promising NTR candidates combined with sophisticated high-throughput screening methods. Encouragingly, these efforts were mostly fruitful, identifying enzymes with up to 45-fold higher catalytic efficiency with respect to CB1954 compared to wild-type nfsB [82].

Nevertheless, the lack of an optimal NTR/prodrug combination was compounded when safety concerns around the use of CB1954 in humans were brought to light; a phase I study in cancer patients revealed dose-limiting diarrhea and hepatotoxicity, with subsequent toxicological studies confirming metabolism of the prodrug by endogenous human liver enzymes [80, 87]. Naturally, research also branched toward the identification of novel prodrugs that are either safer or a better match with candidate NTRs; these include dinitrobenzamide mustards, oxazino-acrinides, nitrobenzyl, and nitroheterocyclic carbamate prodrugs [78, 79]. A subset of these compounds has indeed demonstrated better binding and cytotoxic properties than CB1954 in combination with nfsB or other NTRs, as well as a

Table 3.2 Properties of naturally occurring NTRs with respect to CB1954

Enzyme	Organism	Cofactor	[b]K_{cat} (s^{-1})	[c]K_M^{CB1954} (µM)	[d]K_{cat}/K_M^{CB1954} (s^{-1} μM^{-1})	Products	Refs.
nfsB (EcoNTR)[a] [P38489]	*Escherichia coli*	NADH	6.0	862	0.007	4HX+2HX	[83]
HinNTR[a] [Q4QJZ7]	*Haemophilus influenzae*	NADH	56.2	690	0.081	4HX	[24]
NmeNTR[a] [Q9K022]	*Neisseria meningitis*	NADH NADPH	4.04 15.23	2.47	1.636 6.166	4HX	[41]
YwrO [Q8VSR5]	*Bacillus amyloliquefaciens*	NADH	8.2	617	0.013	4HX	[84]
NfsA [A7ZJR9]	*Escherichia coli*	NADH NADPH	2.60 20.90	18 140	0.15	2HX	[85]
YfkO [Q65MG6]	*Bacillus licheniformis*	NADH	1067	30	35.6	4HX	[86]

[a]Enzymes that have been expressed in clostridial hosts

[b]K_{cat}: The catalytic constant for the conversion of CB1954 to the product, an indication of the reaction turnover

[c]K_M^{CB1954}: The Michaelis constant, defined as the concentration of CB1954 at which the initial rate of the reaction is half of the maximum velocity, an indication of the enzyme affinity for the substrate

[d]K_{cat}/K_M^{CB1954}: The "specificity constant" of the reaction, an indication of the overall catalytic efficiency at low substrate concentrations

more pronounced bystander effect. Most notable and clinically advanced among those is PR-104, a dinitrobenzamide mustard initially developed as a hypoxia-activated prodrug. PR-104 is also the only prodrug apart from CB1954 that has been tested in combination with an NTR-expressing clostridial strain; in fact, Liu *et al.* demonstrated that PR-104 in combination with an sNTR-expressing *C. sporogenes* strain was more efficient than CB1954 in generating a sustained tumor reduction in mice with SiHa xenografts, even at comparatively lower administered doses [40]. Unfortunately, findings from phase I/II clinical trials employing PR-104 have cast doubts on the clinical utility of this prodrug; dose-limiting myelotoxicity attributed to prodrug metabolism by the human aldo-keto reductase 1C3 (AKR1C3) as well as high levels of clearance were common shortcomings responsible for stalling the clinical implementation of PR-104, inside or outside CDEPT [82].

Despite all the aforementioned difficulties encountered along the development path of NTRs as PCEs for CDEPT, this field of research remains the most active, given the large substrate promiscuity of the NTR family and the great number of unexplored possibilities that lie ahead [82]. In support of this, the incorporation of NTRs in clostridial cancer vectors has additional advantages. On one hand, NTRs can be engineered to metabolize not only the desired prodrug but also a suitable imaging probe (as discussed in more detail in Section 3.3.6). On the other hand, NTRs have been found to increase the sensitivity of clostridial strains toward antibiotics routinely used for their clearance (e.g., metronidazole), therefore providing an additional biosafety feature [82].

3.3.2.3 Carboxypeptidase G2

Another enzyme that had been considered for implementation in CDEPT was the zinc-dependent secreted metalloenzyme, carboxypeptidase G2 (CPG2). CPG2 cleaves the C-terminal glutamate moiety of folate-based compounds, which are essential in a number of intracellular functions and primarily in DNA synthesis. To that effect, CPG2 could be paired with glutamated benzoyl nitrogen mustard prodrugs whose CPG2-mediated metabolism would yield cytotoxic nitrogen mustard derivatives [88]. CPG2 may be well suited for CDEPT given the lack of a human enzyme analogue as well as its established clinical use as a rescue therapy in methotrexate-induced toxicities.

CPG2 expression and secretion have been attempted twice in *C. sporogenes* using a codon-optimized version of the CPG2 gene from *Variovorax paradoxus*. The native signal peptide of the protein was substituted for the eglA signal peptide from *C. saccharobutylicum*, which would be more suitable for use in a gram-positive organism. Unfortunately, in both instances, there was almost no CPG2 activity detected in the culture supernatants, presumably due to proteolytic cleavage of the enzyme as a result of proteases secreted by *C. sporogenes*. CPG2 activity was higher in the soluble fraction of cell lysates, indicating that protein export might have been defective [42, 43]. In view of the above shortcomings, the implementation of CPG2 in CDEPT has not been pursued further.

3.3.3 Clostridial-Directed Antibody Therapy

In a fashion similar to CDEPT, clostridial hosts have also been engineered to express antibodies with direct anticancer functions. In the case of CDAT the requirements of the system are fewer, with the only crucial constraint being that the antibody of interest should not interfere with the cellular functions of the host.

3.3.3.1 Anti-hypoxia-inducible factor 1 alpha antibody

Anti-hypoxia-inducible factor 1 alpha (HIF1) is a key transcription alregulator of the adaptive response to hypoxia, responsible for activating multiple genes involved in oxygen delivery and the metabolic adaptation to hypoxic conditions. Consequently, HIF1 plays a crucial role in mediating angiogenesis in solid tumors; in fact, HIF1a subunit overexpression is evident in many tumor types and is associated with conferring selective advantages that promote mutagenesis and tumor growth [89]. Hence, inhibition of HIF1a by the means of an antibody is a rational therapeutic strategy. Delivery of the antibody by CDAT will ensure its tumor-selective action, thereby preventing HIF1a neutralization elsewhere in the body.

The nucleotide sequence for a HIF1a-targeting small antibody fragment (VHH-AG2) was introduced in *C. sporogenes* and *C. novyi*-NT by conjugation. VHHs are naturally occurring, single-chain antibodies from camelids; while being smaller in size (15 kDa) they retain full antigen-binding capacity and specificity. The VHH-AG2 sequence was preceded by the *eglA* signal sequence from *C. saccharobutylicum* in order to enable secretion. Expression of a functional antibody with conserved binding capacity toward the HIF1a antigen was confirmed in both strains [44]. Although the *in vivo* efficacy of these strains was not evaluated, merely the confirmation that clostridial hosts—including proteolytic strains—are capable of expressing functional antibodies was of crucial importance, opening a new range of therapeutic options.

3.3.3.2 Antivascular endothelial growth factor antibody

Vascular endothelial growth factor (VEGF) is a central regulator in the vascular development of growing tumors, often considered as the most important tumor angiogenesis factor. Therefore, it is an attractive drug target, being indispensable to tumor progression and expressed by nearly all malignant tumors. A humanized, recombinant monoclonal antibody against VEGF-A (bevasizumab) has proven effective in decelerating tumor progression in clinical settings. On one hand, VEGF inhibition could assist in the normalization of the tumor vasculature, whereby improved tumor perfusion and oxygenation would render the tumor more accessible to chemotherapy and abate its invasive and metastatic tendencies. On the other hand, it could lead to complete cessation of the tumor vascularization process, in which case oxygen and nutrient deprivation would lead to tumor necrosis, making the tumor even more suitable for clostridial colonization [90].

Expression of a monoclonal anti-VEGF antibody [91] was attempted in *C. sporogenes*. Again, the protein was designed to be expressed in a secreted form by incorporation of the eglA signal peptide from *C. saccharobutylicum*. However, antibody expression proved challenging and was never confirmed. This was attributed to potential toxicity brought about by the overexpression of the antibody in the clostridial host; even implementation of an inducible system was not able to resolve this technical hurdle [42]. Yet, given the fact that the VHH-AG2 antibody was previously successfully expressed in the same host, it is likely that failure of expression in this case is related to antibody-specific factors and as such, it should not discourage the consideration of alternative antibodies in the future.

3.3.4 Immunotherapy

The immune system plays a vital role in identifying and eliminating transformed cells in the early stages of cancer and may even prevent tumor formation altogether [92]. Unfortunately, some cancer cells survive this process and their immunogenicity becomes diminished. New populations of tumor cells derived from these renegade cells maintain the ability to escape the immune system, and as a result, growing tumors can no longer be detected by immune effectors, ultimately leading to outgrowth of cancer. Even stromal components in the tumor microenvironment, including cells of the innate and adaptive arm of the immune system, are often referred to as "immunoignorant" because they abstain from providing "danger signals" to the immune system [93].

Immunosuppression is maintained by a range of signaling molecules that are present in the tumor microenvironment; these molecules may not only inhibit immune responses but also switch responses to inefficient types of immunity [3, 94, 95]. Yet, tumor-antagonizing processes may also take place, with the eventual outcome being dictated by the combination/domination of specific cytokines. Logically, in the context of cancer immunotherapy, the cytokine milieu of the tumor can be perturbed in such a way that the patient's immune system is restimulated and redirected against the tumor, with the ability to eliminate cancer cells in the tumor microenvironment. In this regard, employing clostridia for the delivery of immunotherapeutic functionalities and particularly cytokines is of great interest.

Currently, interleukin-2 (IL-2) and interferon alpha (IFN-α) are the only clinically approved cytokines for immune system stimulation. Granulocyte-macrophage colony-stimulating factor (GM-CSF) and granulocyte colony-stimulating factor (G-CSF) have also been approved for clinical use, but these are mainly employed as a means of accelerating the recovery of neutrophil granulocytes following chemotherapy. Other interleukins, such as IL-7, IL-12, IL-18, and IL21, have not yet reached the clinic but are currently being studied, both as adjuvants and as stand-alone agents [3, 96]. In a clinical setting however, IV administration of cytokines has proved of limited efficacy and relatively toxic, with an array of unwanted side effects [97].

Employing a clostridial vector for *in situ* production of cytokines can improve the safety profile and tolerability of cytokine immunotherapy. Furthermore, it might be advantageous for cytokines that are difficult to produce and purify for administration as protein drugs [98]. In support of this rationale, there is now a body of evidence suggesting that local immunotherapy approaches are indeed effective as well as safe; they have been shown to minimize local immunosuppression and to mediate strong immune responses locally and systemically while minimizing systemic toxicity. They have even been shown to induce tumor regression in metastatic tumor deposits where immunotherapy has not been applied [95]. It is also likely that the delivered immunotherapeutic will act synergistically with any immune stimulation that may arise as a result of the bacterial tumor colonization [2].

The majority of local immunotherapy has so far been pursued via the means of intertumoral (IT) injections—evidently, the use of a clostridial vector that can be administered intravenously is likely to be more widely applicable. Unlike other bacterial species, engineering of clostridia to incorporate immunotherapeutic functionalities has been rather limited. Only three cytokines have been expressed in clostridial hosts: tumor necrosis factor alpha (TNF-α), IL-2, and more recently IL-12. These attempts are described in detail below.

3.3.4.1 Tumor necrosis factor alpha

TNF-α is a pleiotropic anticancer cytokine; in the context of cancer therapy, apart from mediating a direct cytotoxic effect against cancer cells via induction of apoptosis, it also stimulates a T-cell-driven immune response with selective action on tumor neovasculature [99].

Expression and secretion of murine TNF-α (mTNF-α) has been demonstrated in *C. acetobutylicum*. Although the mTNF-α nucleotide sequence was employed without codon optimization, the native signal peptide of the eukaryotic protein would not be recognized by the clostridial host and therefore the *eglA* signal sequence from *C. saccharobutylicum* was used instead. Biologically active mTNF-α protein was detected in both supernatants and lysates of the recombinant bacterial cultures for up to 12 h and 20 h, respectively; loss of activity thereafter was attributed to acidification of the culture media. The protein concentration in and out of the cell paralleled the pattern of cell growth, while a maximum *in vitro* activity of 10^3 U/mL was observed against WEH164 clone 13 cell lines for both supernatants and lysates [45]. This was the first example of successful secretion of a eukaryotic protein from a clostridial host, paving the way for subsequent improvements to the system [49]. Later on, *in vivo* mTNF-α activity was also established in WAG/Rij rats harboring subcutaneously implanted rhabdomyosarcomas; mTNF-α concentrations were considerably higher in tumor homogenates of mice treated with recombinant spores versus in untreated and nonrecombinant controls [46].

Expression of TNF-α has also been paired with a radiation-inducible *recA* promoter, capitalizing on the synergistic effect of TNF-α and radiation in terms of cancer cell killing as well as introducing a temporal control mechanism on gene expression. Promoter induction was achieved at a clinical relevant radiation dose of 2 Gy, generating a maximum increase of 44% in mTNF-α expression and secretion relative to the noninduced state [47]. The responsiveness of the promoter to radiation was further enhanced (up to 412% increase in mTNF-α expression and secretion) by incorporation of an extra Cheo box in the promoter sequence; the Cheo box is the specific operator sequence where the *LexA* repressor is bound in the absence of radiotherapy-induced cell damage [48].

3.3.4.2 Interleukin-2

IL-2 is another pluripotent cytokine with anticancer potential. It is generally regarded as a "T-cell growth factor," fundamental in regulating the survival, proliferation, and/or differentiation of activated T cells as well as natural killer (NK) cells. IL-2 can also upregulate the production of other cytokines involved in immunostimulation, such as TNF-α. In view of its diverse functions, IL-2 was the first method of cancer immunotherapy to reach the clinic [100].

Following the previous successful studies with TNF-α, the same research group attempted expression and secretion of rat IL-2 (rIL2) in *C. acetobutylicum,* once again employing the *eglA* promoter and signal sequence from *C. saccharobutylicum*. Levels of extracellular rIL2 ranged from 85 ng/mL to 800 ng/mL while secretion efficiencies ranged between 77% and 97%, depending on the growth phase. Biological activity of the secreted protein was confirmed using *in vitro* T-cell proliferation assays, whereby extracellular IL-2 levels peaked at 1×10^5 IU/ml. However, the *in vivo* efficacy of this recombinant strain was not assayed, leaving unanswered the question of whether the levels of rIL2 secretion achieved are of clinical significance [50].

3.3.4.3 Interleukin-12

IL-12 is a cytokine involved in both innate and adaptive cell-mediated immune responses, often regarded as an important link between the two branches of immunity. The physiological hallmark of IL-12 is the induction of interferon gamma (IFN-γ) production. In the context of cancer immunotherapy, IL-12 may be of benefit as it significantly enhances the activity of cytotoxic cells (e.g., cytotoxic T lymphocytes and NK cells) as well as directly inhibiting the vascularization processes of growing tumors [101].

Approximately 10 years after the publication of the rIL2 study, Zhao *et al.* reported the successful expression and secretion of murine IL-12 (mIL12) in *C. sporogenes* ATCC 3584 [51]. In line with the previous studies, the group resorted to the use of the *eglA* promoter and signal sequence from *C. saccharobutylicum*. Encouragingly, biologically active IL-12 was detected in culture supernatants with a concentration of approximately 18 pg/mL; it appears that protein export was extremely efficient since no detectable levels of IL-12 were found in cell lysates. It should be noted that the levels of mIL12 in the extracellular portion are much lower than those reported previously with rIL2 (85–800 ng/mL); *ceteris paribus,* this may be attributed to partial enzymatic breakdown of the secreted protein, given the proteolytic character of the strain employed in this study. Nevertheless, treatment of immunocompetent, female BALB/c mice bearing subcutaneous EMT6 mammary carcinomas with recombinant spores generated a statistically significant antitumor efficacy (tumor growth delay ≈ 6 days) compared to sham- or wild-type-treated animals. Complete tumor regression was also observed in 1/7 tumors 26 days after treatment. Finally, IFN-γ plasma levels were elevated in mice treated with the recombinant spores, consistent with the production of IL-12 in the area of the tumor [51].

3.3.5 Various Functionalities

3.3.5.1 Colicin E3

Colicin E3, an *E. coli*–derived antimicrobial peptide with cancerostatic properties, was actually the first heterologous gene to be engineered in a clostridial host with the aim of enhancing its oncolytic properties. Despite the elemental genetic tools available at the time, Schlechte and Elbe managed to successfully introduce the Colicin E3 gene in *C. oncolyticum* M55; expression of active protein was demonstrated by virtue of the formation of inhibitory zones in a soft agar layer containing a Colicin-E3–sensitive *E. coli* strain. Most importantly, their attempt marked the debut of genetic manipulation of clostridial strains in the context of cancer therapy [52].

3.3.5.2 Methionine-γ-lyase

Methionine-γ-lyase (MGL) is a pyridoxal 5′-phosphate (PLP)-dependent enzyme physiologically responsible for the metabolism of L-methionine into a-ketobutyrate, methanethiol, and ammonia [102, 103]. MGL is only present in specific bacterial lineages, parasitic protozoa, and plants while being entirely absent from mammalian cells [104]. Dependence on exogenous methionine appears to be an obligatory and universal characteristic of tumors; unlike normal cells, which are able to synthesize methionine from alternative sources (e.g., from homocysteine), the growth of malignant cells is entirely dependent on the provision of extracellular methionine, a probable Achilles' heel [105]. In fact, methionine depletion has been shown to mediate various anticancer effects, eventually leading to cancer cell death via apoptosis [103, 106]. In a clinical context, methionine depletion has been largely pursued via the means of methionine-restricted diets, but mostly with moderate outcomes [105, 106]. Consequently, the implementation of MGL in the context of cancer therapy is considered a promising approach, given its powerful methionine-depletion capabilities as demonstrated in *in vivo* studies [105].

Besides the obvious role of MGL in methionine depletion, the anticancer effects of the enzyme can be further exploited in combination with suicide prodrugs. For instance, the enzyme has been studied in combination with selenomethionine, generating encouraging preclinical outcomes. MGL has also been found to act synergistically with 5-FU, cisplatin, vincristine, and nitrosourea, assisting in the sensitization of tumor cells toward these chemotherapeutic agents [105, 106]. Preclinical *in vivo* data also suggest that MGL-based anticancer therapy can be used for a wide range of tumors, including those resistant to chemotherapy or radiation [103].

Despite the above considerations, the clinical implementation of MGL has been stalled due to the fact that systemically administered MGL is highly immunogenic, generating severe anaphylactic reactions in primate models [107]. As a result, expression of MGL from a clostridial host may be an ideal solution, enabling MGL targeting at the site of the tumor and minimizing the likelihood of MGL-invoked systemic side effects.

C. sporogenes is one of the few bacterial strains that natively express MGL [108, 109]. Additionally, when compared to MGL homologues from other bacterial species, the purified form of the *C. sporogenes* protein is characterized by a higher catalytic activity with respect to methionine [109]. Being confident about the in-host functionality of the protein, *C. sporogenes* can be engineered to overexpress MGL, for example, by introducing another copy in the genome under the control of a strong constitutive promoter.

3.3.5.3 Panton Valentine Leukocidin

Panton valentine leucocidin (PVL) is a β-pore-forming toxin from *Staphylococcus aureus* that causes leukocyte destruction and has an overall immunosuppressive action [110]. PVL was engineered in a strain of *C. perfringens* with the aim of diminishing host inflammatory responses and facilitating unhindered microbial replication in the tumors. This approach, although entirely opposite to the concept of cancer immunotherapy discussed previously, may be rational in light of the strain employed. *C. perfringens* is a highly pathogenic and phospholipase-C secreting strain with a residual oxygen tolerance that would allow it to germinate in tissues other than tumors [111]. It follows that *C. perfringens* is probably more visible to the immune system than other clostridial strains, eliciting an inflammatory response against itself and therefore minimizing the potential oncolytic benefit of the treatment.

Therefore, alongside the introduction of the PVL gene, the researchers also deleted the superoxide dismutase (sod) gene in order to minimize the oxygen tolerance of the strain and improve its tumor selectivity. Upon treatment of PANC02 tumor-bearing, immunocompetent female C57BL/6 mice with the *C. perfringens* sod^-/PVL^+ spores, IT bacterial titers were elevated, consistent with a reduction in the recruitment of neutrophils and macrophages toward the tumor. This translated into substantially prolonged survival of the mice treated with the sod^-/PVL^+ recombinant spores, compared to those treated with wild-type or sod^- spores. Most importantly, there was no evidence of systemic toxicity [53]. Nevertheless, there are certainly safety concerns with regard to engineering replicating bacterial vectors to express immunosuppressive gene products. (Please note that the present study has been retracted since publication due to a duplication of presented micrographs across different publications of the same research group) [112].

3.3.6 Imaging

The preclinical and clinical development of clostridial cancer therapies would be significantly facilitated by an ability to monitor their *in vivo* journey in a noninvasive manner. Imaging-acquired information could assist in the full *in vivo* characterization of clostridial therapies as well as provide a more accurate insight into aspects where our knowledge to date is limited; these include the extent of tumor necrosis/hypoxia required for colonization and subsequently the degree of colonization required for a clinically relevant tumor reduction. Relevant information is currently inferred using suboptimal and inconclusive methods, such as immunoblotting, Gram–Twort staining, and the determination of CFU per gram of tumor homogenates [2]. Additionally, imaging could provide real-time information on the localization of bacteria after systemic administration, mitigating concerns of off-target effects and verifying safety. In a clinical setting, the imaging functionality of a clostridial vector can be repurposed toward noninvasive tumor detection, cancer diagnosis, and stage classification, as well as toward informing the selection/timing of treatments (e.g., the administration of a prodrug) and monitoring their effectiveness [2, 6].

Most importantly, clostridial vectors can provide an appealing solution in overcoming limitations of other imaging methods, such as the lack of tumor specificity and the need for repeated administration of the imaging probes; the inherent tumor-targeting properties of clostridia will guarantee the first, whereas their IT replication will amplify the imaging signal, naturally enhancing the signal-to-noise ratio and eliminating the need for repeated administration of the tracer. Furthermore, since clostridial spores are systemically delivered they can be used without prior knowledge of tumor location, in theory also being capable of revealing concealed tumors not identified via other means [11, 113]. Evidently, the development of an imaging functionality suitable for both preclinical and clinical settings is highly desirable.

In principle, the imaging functionality can be incorporated *de novo* in the clostridial host of interest (e.g., by introducing a suitable reporter gene) or by harnessing genes already present; these can be either native genes (e.g., endogenous NTRs) or heterologous ones, introduced in the first place for the purpose of delivering an anticancer functionality (e.g., a PCE gene for CDEPT). The latter option seems to be ideal, also enabling the monitoring of the therapeutic functionality via the imaging capability. In the majority of cases, a suitable imaging probe is also required, selected on the basis of its ability to be systemically delivered and subsequently processed by the gene product into a cell-accumulating, imageable form as well as its appropriateness for the imaging technique to be employed.

To date, the only study in which tumor imaging via the means of a clostridial vector has been demonstrated made use of a recombinant strain of *C. sporogenes* engineered to express sNTR (as described previously). This strain was used in combination with 6-chloro-9-nitro-5-oxo-5H-benzo [a]phenoxazine (CNOB), a nonfluorescent compound that is converted by sNTR to a highly fluorescent derivative with excitation and emission wavelengths in the visible spectrum. In this manner, subcutaneous SiHa tumors of female immunodeficient nude mice were successfully imaged *in vivo* using a small-animal imaging system; as expected, localization of the signal was tumor specific and maximum CNOB metabolism was observed in the necrotic centers of the cancerous mass [40].

Although CNOB is currently the only (fluorescent) imaging probe tested in combination with a clostridial-derived NTR, a range of other NTR-activated imaging probes has been developed independently. For instance, CytoCy5s is a cell-permeable quenched probe that upon NTR-mediated reduction is no longer able to diffuse out of the cell and fluoresce in the near-infrared spectrum [114]. Similarly, a nitroreductase caged luciferin (NCL) probe has been developed for NTR-specific bioluminescence imaging. NCL is a caged form of luciferin that can be released and therefore processed by luciferase only, following reduction by an NTR [115]. Both probes have been shown to enable the localization of bacterial populations in mice with high accuracy, including the imaging of tumor masses.

Nevertheless, the use of fluorescence and bioluminescence imaging is restricted to preclinical applications in small animals. Therefore, it would be advantageous to pair the functionalities already present in the clostridial host with probes suitable for imaging techniques of more direct clinical relevance, such as magnetic resonance imaging (MRI), computerized tomography (CT), single-photon emission computed tomography (SPECT), positron emission tomography (PET), and hybrid methods, for example, CT/PET. These techniques are highly sensitive and quantitative, providing adequate spatial resolution and having no clinically impeding depth limit [116].

In this context, significant progress has been made in repurposing existing clinical stage 2-nitroimidazole (2-NI) ^{18}FPET imaging probes from hypoxia-activated to NTR-activated equivalents. Probe optimization is ongoing in order to decrease the responsiveness of these probes to hypoxia and hence improve the signal of NTR imaging. Likewise, NTRs are being engineered into PET-competent counterparts, with the aim of making them able to metabolize the candidate probes but without compromising their ability to metabolize the desired prodrug [82, 117]. In the case of clostridial vectors, it is likely that native clostridial NTRs may also be able to metabolize the imaging probe to a certain extent, therefore contributing to signal amplification [82].

Besides PET imaging, it has also been proposed that CD-expressing strains could be imaged using ^{19}F-MRI, taking advantage of the fact that 5-FC and its metabolites are fluorinated and would generate ^{19}F nuclear magnetic resonance (NMR) of high resolution [118, 119]. Similarly, any other PCE-expressing strain that can be paired with a suitable fluorinated prodrug can be used for ^{19}F-MRI imaging.

In the case where the imaging functionality is introduced *de novo* into the clostridial vector, the options could extend beyond those discussed above. For fluorescence imaging, the clostridial host can be engineered to express oxygen-independent fluorescent proteins, which unlike the green fluorescent protein (GFP) do not require oxygen for chromophore maturation [120, 121]. For bioluminescence imaging, luminescence constructs such as the reshuffled luxABCDE operon optimized for expression in gram-positive strains can be introduced in the clostridial host of interest [122]. Introduction of the entire operon would result in continuous luciferase-catalyzed light emission without the need of exogenous substrates, apart from molecular oxygen [123]. In the context of an anaerobic organism and the hypoxic environment of the tumor, the fulfillment of the oxygen requirement may pose a challenge. Nevertheless, it has been shown that the *lux* operon is functional even at very low oxygen tensions [6]. In support of this, bioluminescence imaging has been successfully applied in this fashion for the imaging of the tumor-colonizing anaerobic *Bifidobacterium breve* [122]. Also, high levels of *Vibrio fischeri* luciferase has been expressed in *C. perfringens* under strictly anaerobic conditions, thereby also providing confidence that the operon can be correctly expressed in a clostridial host [124, 125].

As far as more clinically relevant imaging methods are concerned, clostridial vectors can be made PET (or SPECT) competent by engineering them to express the herpes simplex virus type I thymidine kinase (HSV1-tk), which is currently the mainstay reporter gene for nuclear imaging. HSV1-tk can mediate the phosphorylation of suitable radioactive substrates, such as ^{125}I-2′-fluoro-2′deoxy-5-iodouracil-β-D-arabinofuranoside (^{125}I-FIAU), ^{124}I-FIAU, or ^{18}F-9-(4-fluoro-3-hydroxymethylbutyl)-guanine (^{18}F-FHBG) [113], giving rise to a SPECT/PET-detectable reaction [11]. In fact, Soghomonyan *et al.* have demonstrated FIAU accumulation in tumor tissue in combination with *Salmonella*-expressing HSV1-tk [126]. Endogenous thymidine kinases of *C. novyi*-NT have also been shown to react with radio labelled substrates, enabling the detection of *C. novyi*-NT (and of tumors) using SPECT [87]. Alternatively, HSV1-tk can be fused with any desired NTR, enabling the realization of the therapeutic function by the NTR and at the same time the realization of the imaging functionality by the HSV1-tk [82]; although this option may pose more hurdles from a genetic manipulation point of view, it has the potential of streamlining the noninvasive imaging of nitroreductase-based therapies by harnessing existing know-how in the field of molecular imaging.

It is evident that visualization of tumors using clostridial strains engineered with an imaging functionality is a feasible strategy independently of the way via which it may be pursued.

3.4 Conclusion and Future Opportunities

While significant progress has been achieved in enhancing the oncolytic properties of clostridia via genetic engineering, an exciting set of possibilities still remains to be pursued. Unlike the other bacterial candidates for cancer therapy, clostridia have been engineered to a lesser extent, mostly due to the lack of suitable genetic tools. Nevertheless, on the basis of the efforts undertaken so far, it has become evident that clostridial hosts are capable of tolerating and expressing a variety of prokaryotic as well as eukaryotic proteins. Therefore, clostridial vectors could, in principle, be engineered to deliver *any* desired anticancer agent and turned into a platform technology. Expanding on this, clostridial hosts can also be envisioned as multimodality vectors, simultaneously conveying multiple functionalities with synergistic anticancer effects. For instance, it is possible that the same strain can be engineered to stably deliver multiple therapeutic gene products simultaneously. Considering the multifactorial nature of cancer, the rationale behind multifunctionalizing the clostridial vector is entirely justified, enabling the cotargeting of mechanisms responsible for cancer growth and/or treatment resistance while reducing the drug burden of cancer patients [127]. Thankfully, with the arsenal of genetic tools now available as well as the pace with which new ones are developed, such a prospect seems realistic. The recent implementation of the CRISPR technology in various clostridial strains is expected to facilitate the genomic integration of multiple heterologous genes, without the need of antibiotic resistance markers [64–66].

Besides the new genetic engineering prospects, it is important to note that potential hurdles are presently surmountable, thus bringing clostridial cancer therapies closer to the clinic than ever before. Firstly, biocontainment and biosafety considerations are currently built into the design of the newer generation of clostridial vectors (e.g., uracil auxotrophy, no additional antibiotic markers). Secondly, a substantial body of research is in place underpinning the use of appropriate scientific protocols and preclinical animal models; these facilitate the generation of robust preclinical data, which will be clostridia's passport to clinical studies. The large-scale production of spores adhering to good manufacturing practice (GMP) standards is feasible at an affordable cost, ensuring that future demands can be met successfully. Finally, we anticipate that the forthcoming clinical evaluations will support the regulatory journey of clostridial therapies as well as alleviate potential public fears against and concerns regarding the use of genetically engineered bacteria for cancer therapy.

References

1. National Cancer Institute (NCI). Definition of solid tumor–NCI Dictionary of Cancer Terms. Retrieved from http://www.cancer.gov/publications/dictionaries/cancer-terms, (2015).
2. Mowday A., Guise C., Ackerley D., Minton N., Lambin P., Dubois L., *et al.* Advancing clostridia to clinical trial: past lessons and recent progress. *Cancers,* 8(7) (2016) 63.
3. World Health Organization (WHO). *World Cancer Report* (2014).
4. Bertout J. A., Patel S. A., Simon M. C. The impact of O_2 availability on human cancer. *Nature Reviews Cancer,* 8(12) (2008) 967–975.
5. Dang L. H., Bettegowda C., Huso D. L., Kinzler K. W., Vogelstein B. Combination bacteriolytic therapy for the treatment of experimental tumors. *Proceedings of the National Academy of Sciences of the United States of America,* 98(26) (2001) 15155–15160.
6. Cronin M., Akin A. R., Collins S. A., Meganck J., Kim J.-B., Baban C. K., *et al.* High resolution in vivo bioluminescent imaging for the study of bacterial tumour targeting. *PLOS One,* 7(1) (2012) e30940.

7. Vaupel P., Mayer A. Hypoxia in cancer: significance and impact on clinical outcome. *Cancer and Metastasis Reviews,* 26(2) (2007) 225–239.
8. Wilson W. R., Hay M. P. Targeting hypoxia in cancer therapy. *Nature Reviews Cancer,* 11(6) (2011) 393–410.
9. Forbes N. S. Engineering the perfect (bacterial) cancer therapy. *Nature Reviews Cancer,* 10(11) (2010) 785–794.
10. Cosse J. P., Michiels C. Tumour hypoxia affects the responsiveness of cancer cells to chemotherapy and promotes cancer progression. *Anti-cancer Agents in Medicinal Chemistry,* 8(7) (2008) 790–797.
11. Liu S. C., Minton N. P., Giaccia A. J., Brown J. M. Anticancer efficacy of systemically delivered anaerobic bacteria as gene therapy vectors targeting tumor hypoxia/necrosis. *Gene Therapy,* 9(4) (2002) 291–296.
12. Theys J., Landuyt W., Nuyts S., Van Mellaert L., Bosmans E., Rijnders A., *et al.* Improvement of *Clostridium* tumour targeting vectors evaluated in rat rhabdomyosarcomas. *FEMS Immunology and Medical Microbiology,* 30(1) (2001) 37–41.
13. Kubiak A. M., Poehlein A., Budd P., Kuehne S. A., Winzer K., Theys J., *et al.* Complete genome sequence of the nonpathogenic soil-dwelling bacterium *Clostridium sporogenes* strain NCIMB 10696. *Genome Announcements,* 3(4) (2015) e00942–15.
14. Mengesha A., Dubois L., Paesmans K., Wouters B., Lambin P., Theys J. *Clostridia: Molecular Biology in the Post-genomic Era,* Brüggemann H., Gottschalk G., (eds.) Chapter 11: Clostridia in anti-tumour therapy, (2009), Caister Academic Press, UK, pp. 199–214.
15. Wei M. Q., Ellem K. A., Dunn P., West M. J., Bai C. X., Vogelstein B. Facultative or obligate anaerobic bacteria have the potential for multimodality therapy of solid tumours. *European Journal of Cancer,* 43(3) (2007) 490–496.
16. Fabricius E. M., Schneeweiss U., Schau H. P., Schmidt W., Benedix A. Quantitative investigations into the elimination of in vitro-obtained spores of the non-pathogenic *Clostridium butyricum* strain CNRZ 528, and their persistence in organs of different species following intravenous spore administration. *Research in Microbiology,* 144(9) (1993) 741–753.
17. Zu C., Wang J. S. Tumor-colonizing bacteria: A potential tumor targeting therapy. *Critical Reviews in Microbiology,* 40(3) (2014) 225–235.

18. Fang J., Liao L., Yin H., Nakamura H., Shin T., Maeda H. Enhanced bacterial tumor delivery by modulating the EPR effect and therapeutic potential of *Lactobacillus casei*. *Journal of Pharmaceutical Sciences*, 103(10) (2014) 3235–3243.
19. Minton N. P. Clostridia in cancer therapy. *Nature Reviews Microbiology*, 1(3) (2003) 237–242.
20. Bettegowda C., Huang X., Lin J., Cheong I., Kohli M., Szabo S. A., *et al.* The genome and transcriptomes of the anti-tumor agent *Clostridium novyi-NT*. *Nature Biotechnology*, 24(12) (2006) 1573–1580.
21. Agrawal N., Bettegowda C., Cheong I., Geschwind J. F., Drake C. G., Hipkiss E. L., *et al.* Bacteriolytic therapy can generate a potent immune response against experimental tumors. *Proceedings of the National Academy of Sciences of the United States of America*, 101(42) (2004) 15172–15177.
22. Cheong I., Huang X., Bettegowda C., Diaz L. A. Jr., Kinzler K. W., Zhou S., *et al.* A bacterial protein enhances the release and efficacy of liposomal cancer drugs. *Science*, 314(5803) (2006) 1308–1311.
23. Albert M. L. Death-defying immunity: do apoptotic cells influence antigen processing and presentation? *Nature Reviews Immunology*, 4(3) (2004) 223–231.
24. Theys J., Pennington O., Dubois L., Anlezark G., Vaughan T., Mengesha A., *et al.* Repeated cycles of *Clostridium*-directed enzyme prodrug therapy result in sustained antitumour effects in vivo. *British Journal of Cancer*, 95(9) (2006) 1212–1219.
25. Diaz L. A., Cheong I., Foss C. A., Zhang X., Peters B. A., Agrawal N., *et al.* Pharmacologic and toxicologic evaluation of *C. novyi-NT* spores. *Toxicological Sciences*, 88(2) (2005) 562–575.
26. Bernardes N., Seruca R., Chakrabarty A. M., Fialho A. M. Microbial-based therapy of cancer: Current progress and future prospects. *Bioengineered Bugs*, 1(3) (2010) 178–190.
27. Bettegowda C., Dang L. H., Abrams R., Huso D. L., Dillehay L., Cheong I., *et al.* Overcoming the hypoxic barrier to radiation therapy with anaerobic bacteria. *Proceedings of the National Academy of Sciences of the United States of America*, 100(25) (2003) 15083–15088.
28. Gericke D., Dietzel F., Konig W., Ruster I., Schumacher L. Further progress with oncolysis due to apathogenic clostridia. *Zentralbl Bakteriol Orig A*, 243(1) (1979) 102–112.
29. Mose J. R. Experiments to improve the oncolysis-effect of clostridial-strain M55 (author's transl). *Zentralbl Bakteriol Orig A*, 244(4) (1979) 541–545.

30. Dietzel F., Gericke D., Konig W. Tumor hyperthermia using high frequency for increase of oncolysis by *Clostridium butyricum* (M 55). *Strahlentherapie,* 152(6) (1976) 537–541.

31. Howard S. C., Jones D. P., Pui C.-H. The tumor lysis syndrome. *New England Journal of Medicine,* 364(19) (2011) 1844–1854.

32. Amer M. H. Gene therapy for cancer: present status and future perspective. *Molecular and Cellular Therapies,* 2 (2014) 27.

33. Verma I. M., Somia N. Gene therapy—promises, problems and prospects. *Nature,* 389(6648) (1997) 239–242.

34. Wei M. Q., Ren R., Good D., Anne J. Clostridial spores as live 'Trojan horse' vectors for cancer gene therapy: comparison with viral delivery systems. *Genetic Vaccines and Therapy,* 6 (2008) 8.

35. Lehouritis P., Springer C., Tangney M. Bacterial-directed enzyme prodrug therapy. *Journal of Controlled Release,* 170(1) (2013) 120–131.

36. Wei M. Q., Mengesha A., Good D., Anne J. Bacterial targeted tumour therapy—dawn of a new era. *Cancer Letters,* 259(1) (2008) 16–27.

37. Fox M. E., Lemmon M. J., Mauchline M. L., Davis T. O., Giaccia A. J., Minton N. P., *et al.* Anaerobic bacteria as a delivery system for cancer gene therapy: in vitro activation of 5-fluorocytosine by genetically engineered clostridia. *Gene Therapy,* 3(2) (1996) 173–178.

38. Theys J., Landuyt W., Nuyts S., Van Mellaert L., van Oosterom A., Lambin P., *et al.* Specific targeting of cytosine deaminase to solid tumors by engineered *Clostridium acetobutylicum*. *Cancer Gene Therapy,* 8(4) (2001) 294–297.

39. Lemmon M. J., van Zijl P., Fox M. E., Mauchline M. L., Giaccia A. J., Minton N. P., *et al.* Anaerobic bacteria as a gene delivery system that is controlled by the tumor microenvironment. *Gene Therapy,* 4(8) (1997) 791–796.

40. Liu S.-C., Ahn G.-O., Kioi M., Dorie M.-J., Patterson A. V., Brown J. M. Optimized *Clostridium*-directed enzyme prodrug therapy improves the antitumor activity of the novel DNA Cross-linking agent PR-104. *Cancer Research,* 68(19) (2008) 7995–8003.

41. Heap J. T., Theys J., Ehsaan M., Kubiak A. M., Dubois L., Paesmans K., *et al.* Spores of *Clostridium* engineered for clinical efficacy and safety cause regression and cure of tumors in vivo. *Oncotarget,* 5(7) (2014) 1761–1769.

42. Budd P. G. Implementation and optimisation of alternative therapeutics for use in *Clostridium sporogenes* as a delivery vehicle. PhD thesis, University of Nottingham (2015).

43. Pennington O. The development of molecular tools for the expression of prodrug converting enzymes in *Clostridium sporogenes.* PhD thesis, University of Nottingham (2006).

44. Groot A. J., Mengesha A., van der Wall E., van Diest P. J., Theys J., Vooijs M. Functional antibodies produced by oncolytic clostridia. *Biochemical and Biophysical Research Communications,* 364(4) (2007) 985–989.

45. Theys J., Nuyts S., Landuyt W., Van Mellaert L., Dillen C., Bohringer M., *et al.* Stable *Escherichia coli–Clostridium acetobutylicum* shuttle vector for secretion of murine tumor necrosis factor alpha. *Applied and Environmental Microbiology,* 65(10) (1999) 4295–4300.

46. Theys J., Landuyt A. W., Nuyts S., Van Mellaert L., Lambin P., Anne J. *Clostridium* as a tumor-specific delivery system of therapeutic proteins. *Cancer Detection and Prevention,* 25(6) (2001) 548–557.

47. Nuyts S., Van Mellaert L., Theys J., Landuyt W., Bosmans E., Anne J., *et al.* Radio-responsive recA promoter significantly increases TNFα production in recombinant clostridia after 2 Gy irradiation. *Gene Therapy,* 8(15) (2001) 1197–1201.

48. Nuyts S., Van Mellaert L., Barbe S., Lammertyn E., Theys J., Landuyt W., *et al.* Insertion or deletion of the Cheo box modifies radiation inducibility of *Clostridium* promoters. *Applied and Environmental Microbiology,* 67(10) (2001) 4464–4470.

49. Barbe S., Van Mellaert L., Anne J. *Clostridium*-mediated transfer system of therapeutic proteins to solid tumors: increased heterologous protein production. *Communications in Agricultural and Applied Biological Sciences,* 69(2) (2004) 49–52.

50. Barbe S., Van Mellaert L., Theys J., Geukens N., Lammertyn E., Lambin P., *et al.* Secretory production of biologically active rat interleukin-2 by *Clostridium acetobutylicum* DSM792 as a tool for anti-tumor treatment. *FEMS Microbiology Letters,* 246(1) (2005) 67–73.

51. Zhang Y. L., Lu R., Chang Z. S., Zhang W. Q., Wang Q. B., Ding S. Y., *et al.* *Clostridium sporogenes* delivers interleukin-12 to hypoxic tumours, producing antitumour activity without significant toxicity. *Letters in Applied Microbiology,* 59(6) (2014) 580–586.

52. Schlechte H., Elbe B. Recombinant plasmid DNA variation of *clostridium oncolyticum*—model experiments of cancerostatic gene

transfer. *Zentralblatt Fur Bakteriologie, Mikrobiologie Und Hygiene, Series A*, 268(3) (1988) 347–356.

53. Li Z., Fallon J., Mandeli J., Wetmur J., Woo S. L. A genetically enhanced anaerobic bacterium for oncopathic therapy of pancreatic cancer. *Journal of the National Cancer Institute*, 100(19) (2008) 1389–1400.
54. Heap J. T., Pennington O. J., Cartman S. T., Minton N. P. A modular system for *Clostridium* shuttle plasmids. *Journal of Microbiological Methods*, 78(1) (2009) 79–85.
55. Cartman S. T., Kelly M. L., Heeg D., Heap J. T., Minton N. P. Precise manipulation of the *Clostridium difficile* chromosome reveals a lack of association between the *tcdC* genotype and toxin production. *Applied and Environmental Microbiology*, 78(13) (2012) 4683–4690.
56. Ehsaan M., Kuit W., Zhang Y., Cartman S. T., Heap J. T., Winzer K., *et al.* Mutant generation by allelic exchange and genome resequencing of the biobutanol organism *Clostridium acetobutylicum* ATCC 824. *Biotechnology for Biofuels*, 9(1) (2016) 4.
57. Heap J. T., Kuehne S. A., Ehsaan M., Cartman S. T., Cooksley C. M., Scott J. C., *et al.* The ClosTron: mutagenesis in *Clostridium* refined and streamlined. *Journal of Microbiological Methods*, 80(1) (2010) 49–55.
58. Kuehne S. A., Heap J. T., Cooksley C. M., Cartman S. T., Minton N. P. ClosTron-mediated engineering of *Clostridium*. *Methods in Molecular Biology*, 765 (2011) 389–407.
59. Ng Y. K., Ehsaan M., Philip S., Collery M. M., Janoir C., Collignon A., *et al.* Expanding the repertoire of gene tools for precise manipulation of the *Clostridium difficile* genome: allelic exchange using pyrE alleles. *PLOS One*, 8(2) (2013) e56051.
60. Cartman S. T., Minton N. P. A mariner-based transposon system for in vivo random mutagenesis of *Clostridium difficile*. *Applied and Environmental Microbiology*, 76(4) (2010) 1103–1109.
61. Zhang Y., Grosse-Honebrink A., Minton N. P. A universal mariner transposon system for forward genetic studies in the genus *Clostridium*. *PLOS One*, 10(4) (2015) e0122411.
62. Heap J. T., Ehsaan M., Cooksley C. M., Ng Y.-K., Cartman S. T., Winzer K., *et al.* P. Integration of DNA into bacterial chromosomes from plasmids without a counter-selection marker. *Nucleic Acids Research*, 40(8) (2012) e59–e59.
63. Kovács K., Willson B. J., Schwarz K., Heap J. T., Jackson A., Bolam D. N., *et al.* Secretion and assembly of functional mini-cellulosomes from synthetic chromosomal operons in *Clostridium acetobutylicum* ATCC 824. *Biotechnology for Biofuels*, 6(1) (2013) 117.

64. Huang H., Chai C., Li N., Rowe P., Minton N. P., Yang S., *et al.* CRISPR/Cas9-based efficient genome editing in *Clostridium ljungdahlii*, an autotrophic gas-fermenting bacterium. *ACS Synthetic Biology,* 5(12) (2016) 1355–1361.

65. Li Q., Chen J., Minton N. P., Zhang Y., Wen Z., Liu J., *et al.* CRISPR-based genome editing and expression control systems in *Clostridium acetobutylicum* and *Clostridium beijerinckii. Biotechnology Journal,* 11(7) (2016) 961–972.

66. Wang Y., Zhang Z. T., Seo S. O., Choi K., Lu T., Jin Y. S., *et al.* Markerless chromosomal gene deletion in *Clostridium beijerinckii* using CRISPR/Cas9 system. *Journal of Biotechnology,* 200 (2015) 1–5.

67. Minton N. P., Ehsaan M., Humphreys C. M., Little G. T., Baker J., Henstra A. M., *et al.* A roadmap for gene system development in *Clostridium. Anaerobe,* 41 (2016) 104–112.

68. Morrissey D., O'Sullivan G. C., Tangney M. Tumour targeting with systemically administered bacteria. *Current Gene Therapy,* 10(1) (2010) 3–14.

69. Danino T., Lo J., Prindle A., Hasty J., Bhatia S. N. In vivo gene expression dynamics of tumor-targeted bacteria. *ACS Synthetic Biology,* 1(10) (2012) 465–470.

70. Lee J., Jang Y. S., Papoutsakis E. T., Lee S. Y. Stable and enhanced gene expression in *Clostridium acetobutylicum* using synthetic untranslated regions with a stem-loop. *Journal of Biotechnology,* 230 (2016) 40–43.

71. Kubiak A. M. The use of *Clostridium sporogenes* in directed enzyme pro-drug therapy. PhD thesis, University of Nottingham (2013).

72. Mengesha A., Dubois L., Lambin P., Landuyt W., Chiu R. K., Wouters B. G., *et al.* Development of a flexible and potent hypoxia-inducible promoter for tumor-targeted gene expression in attenuated Salmonella. *Cancer Biology & Therapy,* 5(9) (2006) 1120–1128.

73. St Jean A. T., Zhang M., Forbes N. S. Bacterial therapies: completing the cancer treatment toolbox. *Current Opinion in Biotechnology,* 19(5) (2008) 511–517.

74. Van Mellaert L., Barbé, S., Anné, J. *Clostridium* spores as anti-tumour agents. *Trends in Microbiology,* 14(4) (2006) 190–196.

75. Minton N. P., Mauchline M. L., Lemmon M. J., Brehm J. K., Fox M., Michael N. P., *et al.* Chemotherapeutic tumour targeting using clostridial spores. *FEMS Microbiology Reviews,* 17(3) (1995) 357–364.

76. Zarogoulidis P., Darwiche K., Sakkas A., Yarmus L., Huang H., Li Q., *et al.* Suicide gene therapy for cancer—current strategies. *Journal of Genetic Syndromes and Gene Therapy,* 4: 16849. 2013.

77. Theys J., Lambin P. *Clostridium* to treat cancer: dream or reality? *Annals of Translational Medicine,* 3(Suppl 1) (2015) S21.

78. Roldan M. D., Perez-Reinado E., Castillo F., Moreno-Vivian C. Reduction of polynitroaromatic compounds: the bacterial nitroreductases. *FEMS Microbiology Reviews,* 32(3) (2008) 474–500.

79. Oliveira I. M., Bonatto D., Antonio J., Henriques P. *Current Research, Technology and Education Topics in Applied Microbiology and Microbial Biotechnology* (Vol. 2), Mendez Vilas A. (ed.), Nitroreductases: Enzymes with Environmental, Biotechnological and Clinical Importance., (2010), Formatex Research Center, Badajoz, pp. 1008–1019.

80. Tang M. H. Y., Helsby N. A., Wilson W. R., Tingle M. D. Aerobic 2- and 4-nitroreduction of CB 1954 by human liver. *Toxicology,* 216(2–3) (2005) 129–139.

81. Helsby N. A., Ferry D. M., Patterson A. V., Pullen S. M., Wilson W. R. 2-Amino metabolites are key mediators of CB 1954 and SN 23862 bystander effects in nitroreductase GDEPT. *British Journal of Cancer,* 90(5) (2004) 1084–1092.

82. Williams E. M., Little R. F., Mowday A. M., Rich M. H., Chan-Hyams J. V., *et al.* Nitroreductase gene-directed enzyme prodrug therapy: insights and advances toward clinical utility. *Biochemical Journal,* 471(2) (2015) 131–153.

83. Knox R. J., Friedlos F., Sherwood R. F., Melton R. G., Anlezark G. M. The bioactivation of 5-(aziridin-1-yl)-2,4-dinitrobenzamide (CB1954)–II. A comparison of an *Escherichia coli* nitroreductase and Walker DT diaphorase. *Biochemical Pharmacology,* 44(12) (1992) 2297–2301.

84. Anlezark G. M., Vaughan T., Fashola-Stone E., Michael N. P., Murdoch H., Sims M. A., *et al. Bacillus amyloliquefaciens* orthologue of *Bacillus subtilis* ywrO encodes a nitroreductase enzyme which activates the prodrug CB 1954. *Microbiology,* 148(Pt 1) (2002) 297–306.

85. Vass S. O., Jarrom D., Wilson W. R., Hyde E. I., Searle P. F. *E. coli* NfsA: an alternative nitroreductase for prodrug activation gene therapy in combination with CB1954. *British Journal of Cancer,* 100(12) (2009) 1903–1911.

86. Emptage C. D., Knox R. J., Danson M. J., Hough D. W. Nitroreductase from *Bacillus licheniformis*: a stable enzyme for prodrug activation. *Biochemical Pharmacology,* 77(1) (2009) 21–29.

87. Kubiak A. M., Minton N. P. The potential of clostridial spores as therapeutic delivery vehicles in tumour therapy. *Research in Microbiology,* 166(4) (2015) 244–254.

88. Rowsell S., Pauptit R. A., Tucker A. D., Melton R. G., Blow D. M., Brick P. Crystal structure of carboxypeptidase G2, a bacterial enzyme with applications in cancer therapy. *Structure,* 5(3) (1997) 337–347.

89. Semenza G. L. HIF-1 and tumor progression: pathophysiology and therapeutics. *Trends in Molecular Medicine,* 8(4) (2002) S62–S67.

90. Matsumoto K., Ema M. Roles of VEGF-A signalling in development, regeneration, and tumours. *Journal of Biochemistry,* 156(1) (2014) 1–10.

91. Mabry R., Gilbertson D. G., Frank A., Vu T., Ardourel D., Ostrander C., *et al.* A dual-targeting PDGFRbeta/VEGF-A molecule assembled from stable antibody fragments demonstrates anti-angiogenic activity in vitro and in vivo. *mAbs,* 2(1) (2010) 20–34.

92. Shankaran V., Ikeda H., Bruce A. T., White J. M., Swanson P. E., Old L. J., *et al.* IFN[gamma] and lymphocytes prevent primary tumour development and shape tumour immunogenicity. *Nature,* 410(6832) (2001) 1107–1111.

93. Dunn G. P., Old L. J., Schreiber R. D. The immunobiology of cancer immunosurveillance and immunoediting. *Immunity,* 21(2) (2004) 137–148.

94. Hanahan D., Weinberg Robert A. Hallmarks of cancer: the next generation. *Cell,* 144(5) (2011) 646–674.

95. Nelson D., Fisher S., Robinson B. The “Trojan Horse” approach to tumor immunotherapy: targeting the tumor microenvironment. *Journal of Immunology Research,* 2014 (2014) 789069.

96. Anestakis D., Petanidis S., Kalyvas S., Nday C. M., Tsave O., Kioseoglou E., *et al.* Mechanisms and applications of interleukins in cancer immunotherapy. *International Journal of Molecular Sciences,* 16(1) (2015) 1691–1710.

97. Vial T., Descotes J. Clinical toxicity of interleukin-2. *Drug Safety,* 7(6) (1992) 417–433.

98. Loeffler M., Le’Negrate G., Krajewska M., Reed J. C. Attenuated *Salmonella* engineered to produce human cytokine LIGHT inhibit tumor growth. *Proceedings of the National Academy of Sciences of the United States of America,* 104(31) (2007) 12879–12883.

99. van Horssen R., ten Hagen T. L. M., Eggermont A. M. M. TNF-α in cancer treatment: molecular insights, antitumor effects, and clinical utility. *Oncologist,* 11(4) (2006) 397–408.

100. Sim G. C., Radvanyi L. The IL-2 cytokine family in cancer immunotherapy. *Cytokine & Growth Factor Reviews,* 25(4) (2014) 377–390.

101. Zundler S., Neurath M. F. Interleukin-12: Functional activities and implications for disease. *Cytokine & Growth Factor Reviews,* 26(5) (2015) 559–568.

102. Revtovich S., Anufrieva N., Morozova E., Kulikova V., Nikulin A., Demidkina T. Structure of methionine gamma-lyase from *Clostridium sporogenes. Acta Crystallographica. Section F, Structural Biology Communications,* 72(Pt 1) (2016) 65–71.

103. Sato D., Nozaki T. Methionine gamma-lyase: the unique reaction mechanism, physiological roles, and therapeutic applications against infectious diseases and cancers. *IUBMB Life,* 61(11) (2009) 1019–1028.

104. Sato D., Kobayashi S., Yasui H., Shibata N., Toru T., Yamamoto M., *et al.* Cytotoxic effect of amide derivatives of trifluoromethionine against the enteric protozoan parasite *Entamoeba histolytica. International Journal of Antimicrobial Agents,* 35(1) (2010) 56–61.

105. Tan Y., Xu M., Hoffman R. M. Broad selective efficacy of recombinant methioninase and polyethylene glycol-modified recombinant methioninase on cancer cells in vitro. *AntiCancer Research,* 30(4) (2010) 1041–1046.

106. Yoshioka T., Wada T., Uchida N., Maki H., Yoshida H., Ide N., *et al.* Anticancer efficacy in vivo and in vitro, synergy with 5-fluorouracil, and safety of recombinant methioninase. *Cancer Research,* 58(12) (1998) 2583–2587.

107. Georgiou, G. and Stone, E. (2014). Engineered enzymes with methionine-gamma-lyase enzymes and pharmacological preparations thereof. United States Patent No. *US8709407B2.*

108. Kreis W., Hession C. Isolation and purification of L-methionine-α-deamino-γ-mercaptomethane-lyase (L-methioninase) from *Clostridium sporogenes. Cancer Research,* 33(8) (1973) 1862–1865.

109. Morozova E. A., Kulikova V. V., Yashin D. V., Anufrieva N. V., Anisimova N. Y., Revtovich S. V., *et al.* Kinetic parameters and cytotoxic activity of recombinant methionine γ-lyase from *Clostridium tetani, Clostridium sporogenes, Porphyromonas gingivalis* and *Citrobacter freundii. Acta Naturae,* 5(3) (2013) 92–98.

110. Yoong P. Enhancement of bacterial virulence by antibody neutralization of immune-activating toxins. *Virulence,* 1(5) (2010) 409–413.

111. Li Z., Fallon J., Mandeli J., Wetmur J., Woo S. L. The oncopathic potency of *Clostridium perfringens* is independent of its alpha-toxin gene. *Human Gene Therapy,* 20(7) (2009) 751–758.

112. Li Z., Fallon J., Mandeli J., Wetmur J., Woo S. L. Retraction: A genetically enhanced anaerobic bacterium for oncopathic therapy of pancreatic cancer. *Journal of the National Cancer Institute,* 102(4) (2010) 283.

113. Pawelek J. M., Low K. B., Bermudes D. Bacteria as tumour-targeting vectors. *Lancet Oncology,* 4(9) (2003) 548–556.

114. Stanton M., Cronin M., Lehouritis P., Tangney M. In vivo bacterial imaging without engineering; a novel probe-based strategy facilitated by endogenous nitroreductase enzymes. *Current Gene Therapy,* 15(3) (2015) 277–288.

115. Vorobyeva A. G., Stanton M., Godinat A., Lund K. B., Karateev G. G., Francis K. P., *et al.* Development of a bioluminescent nitroreductase probe for preclinical imaging. *PLOS One,* 10(6) (2015) e0131037.

116. Condeelis J., Weissleder R. In vivo imaging in cancer. *Cold Spring Harbor Perspecties in Biology,* 2(12) (2010) a003848.

117. Guise, C. P., Ackerley, D. F., Ashoorzadeh, A., Copp, J. N., Flanagan, J. U., Mowday, A. M., Patterson, A. V., Prosser, G. A., Smaill, J. B. and Syddall, S. P. (2013). Bacterial nitroreductase enzymes and methods relating thereto. United States Patent No. *US20130295011A1.*

118. Tirandaz H., Salehi-Najafabadi A., Eslamifar A. Cytosine deaminase producing *Clostridium* may be used in detection of tumors. *Medical Hypotheses,* 67(5) (2006) 1257–1258.

119. Ziv K., Plaks V., Neeman M., Granot D., Cohen B. *Molecular and Cellular MR Imaging,* Bulte J. W. M. (ed.), Chapter 11: Molecular Imaging of Reporter Genes, (2007), CRC Press, Taylor & Francis Group, USA, pp. 199–217.

120. Drepper T., Eggert T., Circolone F., Heck A., Krausz U., Guterl J.-K., *et al.* Reporter proteins for in vivo fluorescence without oxygen. *Nature Biotechnology,* 25(4) (2007) 443–445.

121. Li Y., Xu T., Tschaplinski T. J., Engle N. L., Yang Y., Graham D. E., *et al.* Improvement of cellulose catabolism in *Clostridium cellulolyticum* by sporulation abolishment and carbon alleviation. *Biotechnology for Biofuels,* 7(1) (2014) 25.

122. Cronin M., Sleator R. D., Hill C., Fitzgerald G. F., van Sinderen D. Development of a luciferase-based reporter system to monitor *Bifidobacterium breve* UCC2003 persistence in mice. *BMC Microbiology,* 8: 161. 2008.

123. Waidmann M. S., Bleichrodt F. S., Laslo T., Riedel C. U. Bacterial luciferase reporters: the Swiss army knife of molecular biology. *Bioengineered Bugs,* 2(1) (2011) 8–16.

124. Phillips-Jones M. K. Bioluminescence (lux) expression in the anaerobe *Clostridium perfringens*. *FEMS Microbiology Letters,* 106(3) (1993) 265–270.

125. Phillips-Jones M. K. Use of a lux reporter system for monitoring rapid changes in α-toxin gene expression in *Clostridium perfringens* during growth. *FEMS Microbiology Letters,* 188(1) (2000) 29–33.

126. Soghomonyan S. A., Doubrovin M., Pike J., Luo X., Ittensohn M., Runyan J. D., *et al.* Positron emission tomography (PET) imaging of tumor-localized *Salmonella* expressing HSV1-TK. *Cancer Gene Therapy,* 12(1) (2004) 101–108.

127. Hanahan D. Rethinking the war on cancer. *Lancet,* 383(9916) (2013) 558–563.

Chapter 4

Bacteria-Derived Alternatives to Live *Mycobacterium bovis* Bacillus Calmette–Guerin for Nonmuscle Invasive Bladder Cancer Treatment

Esther Julián and Estela Noguera-Ortega

Departament de Genètica i de Microbiologia, Facultat de Biociències, Universitat Autònoma de Barcelona, 08193, Bellaterra, Barcelona, Spain

esther.julian@uab.cat

The most successful immunotherapeutic treatment for nonmuscle invasive bladder cancer (NMIBC) to date is the intravesical instillation of *Mycobacterium bovis* bacillus Calmette–Guérin (BCG). The adverse events associated with this successful therapy have prompted researchers to find safer options. A broad *armamentarium* of bacteria and bacteria-derived components has been studied, seeking to achieve an efficacy similar to or higher than that of live BCG, with only minor adverse events. This chapter covers both the unsuccessful and the encouraging immunotherapeutic agents that can serve as substitutes for live-BCG treatment, from species of microorganisms genealogically distant from mycobacteria, such as lactic bacteria, to purified mycobacteria

Microbial Infections and Cancer Therapy: Recent Advances
Edited by Ananda M. Chakrabarty and Arsénio M. Fialho

ISBN 978-981-4774-86-4 (Hardcover), 978-1-351-04190-4 (eBook)
www.panstanford.com

antigens, nonviable mycobacteria, or nontuberculous mycobacteria. It places particular emphasis on the special characteristics that make mycobacteria different from other microorganisms. Finally, it describes possible future approaches to solving the problems associated with live-BCG treatment.

4.1 Success of BCG in Bladder Cancer Treatment

The intravesical instillation of *Mycobacterium bovis* bacillus Calnette–Guérin (BCG) remains the gold standard treatment of nonmuscle invasive bladder cancer (NMIBC). International guidelines agree that for high-risk patients in whom radical cystectomy is not performed, BCG is the preferred treatment following transurethral resection (TUR) of a bladder tumor and an immediate postoperative dose of chemotherapy [1, 2]. Although which treatment regimens are optimal is still under debate [3–5] and there is no consensus on the exact mechanism of action or on predictive factors of the response to this mycobacterium [6, 7], for over 35 years the administration of this attenuated live mycobacterium has been the mainstay for treating this type of cancer to prevent tumor recurrence and progression [8].

Today, it is not possible to monitor the details of the outcomes of intravesical instillation of BCG in patients, but results from *in vitro*, *ex vivo*, and *in vivo* experiments in bladder cancer (BC) models and, more importantly, snapshots of the immune response and outcomes of BCG-treated patients allow us to draw a picture of the cascade of events initiated by BCG inside the bladder. However, many questions remain to be answered.

The first interaction between the mycobacteria and the human body occurs in the urothelium. BCG is believed to have a direct antitumor effect against residual tumor cells after surgery or against aberrant epithelial cells in the urothelial layer that can develop into new tumors. *In vitro* experiments show that BCG inhibits tumor cell proliferation by inducing apoptosis [9–12] or/and arresting the cell cycle [13, 14]. Various authors have demonstrated that both normal and malignant bladder epithelial cells act as a first-line defense, producing cytokines and chemokines after BCG instillation [15]. Together, these cytokines, as well as those produced by residing dendritic cells (DCs) and macrophages, which are activated after phagocytosis of BCG, induce the infiltration and activation of inflammatory leukocytes, leading to a profound cellular response inside the bladder. In fact, urothelial tumors in nude mice depleted of T cells do not react to BCG [16]. The development of a predominant Th1 cytokine profile, for example, interferon (IFN)-γ, interleukin (IL)-2, and IL-12, is associated with the therapeutic effects of BCG, whereas the presence of a high level of Th2 cytokines (e.g., IL-10) is associated with BCG failure [17]. BCG activity requires an active host immune system to initiate the cascade of immune events that can then prevent the progression of the tumor. Detailed data on the BCG effect are described extensively in numerous excellent reviews [17–19].

4.2 Problems Associated with the Intravesical Instillation of BCG

Although recurrence and progression are successfully prevented at high rates in patients treated with BCG, two major problems are associated with intravesical instillation of BCG and are the focus of research efforts. On the one hand, the efficacy of BCG treatment is approximately 50%–70% [20, 21], which means that some patients, for unknown reasons, do not respond to BCG treatment. To improve the effectiveness of BCG, different strategies are currently under study, such as the combination of chemotherapeutics with BCG [22, 23] and the construction of recombinant BCG strains genetically modified to express cytokines or immunomodulatory molecules that enhance the immune response (i.e., IFN-α) [24, 25] or that block IL-10 production to modulate the tumor microenvironment [17, 26, 27]. On the other hand, other studies are focused on reducing adverse effects to improve the safety of this immunotherapy.

Intravesical BCG therapy has serious side effects. Several reports have described problems associated with BCG instillation. Approximately 30%–40% of patients suffer from high fever, granulomatous prostatitis, pneumonitis, hepatitis, etc. [28–31]. Many patients are advised to stop BCG treatment due to toxicity, which mainly occurs during the first year of BCG therapy [32]. However, the most worrying and alarming problem is the possibility of systemic events. With respect to the cause of systemic adverse events, there is considerable debate in the literature about whether these events are part of a hypersensitivity reaction or due to an ongoing active infection [33], based on the fact that some patients with side effects from BCG respond very well to glucosteroids and/or antituberculosis medication. Intravascular absorption of viable BCG may occur after traumatic intravesical instillation and lead to systemic infection.

Although the training of nurses and urologists lowers the risk of an accident, a large number of instillations, due to the length of the treatment, increase the chances of an accident [34, 35]. The impossibility of demonstrating the presence of the bacilli in most cases has led some authors to argue that a type IV hypersensitivity reaction occurs after the intravesical instillation of BCG in some BC patients [33, 36]. However, in numerous reports in the literature, BCG was detected as the cause of infection [37–51]. Indeed, Bowyer and coworkers (1995) [52] demonstrated the presence of acid-fast bacilli in the bladder 16 months after the completion of intravesical instillations. Even systemic infections have been described three [37, 44] and six [53] years after BCG treatment completion as a result of the reactivation of the bacilli after the patients had become less immunocompetent.

4.3 Alternatives to Viable BCG

To avoid such unfavorable events, different strategies are being used to develop safer alternatives to intravesical installation of live BCG:

- Bacteria-derived components or bacteria other than mycobacteria, such as *Lactobacillus* species, or toxins from gram-positive and gram-negative microorganisms can be used.
- Mycobacteria-based treatments safer than live BCG are being tested, including the following:
    - o The use of mycobacterial components, such as cell extracts or antigens derived from mycobacteria. The

majority of this work is focused on the administration of cell wall (CW) extracts from BCG or *M. phlei*.
  - o The administration of whole mycobacteria in a nonviable form.
  - o The use of live nontuberculous mycobacteria (NTM).
- The effect of BCG can be ameliorated by reducing the occasioned inflammation or by preventing infection. In the first case, anti-inflammatory molecules are given along with the course of instillations; in the second case, antimicrobial agents are given along with the mycobacterial treatment to avoid the administration of other molecules that could influence the beneficial effect of the BCG.
- Recombinant immunostimulatory molecules (such as cytokines or antibodies), molecules derived from eukaryotes (plant or fungi), and chemotherapeutic agents are being assayed in an attempt to improve the current therapeutic options.

We will focus our review on the work done or currently underway using bacteria-derived agents. BC treatments using recombinant cytokines or antibodies, agents derived from plants or fungi, and oncolytic viruses are beyond the scope of our review.

4.3.1 Bacteria Other Than Mycobacteria

Part of the efficacy of BCG therapy for BC treatment is attributed to the immune response triggered by BCG, and therefore, it is assumed that other bacteria also possess immunostimulatory components that could induce a response favoring tumor clearance. In fact, bacteria that belong to genera distantly related to *Mycobacterium* have been assayed for their antitumor activity in different BC models. The disadvantage of their use is that these bacteria do not share the immunostimulatory antigens (described in Table 4.1) exclusive to mycobacteria, but, in contrast to mycobacteria, other bacteria are easily manipulated to design recombinant strains that are able to overexpress molecules of interest. Furthermore, their use can prevent not only the possibility of infections but also the hypersensitivity reaction described in some patients due to BCG treatment.

Table 4.1 Safety bacteria–based alternatives to life BCG: Bacteria and bacteria-derived components used for bladder cancer treatment

		***In vitro* studies; growth inhibition bladder cancer cell lines**	***In vivo* studies in animal models**	***In vivo* studies in human clinical assays**
Purified mycobacteria antigens				
	MPT-64 antigen		[139]	
	PstS antigen-1	[140]	[140]	
	Naked DNA		[147–150]	
	Ag85		[154, 155]	
	Purified BCG antigens	[156]		
Mycobacteria cell extracts				
	BCG cell wall		[161]	
	R8 BCG cell wall	[165, 167, 170, 171]	[170, 171]	
	M. phlei cell wall		[172]	[174]
	M. phlei cell wall plus DNA	[151, 153]		
Nonviable mycobacteria				
	Hk MIP	[195]		[193, 194]

		In vitro studies; growth inhibition bladder cancer cell lines	*In vivo* studies in animal models	*In vivo* studies in human clinical assays
	Hk-BCG	[167, 178, 181, 182, 185, 198]	[78, 161, 188–190]	[191]
	Hk-*M. phlei*	[185]		
	Hk-*M. brumae*	[185]		
	Hk-*M. vaccae*	[185]		
	Gamma-irradiated BCG	[178, 185, 198]	[198]	
	Gamma-irradiated *M. phlei*	[185, 198]		
	Gamma-irradiated *M. brumae*	[185, 198]	[198]	
	Gamma-irradiated *M. vaccae*	[185]		
	Sonicated BCG	[197]		
Live mycobacteria				
	M. phlei	[185, 192]		
	M. vaccae	[185, 192, 199]		
	M. smegmatis	[26]	[206]	
	TNF-α recombinant *M. smegmatis*	[26]	[206]	
	M. kansasii		[207]	
	M. brumae	[163, 185, 192]	[163, 192]	

(*Continued*)

Table 4.1 (*Continued*)

		***In vitro* studies; growth inhibition bladder cancer cell lines**	***In vivo* studies in animal models**	***In vivo* studies in human clinical assays**
Bacteria other than mycobacteria				
	Salmonella choleraesuis carrying endostatin gene		[55]	
	E7 antigen + Ty21a		[56]	
	Corynebacterium parvum		[63–65]	[66, 67]
	LGG	[75]	[20, 81]	
	Lactobacillus casei strain Shirota	[75]	[80]	[82–84]
Other bacteria components				
	HP-NAP		[90, 91]	
	SEB	[92]	[93]	
	PPE-SEA	[94]	[94]	
	Clostridium perfringens endotoxin	[95]		
	TP-40			[97]
	OM			[99, 100] (NCT02449239)
	OK-432	[101, 102]	[102]	

4.3.1.1 Live bacteria

Since the tumor microenvironment is highly hypoxic, some strategies for immunotherapy have been based on the use of anaerobic or facultative bacteria that can easily survive inside tumors [54].

4.3.1.2 *Salmonella*

Salmonella is advantageous in that the systemic administration of *Salmonella choleraesuis* carrying the endostatin gene resulted in the preferential accumulation of the bacteria in tumors, which in turn led to the inhibition of BC tumors, likely mediated by the massive infiltration of $CD8^+$ cells at the tumor site. As a result, an increase in mouse survival rates was observed [55].

Ty21a, the live attenuated *S. enterica* serovar Typhi vaccine against typhoid fever, was intravesically administered to tumor-bearing mice that had been previously vaccinated with the E7 antigen from human papillomavirus type-16. These mice showed higher survival rates than control tumor-bearing mice [56]. However, in these experiments, lung cancer cells were inoculated into the mouse bladders to induce tumors and no comparison with BCG treatment was made.

4.3.1.3 *Corynebacterium*

Corynebacterium parvum, now denominated *Propionibacterium acnes* [57], was known to be one of the causative agents of acne vulgaris [58], to be a potent immunostimulatory adjuvant [59], and to possess antitumor potential [60]. At the end of the 1970s, some authors began to use *C. parvum* for the treatment of BC in mouse models [61] or as a subcutaneous adjuvant in the treatment of BC patients [62]. During the 1980s, several studies evaluated the antitumor effect and the immunostimulatory capacity of *C. parvum* in different BC models: in subcutaneous tumors when intralesionally administered [63], in grown tumors surgically removed before *C. parvum* and cisplatin combination treatment to simulate the clinical situation [64], and in intravesical tumors when *C. parvum* was administered one and six days after tumor implantation [65]. The results obtained in all these studies suggested that *C. parvum* could be used for the treatment of BC. Moreover, in two small clinical trials, *C. parvum* showed the capacity to induce the infiltration of lymphocytes and plasma cells into the bladder [66] and to prevent recurrence [67]. Despite the promising results obtained during that time, no more studies have been published on this strategy. Later, some *Corynebacterium* species were described to be the cause of some cancers [68] and to be opportunistic infectious agents in cancer patients [69, 70].

4.3.1.4 Lactic bacteria

In contrast to *Corynebacterium*, *Lactobacillus* species are generally regarded as safe. Ohashi *et al.* (2002) [71] demonstrated that these gram-positive lactic acid bacteria, usually used as food supplements, reduce the risk of BC when repeatedly consumed via fermented milk products. Later, Feyisetan *et al.* (2012) [72] presented a possible explanation for this phenomenon. Since DC-activated natural killer (NK) cells are one of the final effector cells that act on BC cells and lactobacilli are known to activate DCs and neutrophils [73] and to induce a Th1-polarized response [74], the consumption of probiotics may establish a positive milieu in the BC patient's body that allows the patient to expel the BC [72]. For the past 20 years, studies of the antitumor therapeutic potential of lactic bacteria have focused on two different treatment strategies: local administration at the tumor site and oral administration.

4.3.1.5 Local administration to the tumor

Both *Lactobacillus rhamnosus* GG (LGG) and *L. casei* strain Shirota exhibited cytotoxic activity on MGH (grade 3 tumor) and RT112 (grade 2) BC cell lines. This toxicity was similar to the toxicity exerted by BCG in MGH but higher than that of BCG in RT112 [75].

In vivo studies revealed that six weekly instillations of either BCG or LGG induced significant infiltration of NK cells into healthy mouse bladders [76]. In an orthotopic murine model of BC, a significant percentage (89%) of tumor-bearing mice intravesically treated with LGG cleared their tumors compared with 77% of BCG-treated mice [20]. However, the orthotopic model used in this study is not ideal for comparing a new therapy to BCG because treatments were started four days after tumor implantation, and because MB49 cells grow aggressively in the bladder, it is recommended to start the treatments 24–48 h after tumor induction, which improves survival rates in BCG-treated mice [77–79].

4.3.1.6 Oral administration

Further studies evaluated the antitumor activity of orally administered lactobacilli. In a murine transplantable model of BC, *L. casei* demonstrated an antitumor effect when animals were fed this bacterium [80]. In a subcutaneous murine model of BC, LGG-fed mice developed smaller tumors because the local and systemic immune response that was induced was greater than that in nontreated mice [81].

A small clinical trial revealed that after TUR of the tumor, the oral administration of *L. casei* prolonged the recurrence-free interval compared with that in patients who received a placebo [82]. In another clinical trial, with more enrolled patients, the oral administration of *L. casei* significantly prevented recurrences in patients with multiple primary tumors and with recurrent single tumors; however, it had no effect on patients with multiple recurrent tumors. Furthermore, no significant differences were found in the side effect profile when comparing *L. casei* treated–patients with patients who received a placebo [83]. In another clinical study, BC patients after TUR were randomly selected to receive either intravesical epirubicin (a chemotherapeutic drug) or intravesical epirubicin along with oral *L. casei*. The three-year recurrence-free survival rates were higher in patients treated with the combination therapy, and no differences were observed in either the side effects, the progression-free rates, or the overall survival [84].

Recombinant lactic bacteria have also been used. For instance, a *Bifidobacterium infantis*–mediated thymidine kinase (BI-TK) suicide gene therapy system injected intravenously together with intraperitoneal ganciclovir therapy showed an antitumor effect on bladder tumor–bearing rats by inducing apoptosis of BC cells [85]. *Lactococcus lactis* expressing the staphylococcal enterotoxin B (SEB), which we will discuss in more detail in the next section, showed improved antitumor and immunostimulatory effects on chemically induced BC tumors in rats [86].

4.3.2 Bacterial Toxins

4.3.2.1 Lipid A from *Salmonella*

There are some published studies on the role of *Salmonella* components in BC treatment, but they are stories of failures. In 1982, Lamm *et al.* demonstrated that Re mutant glycolipid (ReG) from *S. typhimurium* had no antitumor effect on murine BC tumors [87]. In 1989, different preparations of lipopolysaccharide (LPS) from *S. minnesota* and also from other gram-negative microorganisms, such as *Escherichia coli, Klebsiella pneumonia, Pseudomonas aeruginosa, and Serratia,* were shown to be necrotic to intradermal murine BC tumors; however, the severe toxicity was associated with successful therapy [88].

4.3.2.2 *Helicobacter* toxins

Since the time of the studies using lipid A, other less toxic components have been tested as antitumor agents to treat BC. For instance, the toll-like receptor (TLR) 2 ligand *Helicobacter pylori* protein (HP-NAP) has shown the capacity to activate neutrophils to secrete reactive oxygen species and to shift the balance of the immune response toward a Th1 response [89, 90]. This protein has been tested on two BC models, one of them orthotopic, for its antitumor and immunostimulatory effect. HP-NAP treatment reduced tumor growth by inducing necrosis, triggering infiltration of $CD4^+$ and $CD8^+$ IFN-γ-secreting cells into the tumor, and decreasing the vascularization of the tumor compared with that in nontreated tumor-bearing animals [90, 91]. Notably, none of these studies compared HP-NAP to the gold standard BCG treatment.

4.3.2.3 *Staphylococcus aureus* toxins

Other proteins have also been proven to be effective in BC models, including SEA and staphylococcal enterotoxins B (SEB). A first study on the activating potential of SEB on peripheral blood mononuclear cells (PBMCs) showed that coculturing SEB-activated PBMCs with BC cells induced apoptosis of BC cells; however, the soluble factors secreted by SEB-activated PBMCs showed a minor effect on BC cells [92]. In a carcinogen-induced rat model of BC, SEB had antitumor activity similar to that of BCG. Moreover, the group in which both therapies were simultaneously intravesically administered had an advantage compared to the groups receiving single-treatment therapies [93]. Regarding SEA, an engineered oncolytic virus expressing SEA (PPE3-SEA) showed antitumor activity in *in vitro* studies and *in vivo* when intratumorally injected into a subcutaneous murine BC model [94].

4.3.2.4 *Clostridium endotoxin*

A recent publication studied the effect of the *Clostridium perfringens* endotoxin on different low-grade BC cell lines, high-grade BC cell lines, primary 3D cultures derived from NMIBC patients, and normal (nontumor) urothelial cells. This toxin, which specifically binds to claudins that are overexpressed in BC cells, was cytotoxic to low-grade cell lines but not to normal epithelial cells or high-grade T24 cells [95].

4.3.2.5 *Pseudomonas* toxin

A fusion protein combining *Pseudomonas* exotoxin A and transforming growth factor alpha (TP-40) was designed to specifically bind the epidermal growth factor receptor (EGFR), which is overexpressed on BC cells [96]. Although no treatment-associated toxicity was observed in a phase I clinical trial, this fusion protein only conferred advantageous outcomes in carcinoma *in situ* (CIS) patients and not in Ta/T1 patients [97]. Following a similar strategy, oportuzumab monatox (OM) was created as a fusion of the humanized antibody against the epithelial cell adhesion molecule (EpCAM) and the *Pseudomonas* exotoxin A. This fusion protein binds to the BC cell surface, is internalized, and drives apoptosis of BC cells [98]. Since EpCAM is mainly expressed in malignant cells and its expression correlates with BC cell grade, as more EpCAM is expressed in higher-grade cells [99], this therapy specifically targets BC cells. This therapy has been administered to BCG-refractory or BCG-intolerant patients in phase I and II trials. The results of the phase I trial showed that the therapy did not cause severe side effects and that it was more effective in T1 and Ta patients than in CIS patients [99]. In the phase II trial, 44% of the patients completely responded but some of them experienced recurrences [100]. In view of these promising results, in May of 2015, a phase III study started to recruit patients in whom BCG failed (NCT02449239).

4.3.2.6 *Streptococcus*

The *Streptococcus*-derived immunomodulator OK-432 showed the capacity to induce the release of cytokines by BC cells T24 and KK-47 and the capacity to activate PBMCs, as conditioned PBMC supernatant media were cytotoxic to BC cells. Most of this cytotoxic activity was exerted by the tumor necrosis factor (TNF) present in these media [101]. Recently, this agent has been shown to induce apoptosis in T24 and EJ BC cells and to inhibit tumor cell migration and invasion [102]. In an *in vivo* rat model, OK-432 reduced tumor size and metastasis through the action of tumor-associated macrophages (TAMs) [102].

4.3.3 Other Mycobacteria and/or Mycobacterial Components

Due to the long history of success of BCG, most of the work to find alternative therapies to BCG has been done using mycobacteria or mycobacteria-derived components. However, why are mycobacteria used? What makes mycobacteria special compared with other bacteria? Why is BCG therapy so successful?

4.3.3.1 The peculiarities of mycobacteria

Mycobacterium is the only genus in the Mycobacteriaceae family, which belongs to the phylum Actinobacteria. To date, approximately 175 members of this genus have been described (http://www.bacterio.net/mycobacterium.html). Mycobacteria include obligate pathogens as well as ubiquitous environmental nonpathogenic bacilli [103–106]. The principal pathogens are members of the *M, tuberculosis* complex and *M. leprae* (Fig. 4.1), but a small group of nontuberculous environmental mycobacteria can also cause infections, mainly in immunosuppressed individuals but also in immunocompetent individuals. The most frequently isolated opportunistic mycobacteria are the slow-growing members of the *M. avium* complex, *M. kansasii*, *M. xenopi*, and *M. simiae*, and the rapid growers *M. abscessus*, *M. fortuitum*, *M. marinum*, and *M. chelonae* [107–109]. Exposure to aerosolized NTM in water droplets and the detachment of NTM from biofilms that form on catheters are the principal methods of exposure and acquisition of pulmonary or bloodstream infections. Although this group of pathogenic mycobacteria is capable of causing infections, the majority of species are common environmental microorganisms that rarely or never cause infection (Fig. 4.1).

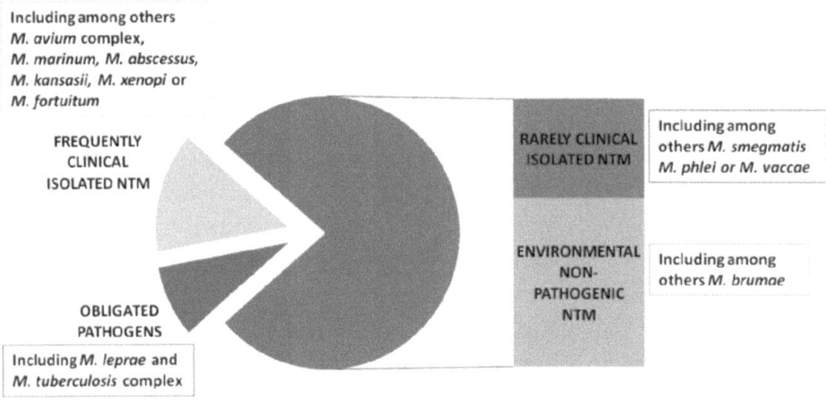

Figure 4.1 Pathogenic and nonpathogenic mycobacteria species: distribution of the described mycobacteria species in terms of their pathogenicity.

The spectrum of characteristics among mycobacteria species extensively varies, with differences in the rate of growth (from four days to four weeks in solid culture medium), colony morphology, the presence of pigmentation, and various biochemical characteristics. Despite this variability, mycobacteria are easily distinguished from other bacteria due to their peculiar CW. In contrast to gram-positive and gram-negative bacteria, mycobacteria have CWs with layers of unique lipids, glycolipids, and lipoproteins covering the cellular membrane. The majority of these molecules are exclusive to mycobacteria, being present neither in other bacteria nor in mammals. All mycobacterial species have in common the arabinogalactan-peptidoglycan-mycolic acid complex (MAPc) [110], but the rest of the CW composition can differ among species and even among similar strains of the same species. Thus, the spectrum of antigenic determinants varies, as we and other authors have previously shown [111, 112].

Most of the molecules present in the mycobacterial CW provide clues regarding the interaction with the host cell, as they are agonists of immune receptors (Table 4.1). Moreover, other molecules located inside the cell, such as proteins, for example, heat-shock proteins, or unmethylated cytosine-guanosine nucleotide (CpG) DNA motifs have been described as potent activators of the immune system (Table 4.1) [113]. Mycobacterial antigens can activate host cells via lectins (Mincle, Dectin 1, or mannose receptor [MR]) [114, 115], TLRs (TLR1, TLR2, TLR6, or TLR 9) [116–119], or T cell receptors via CD1 [120–122]. Receptors such as TLR2 are directly related to antitumor immunity [123–125], being involved in the processing and presentation of tumor peptides and in triggering the production of the cytokines that are essential to antitumoral immunotherapy [126].

The variability of molecules that interact with immune receptors therefore makes mycobacteria a fruitful source of immunostimulatory components for immunotherapeutic treatments, but the whole mycobacteria itself can also be used. It is reasonable to hypothesize that these antigens are also involved in the induction of cytokines in bladder epithelial cells or in resident macrophages and DC after BCG infection.

The understanding of the repertoire of antigenic compounds and their location in each species of mycobacteria is relevant not only because of their possible immunostimulatory effect but also because some of them could interfere with the interaction of mycobacteria with host cells or mask the effect of the other antigenic molecules. Different examples illustrate these two aspects. Regarding the immunostimulatory effect of each strain/species, lipoarabinomannan (LAM) with mannose caps (Man-LAM) is present in pathogenic species and binds to the MR or DC-SIGN receptor, reducing IL-2 and TNF secretion and increasing the secretion of anti-inflammatory cytokines [127, 128]; fast-growing nonpathogenic mycobacteria have terminal arabinose (Ara-LAM) or phosphatidylinositol (PILAM) LAM, which binds to TLR2, triggering a robust immunostimulatory effect with increased IL-12 and TNF production [129–131]. Another example is the case of BCG strains. Deletions and insertions in the genome of BCG after the serial passage of BCG in each laboratory after the initial seed distribution from the Pasteur Institute have resulted in differences in the antigenic pattern (Table 4.1) and consequently in the immunological activities. Even considering members of the same species, BCG strains differ in the presence of phenol glycolipid (PGL), phthiocerol dimycocerosates (PDIM), or MPT64 or in mycolic acid composition [6, 111, 132–135]). All these antigens are related to the BCG-induced immune response [132, 133].

With regard to the masking ability of some molecules or, as it is the same, the hidden position of the antigenic molecules, TLR2 ligands in native BCG or *M. indicus pranii* (MIP) are not well exposed and sonication of the mycobacteria increases the availability of ligands, leading to substantial IL-8 production, while autoclaving mycobacteria decreases the level of exposed TLR2 ligands [136]. Another example is the case of *M. abscessus* strains. From the exact same *M. abscessus* strain, the two possible variants, differing in the presence of glycopeptidolipids (GPLs) in their CW (the smooth colony morphology variant contains GPLs, and the rough variant is devoid of GPLs), have different outcomes in their interaction with immune cells. While smooth colony variants are roughly phagocytosed, rough colony variants are internalized and trigger a high production of TNF-α by macrophages [137]. It has been hypothesized that the presence of GPLs could mask determinant molecules that are able to induce this response.

In the following sections, attempts to substitute viable BCG in BC treatment using either mycobacteria or mycobacteria-derived components are described.

4.3.3.2 Mycobacteria antigens and cell extracts

4.3.3.2.1 *Purified antigens*

As previously discussed, all mycobacteria possess the ability to trigger an immune response. The known capacity of some molecules to induce the release of proinflammatory cytokines to drive a Th1 response in the context of tuberculosis has motivated research into their potential use as immunotherapeutic agents in BC treatment. Components of the mycobacterial CW, cytosol, or secreted antigens have been evaluated in preclinical studies for their application in BC treatment.

MPT-64 antigen from *Mycobacterium bovis* BCG

MPT-64 is an antigenic protein present in pathogenic species of mycobacteria, mainly *M. bovis* and some strains of *M. bovis* BCG [138]. In 2007, Yu and collaborators studied the efficacy of the recombinant BCG subunit protein vaccine MPT-64 in inducing cytokine production and suppressing tumor growth in mice [139]. Various doses of recombinant MPT-64 protein were intravesically instilled six times over two weeks after the implantation of MBT-2 tumor cells in an orthotopic model of the disease. A dose-dependent response was observed, with the highest doses achieving higher survival rates for tumor-bearing mice than for control animals while inducing systemic IFN-γ levels in treated animals. Nevertheless, no comparison with BCG-treated animals was made [139].

38 kDa protein or PstS antigen-1

PstS1 is a *M. tuberculosis* glycosylated lipoprotein that is known by different names in the literature, including protein antigen b (Pab), antigen 5, antigen 78, 38-kDa protein, PhoS, and PstS. This antigen has been widely studied in tuberculosis research because of its high immunogenicity. Only one study described the potential of PstS1 as an immunotherapeutic agent [140]. In this study, PstS1 was able to activate human PBMCs to kill T24 cells in a dose-dependent manner and to induce the production of IFN-γ in these cells. In addition, PstS1 induced DC activation, detected by an increase in CD83 and CD86 and the release of TNF-α and IL-12 p70. In a murine model of BC, four weekly intravesical instillations of PstS1 prolonged survival rates in tumor-bearing mice compared with untreated tumor-bearing mice. Regarding the systemic immune response triggered by this immunostimulatory molecule, splenocytes from PstS1-treated mice specifically responded to the molecule [140].

Mycobacteria DNA

Several studies have shown that BCG DNA is immunostimulatory. This activity has been related to the capacity of the DNA to stimulate NK cells and to induce the release of IFN-α, IFN-β, and IFN-γ in splenocytes [141–143]. In particular, unmethylated CpG motifs are responsible for this activity [144, 145] by interacting with TLR9, which is primarily expressed on B cells and DC. Activated DCs, in turn, express IL-12, which shifts the balance toward a Th1 response. This makes CpG a good candidate for BC therapy [146]. Not only did CpG show antitumor activity in the MB49 subcutaneous model [147, 148], it also showed a higher antitumor effect than BCG in an orthotopic murine BC model. As in BCG immunotherapy to clear tumors, for the mode of action of CpG, T cells are a key piece [148, 149]. Furthermore, when CpG-treated animals that were cured were rechallenged with MB49, the previous treatment protected them from recurrence. Therefore, CpG has both therapeutic effects directly on the tumor and a long-lasting effect [148]. In another study, it was observed that the antineoplastic effect of the combination therapy with CpG together with checkpoint inhibitors, such as blocking antibodies against cytotoxic T lymphocyte antigen-4 (aCTLA-4) and antiprogrammed death receptor-1 (aPD-1), was even superior to that of CpG monotherapy [150].

DNA from *M. phlei* deserves special attention. The DNA of *M. phlei* complexed with *M. phlei* CWs was shown to be a potent BC immunotherapeutic agent, as will be detailed in the next section. The DNA part of the complex has been proven to be responsible for the induction of cytokine release by monocytes and macrophages and to inhibit BC cell proliferation by triggering apoptosis [151–153]. However, the CpG motifs are not responsible for this activity [151].

Alpha-crystallin antigen (fibronectin-binding protein) Ag85 complex

Mycolyl transferases are a complex of three antigenic proteins (Ag85 A, B, and C) present in both the cytosol and the CW of all mycobacteria species. This Ag85 complex has been identified as a major secreted protein of actively replicating *M. tuberculosis*. Their function is the transport of trehalose monomycolate to trehalose dimycolate (TDM) and arabinogalactan mycolate (AGM). The antigen 85B (also known as alpha antigen, MPT59, or antigen 6) triggers a strong Th1 immune response when used to stimulate immune cells. Its immunological properties led to the use of this antigen as the basis for subunit vaccines to prevent tuberculosis. Moreover, Ag85 is a fibronectin-binding protein.

Ag85 cDNA obtained from *M. kansasii* was extracted and transferred to murine tumor cells (MBT-2 BC cells), which were injected into mice. Analysis of the immune response generated indicates that the mycobacterial antigen induces an antitumor response at different levels, eliciting the generation of specific cytolytic $CD8^+$ cells [154].

As DCs are key to the T cell–mediated immune response. Zhang *et al.* [155] engineered DCs to express Ag85A (Ag85A-DC). Ag85A-DCs demonstrated antitumor activity in BC models: after being sensitized with tumor lysates, Ag85A-DCs were able to activate T cells to be cytotoxic to those tumors. Moreover, Ag85A-DCs inhibit BC tumors growth *in vivo* and induce the infiltration of $CD4^+$ and $DC8^+$ T cells into the tumor site.

BCG antigens: Subcellular components

To identify the antigen(s) responsible for the BCG antitumor effect on BC, Zlotta and collaborators [156] fractionated a particular BCG strain, GL-2, a variant of the Paris strain, obtaining the BCG cell wall (BCG-CW), plasma membrane, cytosol, purified polysaccharides as glucans or arabinomannans, purified native proteins from the BCG culture filtrate, a recombinant 22-kDa protein, and the phosphate transporter PstS-2 and -3 proteins. When PBMCs from healthy subjects were treated with the whole bacterium or each fraction, they found that the majority of the components induce the production of IFN-γ, IL-12, IL-2, and IL-6. Live BCG and most of its subcomponents (with the exception of the cytosol and PstS-2 and -3) significantly enhanced IFN-γ and IL-12 secretion, caused expansion of CD3–CD561 cells, and led to non-MHC-restricted cytotoxicity against T24 bladder tumor cells compared with unstimulated controls [156].

4.3.3.2.2 *Cell extracts*

Early work in the last century (1960s–1980s) demonstrated that the whole CW extract and even some purified CW fractions of BCG, *M. kansasii*, *M. smegmatis*, and *M. phlei* (in some initial studies misidentified as *M. smegmatis* [157]) possess antitumor activity when intralesionally administered with irradiated tumor cells in different animal models of cancer [157–160]. CW extracts were formulated into oil droplets, and all of them caused tumor regression. In all these studies, it was necessary for mycobacterial extracts to be delivered intratumorally or close to the tumor for an effective antitumor response. A lipid-rich fraction was shown to be responsible for the antitumor activity of the whole mycobacteria [158]. This was the basis for the discovery of the adjuvant activity of mycobacterial CW components.

After these initial studies, the use of the antitumor activity of mycobacteria cell extracts specifically as a tool for BC treatment has focused on preparations obtained from BCG or *M. phlei*.

BCG cell extracts

Regarding the use of BCG-CW extracts for BC treatment, Akaza *et al.* [161] showed that the coexistence of BCG with tumor cells activated local immunity in a syngeneic mouse subcutaneous tumor model of BC. The critical role of the attachment of BCG preparations to host cells in internalization and induction of a proper effect was also demonstrated [161]. Continuation of this work is challenging due to the difficulty of preparing stable and properly soluble preparations of mycobacterial CWs. As previously explained, the CW of mycobacteria has a highly rich lipid content, which provides a strong hydrophobic character and makes the preparation of stable aqueous solutions difficult. Moreover, the fact that both the mycobacterial CW and the urothelium surface are negatively charged causes them to repel each other, avoiding contact and internalization of mycobacterial CW [162, 163].

To improve the contact of the BCG-CW extract with bladder cells and the internalization into them, Japanese researchers developed a vehicle consisting of nanoparticles in which the surface of liposomes, resembling an envelope-type virus, was modified by an octa-arginine (R8) anchor, a well-known and efficient cell-penetrating peptide [164–166]. Two different formulations have been made using R8 liposomes, involving BCG-CW, which consists of heat-killed (Hk) BCG cells, and BCG CW skeleton (BCG-CWS), which consists of the covalent membrane-attached fraction of the mycobacterial CW, that is, the MAPc. The strain used to prepare the formulation was the Japan BCG strain. Different studies from the same group demonstrated previously that either live or Hk bacteria or the CWS fraction is able to inhibit BC cell growth *in vitro* [167]. Moreover, the accurate composition and immunostimulatory capacity of this fraction was determined in previous studies [168, 169], in which the authors referred to CWS as SPM-105.

R8-liposome-BCG-CW is able to successfully attach to MBT-2 murine BC cells, driving the BCG-CW to lysosomes [170], and to inhibit MBT-2 growth in a syngeneic subcutaneous tumor model.

When the CWS was incorporated into R8-liposomes, a wide range of antitumor activity *in vitro*, *ex vivo*, and *in vivo* was achieved. The nanoparticulate CWS was able to be internalized and inhibit proliferation of human BC cell growth *in vitro* [165]; activated immune cells, leading to their cytotoxic activity against T24 and RT112 BC tumor cells [171]; enhanced Th1 differentiation in naïve $CD4^+$ human cells; and showed potent antitumor activity in an intravesical BC rat model of the disease [171].

M. phlei cell extracts

M. phlei is the long-standing and most prosperous "challenger" of live BCG in the search for mycobacteria-derived agents for use in BC treatment. Similar to *M. smegmatis, M. phlei* is considered "nonpathogenic" (Fig. 4.1). Various cases of *M. phlei* infections have been reported in the literature, but it has nevertheless always been studied as a nonviable therapy.

As explained before, the study of the immunotherapeutic properties of CW extracts of *M. phlei* was initiated at approximately the same time as the study of BCG cell extracts. Additionally, the extracts of *M. phlei* were modified to improve its immunotherapeutic properties, leading to a phase III clinical trial that is currently underway. Initially, Chin *et al.* demonstrated that the CW of *M. phlei* (called MCWE or Regressin™) has an antitumor effect both in orthotopic and heterotopic bladder tumors in mouse models, although the effect was still smaller than that triggered by the instillation of live BCG [172]. The immune response induced after treatment with MCWE or live BCG was similar and significantly higher than that in nontreated mice. MCWE consists of a preparation containing mainly the CW, including TDM and muramyl dipeptide (MDP), which represents the minimal structure of the CW peptidoglycan, among other antigens [173]. CW components of *M. phlei* also led to the apoptosis of BC cells [152]. As explained in regard to BCG-CW extracts, the mycobacterial CW is hydrophobic, resulting in aqueous solutions that are difficult to prepare. To solve this problem, MCWE was formulated in an emulsion of mineral oil in water with thimerosal as a preservative. In 2001, a first small clinical trial using MCWE in high-risk NMIBC showed a rate of response over 62.5% at one year and 49.3% at two years, but almost all patients discontinued the treatment due to adverse events or treatment failure [174]. Since patients previously given BCG treatment responded similarly to those without previous BCG, *M. phlei* extract was proposed as a second-line drug in cases of refractory BCG.

The same authors demonstrated that the CW along with *M. phlei* DNA can inhibit BC cell growth, have an immunostimulatory effect by triggering the production of cytokines, and cause an apoptotic effect on tumor cells [151, 153]. Thus, the composition was improved by adding an *M. phlei* DNA coating to the CW in the formulation and by eliminating thimerosal for its possible toxic effects, and it was called MCNA (Urodicin^{TM}).

The efficacy of MCNA has been evaluated in phase II and III clinical trials. In the first clinical trial, no conclusive results were obtained because the number of patients was low in the different groups and no 12-month follow-up was available for more than half of the treated patients. Nevertheless, approximately 30% of the patients (for both of the doses evaluated) suffered from serious adverse events. Interestingly, the response was similar among patients with and without prior BCG treatment [175].

Results from a phase III study were recently reported [176]. In this study, which included 129 patients, there was no evidence of residual cancer in 25% of the patients after one year and in 19% of patients after two years. A total of 2.3% of the patients experienced adverse events, leading to discontinuation of therapy, and 66% of the patients experienced mild drug-related adverse events. Although the number of patients included in the study was low, the results showed a potential role for MCNA in treating BCG-refractory patients. The number of side effects, as expected, was lower, and the rate of cancer-free survival was similar to that after BCG. However, no simultaneous comparison was made with other therapies.

At the moment, the niche for MCNA seems to be BCG-refractory patients. In these patients, no therapeutic options exist except cystectomy. Due to the lack of risk of infection, the possibility of instillation immediately after TUR has also been proposed [177].

4.3.3.3 Whole nonviable mycobacteria

In 1985, Kelley *et al.* reported the correlation of BCG therapy failure with low levels of BCG viability in the ampule administered to BC patients [178]. Nevertheless, many authors, with the aim of finding safer alternatives to live BCG, have studied the efficacy of the use of mycobacteria killed using different methodologies with varying outcomes, depending on the inactivation methodology and the mycobacteria species used. Unlike CW extracts, nonviable mycobacteria possess the whole antigenic pattern of mycobacteria, but, depending on the inactivation method, some of the possible crucial antigens can be altered or lost.

4.3.3.3.1 *Heat-killed mycobacteria*

Heat-killed BCG

The most widely studied method is heat inactivation, such as autoclaving, which would alter, damage, or destroy thermolabile antigenic components [179, 180]. Various BCG strains and cells lines have been used in different studies [181]. The autoclave-killed BCG Connaught strain was demonstrated to inhibit BC cell growth to the same extent as live BCG in two BC high-grade cell lines (T24 and J82) [179]. Similar results were obtained for the high-grade T24 and HT1376 BC cell lines by infecting them with the Tokyo 172 strain [167]. By contrast, Shah *et al.* found that live-BCG TICE® inhibited 253J and T24 cells significantly more than the Hk form [182]. Unlike the observations made by the above-mentioned authors, other authors found that Hk BCG had no inhibitory effect in MGH BC cells [183].

Regarding the response induced in Hk BCG–infected BC cells, lower levels of IL-6 and IL-8 production were observed in T24, J82, and RT4 cells than in live BCG–infected cells [179]; mRNA expression of IL-6, IL-8 and GM-CSF was lower in MGH cells [183]; and nitric oxide (NO) was lower in T24 cells [182]. By contrast, Zhang *et al.* found that similar mRNA levels of IL-6 and TNF-α were released due to live- and Hk-BCG infection [183] in J82 cells and similar levels of inducible NO synthase (iNOS) were found in T24 BC cells [182]. Thus, in general, Hk BCG induces a direct immune response in BC cells but the response is not as strong as that induced by live BCG.

Regarding the indirect immunostimulatory capacity of Hk BCG *in vitro*, as increased levels of TNF-related apoptosis-inducing ligand (TRAIL/Apo-2L) are present in the urine of BCG-responsive BC patients, Kemp *et al.* studied the TRAIL released by live or Hk BCG–infected neutrophils and did not find significant differences [184]. Yamada *et al.* demonstrated that the cytotoxic capacity of Hk BCG–activated peritoneal exudate cells (PECs) on BC cells was lower than that of cells induced by live BCG due to a lower capacity to induce IFN-γ, TNF-α, and PGE_2 in these cultures [185].

Moreover, Hk BCG induced significantly lower expression of surface activation markers (cluster of differentiation (CD) 80, CD86, and CD40) on the murine macrophage cell line J774 than did the live form [186] and poorly induced the expression of CD80, CD1D, greater intracellular adhesion molecule (ICAM)-1, and IA^K (major histocompatibility complex (MHC) class II) on the MBT-2 murine BC cell line and HLA-DR (MHC class II) on T24 and J82 human BC cell lines [187]. In contrast, in immature DCs, no differences were observed in the activation capacity of live or Hk forms of BCG (CD80, CD83, CD86, and CD40) [188]. The indirect response triggered by Hk BCG is weaker than that triggered by the live form.

Regarding the antitumor effect *in vivo*, Shapiro *et al.* observed greater inhibition of tumors implanted into mice treated with live BCG, which was correlated with high amounts of NK cells and positive footpad tests, compared with the effects of Hk BCG [189]. Although the Hk Tokio 172 strain of BCG showed no ability to attach to MBT-2 murine BC cells, it showed tumor inhibition in a mouse BC model when mixed with the tumor cells prior to implantation due to the induction of a local immune response [161].

At the intravesical level, Günther *et al.* demonstrated no efficacy of Hk BCG for treating tumor-bearing mice, obtaining survival rates similar to those of untreated animals [190]. It was also observed that both Hk and live BCG induce similar production levels of Th2 cytokines (IL-10 and IL-4) but live BCG induces higher production levels of Th1 cytokines (IFN-γ, IL-2, IL-12p40, or TNF-α) than the killed form. Thus, Hk BCG fails to trigger a Th1-balanced response (Fig. 4.2). Regarding this unfavorable milieu, Biot and collaborators observed that Hk BCG was unable to trigger T cell infiltration into the mouse bladder [78]. It was reported that to achieve a favorable shift to a Th1 response, live BCG was required for at least the first instillations [191]. At the clinical level, patients with a history of poor response to BCG who were treated later with Hk BCG showed reduced toxicity and no increase in the risk of tumor recurrence [192].

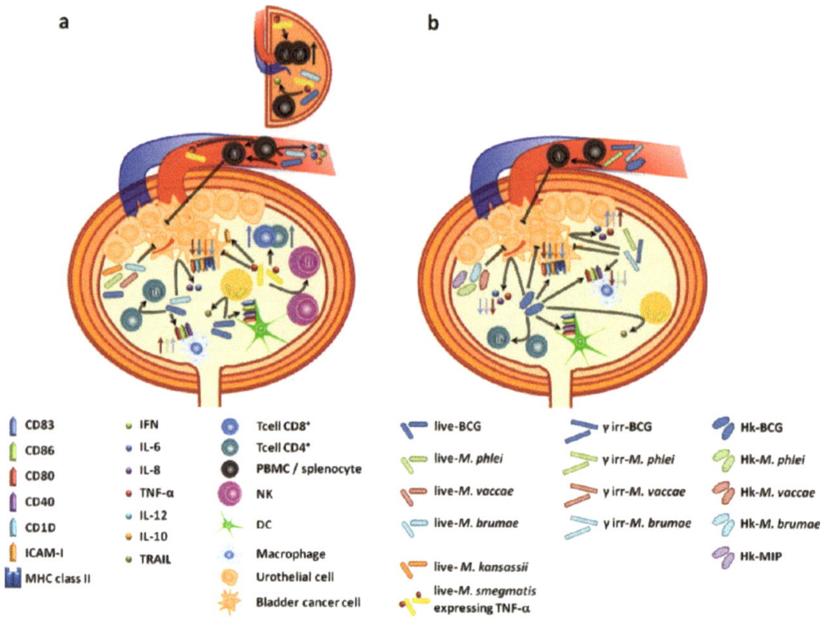

Figure 4.2 Mode of action of live or nonviable mycobacteria in bladder cancer treatment. At the bottom the bladder and the vascularization of the tumor are represented. "AK" stands for activated killer. Inside the lumen of the bladder the mechanisms related to the antitumor response triggered by mycobacteria-based treatment are represented. Splenocytes containing the letter "M" indicate the presence of memory cells. T cells containing Th1 or Th2 indicate the type of response triggered by the intravesically instillated agent.

Other Hk mycobacteria

Other mycobacteria than BCG have also been studied for their antitumor activity in BC. Hk *M. brumae, M. vaccae*, and *M. phlei*, all environmental mycobacteria with proven antitumor efficacy on BC cells [193], were shown to be effective *in vitro* in inhibiting BC cell growth to the same extent as their live forms in T24, J82, and RT4 cell lines [186].

Another environmental mycobacterium, Hk MIP, previously known as *Mycobacterium w*, was demonstrated to maintain 100% survival rates and recurrence-free rates in a small clinical trial that included five BC patients undergoing radiation therapy [194] and was also tested in the treatment of BCG-refractory patients [195]. Recently, MIP was shown to have the capacity to inhibit proliferation *in vitro* of the RT112 and EJ28 BC cell lines [196].

4.3.3.3.2 *Other inactivation methods*

Other inactivation methods have shown different results. Some of them, such as ultraviolet (UV) irradiation or sonication, did not solve the problem of replicative ability, which indicates that UV-irradiated BCG and sonicated BCG were able to grow to a certain degree [197]. Moreover, sonicated BCG was unable to activate human PBMCs to be cytotoxic to BC cells directly established from a patient [198].

Other inactivation methods, such as γ-irradiation, did reduce the mycobacteria viability to zero. In fact, γ-irradiated mycobacteria have shown the most promising results in the treatment of BC because γ-irradiated BCG exerts a similar inhibitory effect on different BC cell lines and induces higher levels of proinflammatory cytokines among all the inactivation methods studied (UV irradiation and three different heat-inactivation methods). Both live and γ-irradiated BCG–activated PBMCs were cytotoxic to the T24 BC cell line [179, 186]. Moreover, unlike Hk BCG, γ-irradiated mycobacterial CWs remain less altered and also retain certain metabolic activity that might be necessary for them to exert their antitumor effect [179]. In contrast, as with Hk BCG, γ-irradiated forms were unable to induce the expression of the activation markers CD80, CD86, or CD40 on the surface of J774 macrophages [186, 199].

For all the parameters explained above, γ-irradiated *M. brumae*, γ-irradiated *M. phlei*, and γ-irradiated *M. vaccae* showed results similar to those of BCG. It must be noted that in all cases, *M. vaccae* showed the weakest effect [186, 199]. Using an orthotopic mouse BC model, tumor-bearing animals were treated with a first course of live BCG and three subsequent courses of γ-irradiated mycobacteria. Following this schedule, both γ-irradiated BCG and *M. brumae* significantly prolonged survival of tumor-bearing mice compared to untreated mice, but γ-irradiated BCG-treated mice survived for a shorter time than mice treated with only live BCG [199].

4.3.3.4 Live nontuberculous mycobacteria

An attractive approach to overcoming adverse BCG-induced effects is to consider the use of nonpathogenic mycobacteria. As explained above, the vast majority of mycobacteria are environmental microorganisms with no history of infection in humans, animal, or plants and they potentially share immunomodulatory antigens with BCG (Table 4.2 and Fig. 4.3). However, few mycobacteria have been evaluated for their antitumor capacity in BC. The next section will cover the preclinical studies carried out with live mycobacteria other than BCG.

Table 4.2 Relevant mycobacteria antigens that are recognized by immune system receptors

Antigen	Immune receptor	Presence in mycobacteria species	Refs.
Ag85C	CR3	All mycobacteria species	[217]
DAT, PAT, SL, TAT	Unknown	Mainly in *M. tuberculosis*; absent in BCG strains; some environmental mycobacteria, such as *M. fortuitum*, have DAT and TAT antigens	[218–220]
CpG DNA	TLR9	All mycobacteria species	[221]
GMM	CD1b; CD1c; Mincle	All mycobacteria species but different structures	[222–225]
GPL	TLR2	Some mycobacteria species, such as *M. abscessus*, *M. phlei*, and *M. smegmatis*; absent in *M. tuberculosis* and in BCG strains	[226, 227]
GroMM	CD1b; Mincle	All mycobacteria species but different structures	[228, 229]
LAM	MR, DC-SIGN (human)/SIGNR3 (mice), Dectin-2, CR3, CD1b	All mycobacteria species but different structures	[230–233]
Lipoproteins (19 kDa)	TLR2	Some mycobacteria species	[234, 235]
LM	TLR2 TLR4 DC-SIGN (human)/ SIGNR3 (mice)	All mycobacteria species	[220, 232, 236, 237]

Antigen	Immune receptor	Presence in mycobacteria species	Refs.
LOS	Unknown	Some mycobacteria species; absent in BCG strains	[238]
MPT64	Unknown	Mainly in pathogenic mycobacteria; only in some BCG strains	[139, 239]
MA	CD1b	All mycobacteria, but different patterns of mycolic acid composition; different composition between BCG strains; *Nocardia* and *Corynebacterium* genera have different mycolic acids	[228]
PDIM	Unknown	Mainly in pathogenic mycobacteria; only in some BCG strains	[220, 236]
PGL	Unknown	Mainly in pathogenic mycobacteria; only in some BCG strains	[220, 236]
PIMs	TLR2, TLR4, MR, DCAR, CD1b, CD14	All mycobacteria species	[119, 240, 241]
PstS1	TLR2, TLR4	*M. tuberculosis* and BCG	[116–118]
TDM	MARCO, Mincle, MCL	All mycobacteria species but different structures	[242–244]
TMM	Mincle; CD1b	All mycobacteria species but different structures	[222]
Cytosolic DNA	cGAS	All mycobacteria species	[245]
MDP	NOD2	All mycobacteria species	[246]

Mycobacterium vaccae

Only two studies have investigated the potential of live *M. vaccae* to inhibit BC. Baran and collaborators showed the differing abilities of different strains of *M. vaccae* to inhibit BC cells *in vitro*. None of the *M. vaccae* strains showed a better antitumor capacity than BCG [200]. The authors also showed the inability of all *M. vaccae* strains to reverse the tolerance response induced in monocytes by tumor cells. The cytotoxicity of *M. vaccae*-stimulated monocytes is lower than that of cells induced by BCG infection [200].

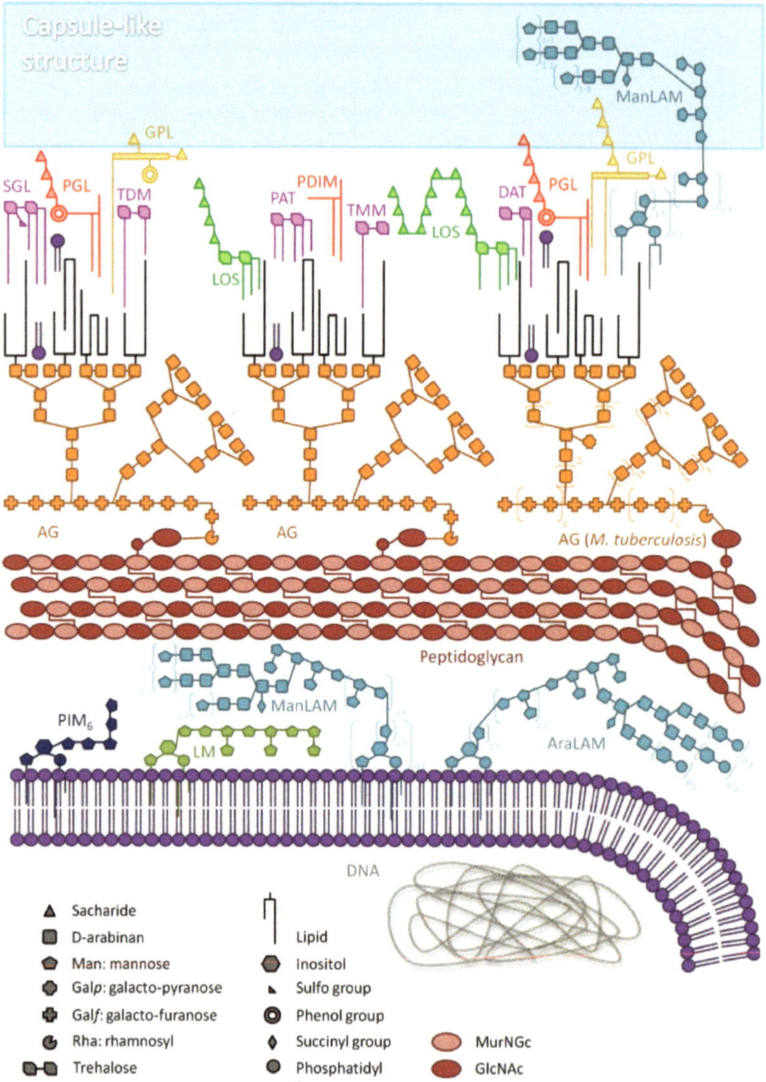

Figure 4.3 Schematic representation of the mycobacterium cell structure: The scheme shows molecules shared by all mycobacteria species and cell wall molecules present in only some mycobacteria species, as is explained in Table 4.2. Neither the structures nor the whole cell wall is drawn to scale.

Recent work in our group also demonstrated the ability of live *M. vaccae* to inhibit BC cell proliferation *in vitro*. In these experiments [186, 193], two different *M. vaccae* colony morphology variants were tested, the smooth variant and its natural rough colony mutant [201], which morphologically differ only in the presence of a polyester on the cell surface of the smooth variant. The results indicated that the smooth variant was more efficacious than the rough one. Nevertheless, as in the previous study, none of them was more efficacious than the BCG Connaught strain in any of the BC cell lines evaluated. Few cases of *M. vaccae* infection in humans have been described in the literature [202].

Mycobacterium smegmatis

M. smegmatis is potentially interesting as an immunostimulatory agent for BC treatment for several reasons. First, as explained before, early studies demonstrated the immunotherapeutic effect of CW extracts of *M. smegmatis* in different tumor models; second, *M. smegmatis* is a rapidly growing mycobacterium, which implies that it is easier to work with than BCG, a slow grower; third, more extensive molecular biology tools are available to work with *M. smegmatis* than with other mycobacteria species. The drawback of the use of *M. smegmatis* is that although considered a nonpathogenic mycobacterium, it has been responsible of various cases of infection [203–206], limiting its use in a live form. Nevertheless, a couple of articles have demonstrated its capacity to inhibit BC cell growth *in vitro* [26] and its ability to express recombinant cytokine to improve *in vivo* BC immunotherapy [207].

Haley *et al.* demonstrated that recombinant *M. smegmatis*–expressing human TNF-α appears to trigger a higher production of proinflammatory cytokines, ICAM-1 expression, and growth inhibition in EJ18, MGH-U1, RT4, and RT112 human BC cells than nontransformed *M. smegmatis*. Both the TNF-α-recombinant and the original *M. smegmatis* induced similar levels of cytotoxic PBMCs after infection [26]. No comparison with BCG, however, was made in the same study. Moreover, Young *et al.* demonstrated that TNF-α-recombinant *M. smegmatis* activates NK cells when inoculated close to MB49 BC cells in a heterotopic syngeneic mouse model. Mouse survival increased to 70% in TNF-α-recombinant *M. smegmatis*–treated mice, in contrast to those treated with parental *M. smegmatis* or BCG, together with high infiltration of CD3 cells at the injection site. Splenocytes from TNF/smegmatis-treated tumor-bearing mice elicit higher IFN-α levels in response to mycobacterial antigen and an increased proliferative response from lymphocytes than those treated with wild-type *M. smegmatis.* The study also suggests an NK-dependent and a T cell–independent role in initial tumor destruction when tumor-bearing mice were treated with TNF/smegmatis [207].

Mycobacterium kansasii

Only one study evaluated the capacity of *M. kansasii* to reduce tumor burden in an orthotopic murine model of the disease [208]. The improved tumor growth reduction of *M. Kansasii* compared to a range of BCG strains was related to the high binding capacity of *M. kansasii* with fibronectin in the injured bladder wall. However, *M. kansasii* is one of the most frequent isolates in pulmonary infections due to NTM, which makes it impossible to use it for cancer treatment in its live form [209].

The case of *Mycobacterium brumae*

Finally, the immunotherapeutic potential of *M. brumae* has recently been described [193]. *M. brumae* was first described in 1993 by Luquin and collaborators from 11 isolates obtained from soil and water samples and one isolate obtained from a sputum sample of an individual without clinical significance [210].

M. brumae was initially studied, in parallel with other selected mycobacteria species (BCG Connaught, *M. confluentis, M. chitae, M. chubuense, M. fallax, M. gastri, M. hiberniae, M. mageritense, M. obuense, M. phlei,* and two strains of *M. vaccae*) for its capacity to inhibit bladder tumor cell lines. These species and strains were selected because of their pathogenicity, their previously described immunostimulatory capacity [112, 201, 211], their growth rate, their phylogenetic relationship, or the differences and similarities between their lipidic and glycolipid CW contents and those of the BCG-CW [193]. After the infection of seven different BC cell lines, covering a range representing different histopathological grades of BC (from high to low grade: T24, J82, RT112, SW780, HG-MG3, and RT4), measurements of cell proliferation revealed that *M. brumae* is able to inhibit cell growth similarly to BCG in high-grade cell lines and even to a greater extent than BCG in BC low-grade cell lines [193].

Further experiments have demonstrated that *M. brumae* triggers macrophage activation by inducing cytokine production and the expression of activation markers such as CD40, CD80, and CD86 to a greater extent than *M. phlei* and the *M. vaccae* smooth strain. In particular, the expression of CD80 and CD86 is superior in *M. brumae*-infected macrophages than in BCG-infected macrophages [186, 193]. *M. brumae* also induces BC tumor cell cytotoxicity in infected human PBMCs. Similar to BCG, *M. brumae* activates *ex vivo* PBMC cytotoxicity via direct contact with tumor cells and by inducing the secretion of soluble factors released by *M. brumae*-activated PBMCs. Furthermore, *M. brumae* was found to significantly induce the secretion of proinflammatory cytokines, such as IL-12p70, IFN-γ and TNF-α, Th1-polarizing cytokines, and the regulatory cytokines IL-10 and IL-6 [186, 193]. When an orthotopic murine model of the disease is used, *M. brumae*-treated tumor-bearing mice survive statistically significantly longer than untreated mice and BCG-treated tumor-bearing mice, although the differences are not statistically significant compared to BCG [193]. Moreover, splenocytes from *M. brumae*-treated tumor-bearing mice elicit a significant mycobacteria-specific Th1-biased response (high IFN-γ levels but no IL-4) compared with splenocytes from untreated mice.

M. brumae does not persist either inside macrophages or inside bladder tumor cells. Moreover, when splenocytes from *M. brumae*-treated mice were cultured, no cells were isolated, indicating than *M. brumae* does not remain inside the animals [193]. However, no episodes of infection related to *M. brumae* have been described, demonstrating that nonpathogenicity of *M. brumae* is crucial for it to be considered a safer alternative to BCG [212, 213]. Therefore, further experiments related to safety are needed to corroborate these data and to consider the use of NTM a safer approach to, and a substitute for, the use of live BCG.

These preclinical studies demonstrate that *M. brumae* has an effect comparable to that of BCG and even potentially superior to that of BGC in inhibiting low-grade tumor cells. Nevertheless, in all experiments, BCG triggers a greater release of cytokines than *M. brumae* [163, 193]. The cytokine expression profiles of *M. brumae* and BCG in PBMCs and macrophages and the cytotoxicity of mycobacteria-activated cells on T24 cells may raise doubt about whether there will be fewer side effects and less toxicity in treated patients. Although it seems that the different patterns of cytokines induced do not have implications regarding mouse survival, further studies are needed to fully investigate this parameter. In conclusion, *M. brumae* is, at least at the moment, the one mycobacterium that has been demonstrated to be as efficacious as or even better than BCG in preclinical studies.

4.3.3.5 Future contributions of mycobacteria to BC treatment

4.3.3.5.1 *Modification of treatment schedule for increased safety*

As previously discussed, the results from the *in vivo* model of the disease indicate that instillations of live mycobacteria are needed, at least during the first instillation, to obtain a favorable antitumor microenvironment. Whereas early studies show that Hk BCG does not protect from the disease in mouse models, de Boer *et al.* later demonstrated in a mouse model of the disease that three initial instillations with live BCG followed by three more instillations of Hk BCG trigger a similar immune response to that triggered using only live BCG [191]. The infiltration of immune cells into the bladder in the orthotopic BC mouse model is initiated after three or four live-BCG instillations [78]. This fact is also observed in BC patients: the presence of cytokines in the urine of BCG-treated patients is detected after the third or fourth instillation of live BCG [214, 215]. This schedule strategy, starting first with live mycobacteria and then using nonviable mycobacteria, is also a valid method to try to reduce the adverse events of BCG. In fact, as mentioned before, a recent study by Lamm and coworkers [192], although in a reduced number of patients, demonstrated fewer side effects but similar efficacy in terms of the risk of recurrence in high-risk patients treated initially with live BCG and, due to BCG infection or BCG intolerance, treated later with Hk BCG.

Recent work using *M. brumae* to treat tumor-bearing mice supports this idea. On the one hand, in contrast to live BCG–treated mice, no live *M. brumae* cells are recovered from the surviving mice, reinforcing the idea that active live bacteria is not always needed [193]. On the other hand, the high survival rates obtained in γ-irradiated *M. brumae*–treated tumor-bearing mice, in which a single first instillation was done with live *M. brumae*, also supports this idea [199]. It could be that live mycobacteria would only be needed for the first instillation and that subsequent treatment with γ-irradiated mycobacteria or properly formulated cell extracts or purified antigens will be sufficient. Further research is needed to clarify this point.

4.3.3.5.2 *Diminished adverse events*

Whether nonviable BCG (irradiated or Hk) or some mycobacteria components are used for BC treatment, the possibility of a hypersensitivity reaction, a systemic adverse event, probably cannot be avoided. An accurate study of the antigen(s) responsible for this reaction, along with a study of the pattern of antigens present in each mycobacterium used, will permit the design of an appropriate tool and also prevent this possible adverse event. Regardless, the availability of a nonviable immunotherapeutic agent, which carries no risk of BCG infection, would make clinicians sure of the origin of the systemic reaction. Importantly, in these hypothetical cases, clinicians would be certain about the treatment they should administer, namely glucocorticoids instead of antituberculosis antibiotics.

4.3.3.5.3 *Improved intravesical delivery*

Another area of research is the adequate delivery of any mycobacteria or mycobacteria component into the bladder. As has been previously mentioned, the antitumor abilities of *M. phlei* and BCG cell extracts are different depending on the formulation used for intravesical instillation. In agreement with these results, recent work using BCG and *M. brumae* has demonstrated that mouse survival and the immune response elicited increase when mycobacteria are instilled in tumor-bearing mice in an emulsion of olive oil in water [163]. Using this emulsion, cells were mainly present as single cells or as small clumps as assessed by microscopy, while mycobacteria viability was preserved. Furthermore, the physicochemical characteristics of olive oil in water–emulsified mycobacteria favor attachment to the bladder wall, including lower pH and hydrophobicity (water-repelling properties) and increased attachment to the extracellular matrix protein fibronectin, previously shown to be crucial for inducing an antitumor immune response [162, 163]. Therefore, the use of adequate formulations that enhance contact between the mycobacteria and the target cells could improve their antitumor efficacy.

Moreover, the implantation of new strategies to improve intravesical delivery of chemotherapeutic agents—photochemical internalization, photodynamic therapy, microwave-induced hyperthermia (thermochemotherapy), electromotive drug administration (EMDA), and device-assisted therapies that facilitate transport into the urothelium [216]—could also be applied to immunotherapeutic agents.

4.3.3.5.4 *Complementary mycobacterial treatments*

Another point of discussion is the different mechanisms of tumor inhibition by different mycobacterial species. It has been demonstrated *in vitro* that BCG and *M. phlei* do not share the same mechanism regulating the inhibition of tumor cell proliferation. This point paves the way for the possibility of using complementary actions of different mycobacteria and justifies the use of other mycobacteria in the same patient if the first instillation does not work properly, that is the case in the trials in which a CW-DNA complex of *M. phlei* has been instilled in BCG-refractory patients. An accurate investigation of the mechanism by which each mycobacterium interacts with tumor cells or immune cells will permit these new combinations. To achieve this aim, precise knowledge of the antigenic composition of each mycobacterium is needed.

4.3.3.5.5 *Constructing the perfect bug*

The greater ease of working with nonpathogenic, rapidly growing mycobacteria instead of BCG, together with their potential antitumor capacity, makes them an ideal tool to manipulate the expression of immunomodulatory cytokines, other immunomodulatory antigens, or key agonists for immune receptors not present in the mother strain. The example of recombinant strains of *M. smegmatis* [207] expressing heterologous antigens with different therapeutic properties suggests the potential of nonpathogenic mycobacteria as carriers or vehicles for immunostimulatory antigens apart from their own and provides an attractive alternative method for making the perfect bug.

4.4 Future Perspectives

The recent shortage of BCG, which has been worsened by the announcement that the main supplier to date has stopped its production, has revealed the scarcity of tools with which to treat NMIBC patients. Although several studies have been carried out throughout the last 40 years, until now, no substitute to BCG is available for treating patients. The dependence on a single treatment has to be solved. Not only are alternatives to improve BCG efficacy needed, but also new agents that are as efficient as BCG but safer are needed. Further research is thus necessary to know the real potential applicability of safer alternatives to BCG.

In the context of the current knowledge about BCG, future directions include the following:

- The identification of the different characteristics at various "omic" levels among different species or even strains of the same species that have shown similar, or even different, antitumor abilities will provide us with a highly valuable tool to further unravel the mechanism(s) responsible for BCG activity in BC.
- The identification of the specific antigens involved in the modulation of important immune responses should provide a straightforward and rational approach for choosing more immunogenic strains, perhaps ultimately yielding a more effective immunotherapy. This will allow the design of specific personalized agents with doses and durations based on patient tolerance and tumor characteristics.
- Knowledge of the mechanism will enable the combination of different antitumor treatments. Finding a battery of tools on the basis of microorganisms could increase the armamentarium of immunotherapeutic agents that can facilitate synergy with other types of agents, such as specific checkpoint inhibitors or chemotherapeutic agents, in order to increase the efficacy and, in turn, reduce the toxicity and resistance to a single treatment.

- Discovery of new mycobacteria species, mycobacterial components, or other bacteria-derived products with antitumor effects would make possible, for instance, the ability to treat patients with low-grade disease, for whom BCG would today be considered and who would be overtreated due to the negative balance between effectiveness and adverse events; to treat patients immediately after tumor resection; or to treat patients in whom BCG has failed.

In conclusion, further exciting research into the bacterial world would provide us with efficacious immunotherapeutic options for BC patients that are safer than BCG.

Acknowledgment

This work was supported by funding from the Spanish Ministry of Economy and Competitiveness (SAF2015-63867-R) and FEDER Funds.

References

1. Lamm D. L., Colombel M., Persad R., Soloway M., Böhle A., Palou J., *et al.* Clinical practice recommendations for the management of non-muscle invasive bladder cancer. *European Urology Supplements,* 7 (2008) 651–666, doi:10.1016/j.eursup.2008.07.009.
2. Babjuk M., Burger M., Zigeuner R., Shariat S. F., Van Rhijn B. W. G., Compérat E., *et al.* EAU guidelines on non-muscle-invasive urothelial carcinoma of the bladder: Update 2013, *European Urology,* 64 (2013) 639–653, doi:10.1016/j.eururo.2013.06.003.
3. Martínez-Piñeiro L., Portillo J. A., Fernández J. M., Zabala J. A., Cadierno I., Moyano J. L., *et al.* Maintenance Therapy with 3-monthly Bacillus Calmette–Guérin for 3 years is not superior to standard induction therapy in high-risk non-muscle-invasive urothelial bladder carcinoma: Final results of randomised CUETO study 98013. *European Urology,* 68 (2015) 256–262, doi:10.1016/j.eururo.2015.02.040.
4. Kamat A. M., Flaig T. W., Grossman H. B., Konety B., Lamm D. L., O'Donnell M. A., *et al.* Expert consensus document: Consensus statement on best practice management regarding the use of intravesical immunotherapy with BCG for bladder cancer. *Nature Reviews Urology,* 12 (2015) 225–235, doi:10.1038/nrurol.2015.58.

5. Oddens J. R., Brausi M., Sylvester R. J., Bono A., Van De Beek C., Van Andel G., *et al.* Final results of an EORTC-GU cancers group randomized study of maintenance Bacillus Calmette–Guérin in intermediate- and high-risk Ta, T1 papillary carcinoma of the urinary bladder: One-third dose versus full dose and 1 year versus 3 years of maintenance. *European Urology,* 63 (2013) 462–472, doi:10.1016/j.eururo.2012.10.039.
6. Redelman-Sidi G., Glickman M. S., Bochner B. H. The mechanism of action of BCG therapy for bladder cancer–a current perspective. *Nature Reviews Urology,* 11 (2014) 153–162, doi:10.1038/nrurol.2014.15.
7. Sylvester R. J., van der Meijden A. P. M., Oosterlinck W., Witjes J. A., Bouffioux C., Denis L., *et al.* Predicting recurrence and progression in individual patients with stage Ta T1 bladder cancer using EORTC risk tables: A combined analysis of 2596 patients from seven EORTC trials. *European Urology,* 49 (2006) 466-5-7, doi:10.1016/j.eururo.2005.12.031.
8. Cambier S., Sylvester R. J., Collette L., Gontero P., Brausi M. A., van Andel G., *et al.* EORTC nomograms and risk groups for predicting recurrence, progression, and disease-specific and overall survival in non-muscle-invasive stage Ta-T1 urothelial bladder cancer patients treated with 1–3 years of maintenance Bacillus Calmette–Guérin. *European Urology,* in press (2015), doi:10.1016/j.eururo.2015.06.045.
9. Shemtov M. M., Cheng D. L., Kong L., Shu W. P., Sassaroli M., Droller M. J., *et al.* LAK cell mediated apoptosis of human bladder cancer cells involves a pH-dependent endonuclease system in the cancer cell: Possible mechanism of BCG therapy. *Journal of Urology,* 154 (1995) 269–274. http://www.ncbi.nlm.nih.gov/pubmed/7776443 (accessed December 12, 2016).
10. Papageorgiou A., Lashinger L., Millikan R., Grossman H. B., Benedict W., Dinney C. P. N., *et al.* Role of tumor necrosis factor-related apoptosis-inducing ligand in interferon-induced apoptosis in human bladder cancer cells. *Cancer Research,* 64 (2004) 8973–8979, doi:10.1158/0008-5472.CAN-04-1909.
11. Sandes E., Lodillinsky C., Cwirenbaum R., Argüelles C., Casabé A., Eiján A. M. Cathepsin B is involved in the apoptosis intrinsic pathway induced by bacillus Calmette–Guérin in transitional cancer cell lines. *International Journal of Molecular Medicine,* 20 (2007) 823–828. http://www.ncbi.nlm.nih.gov/pubmed/17982689 (accessed December 12, 2016).

12. Schwarzer K., Foerster M., Steiner T., Hermann I.-M., Straube E. BCG strain S4-Jena: An early BCG strain is capable to reduce the proliferation of bladder cancer cells by induction of apoptosis. *Cancer Cell International,* 10 (2010) 21, doi:10.1186/1475-2867-10-21.

13. Chen F., Zhang G., Iwamoto Y., See W. A. BCG directly induces cell cycle arrest in human transitional carcinoma cell lines as a consequence of integrin cross-linking. *BMC Urology,* 5 (2005) 8, doi:10.1186/1471-2490-5-8.

14. See W. A., Zhang G., Chen F., Cao Y. p21 Expression by human urothelial carcinoma cells modulates the phenotypic response to BCG. *Urologic Oncology: Seminars and Original Investigations,* 28 (2010) 526–533, doi:10.1016/j.urolonc.2008.12.023.

15. Luo Y., Chen X., O'Donnell M. A. *Mycobacterium bovis* bacillus Calmette–Guérin (BCG) induces human CC- and CXC-chemokines in vitro and in vivo. *Clinical and Experimental Immunology,* 147 (2007) 370–378, doi:10.1111/j.1365-2249.2006.03288.x.

16. Ratliff T. L., Ritchey J. K., Yuan J. J., Andriole G. L., Catalona W. J. T-cell subsets required for intravesical BCG immunotherapy for bladder cancer. *Journal of Urology,* 150 (1993) 1018–1023. http://europepmc.org/abstract/med/8102183 (accessed August 5, 2015).

17. Luo Y., Askeland E. J., Newton M. R., Henning J. R., O'Donnell M. A. Immunotherapy of Urinary bladder carcinoma: BCG and beyond, Prof. Letícia Rangel (ed.), *Cancer Treatment: Conventional and Innovative Approaches,* InTech (2013) doi:10.5772/55283.

18. Kawai K., Miyazaki J., Joraku A., Nishiyama H., Akaza H. Bacillus Calmette–Guérin (BCG) immunotherapy for bladder cancer: Current understanding and perspectives on engineered BCG vaccine. *Cancer Science,* 104 (2013) 22–27, doi:10.1111/cas.12075.

19. Ho P. L., Williams S. B., Kamat A. M. Immune therapies in non-muscle invasive bladder cancer. *Current Treatment Options in Oncology,* 16 (2015), doi:10.1007/s11864-014-0315-3.

20. Seow S. W., Cai S., Rahmat J. N., Bay B. H., Lee Y. K., Chan Y. H., *et al. Lactobacillus rhamnosus* GG induces tumor regression in mice bearing orthotopic bladder tumors, *Cancer Science,* 101 (2010) 751–758, doi:10.1111/j.1349-7006.2009.01426.x.

21. Alexandroff A. B., Jackson A. M., O'Donnell M. A., James K. Review BCG immunotherapy of bladder cancer: 20 years on. *Lancet,* 353 (1999) 1689–1694.

22. Solsona E., Madero R., Chantada V., Fernández J. M., Zabala J. A., Portillo J. A., *et al.* Sequential combination of mitomycin C plus bacillus Calmette–Guérin (BCG) is more effective but more toxic than BCG alone in patients with non–muscle-invasive bladder cancer in intermediate- and high-risk patients: Final outcome of CUETO 93009, a randomized prospective trial. *European Urology,* 67 (2015) 508–516, doi:10.1016/j.eururo.2014.09.026.

23. Di Stasi S. M., Giannantoni A., Giurioli A., Valenti M., Zampa G., Storti L., *et al.* Sequential BCG and electromotive mitomycin versus BCG alone for high-risk superficial bladder cancer: A randomised controlled trial. *Lancet Oncology,* 7 (2006) 43–51, doi:10.1016/S1470-2045(05)70472-1.

24. Askeland E. J., Newton M. R., O'Donnell M. A., Luo Y. Bladder cancer immunotherapy: BCG and beyond. *Advances in Urology,* 2012 (2012), doi:10.1155/2012/181987.

25. Takeuchi A., Eto M., Tatsugami K., Shiota M., Yamada H., Kamiryo Y., *et al.* Antitumor activity of recombinant Bacille Calmette–Guérin secreting interleukin-15-Ag85B fusion protein against bladder cancer. *International Immunopharmacology,* 35 (2016) 327–331, doi:10.1016/j.intimp.2016.03.007.

26. Haley J. L., Young D. G., Alexandroff A., James K., Jackson A. M. Enhancing the immunotherapeutic potential of mycobacteria by transfection with tumour necrosis factor-alpha. *Immunology,* 96 (1999) 114–121. http://www.ncbi.nlm.nih.gov/pubmed/10233685 (accessed December 12, 2016).

27. Luo Y., Chen X., O'Donnell M. A. Role of Th1 and Th2 cytokines in BCG-induced IFN-γ production: Cytokine promotion and simulation of BCG effect. *Cytokine,* 21 (2003) 17–26, doi:10.1016/S1043-4666(02)00490-8.

28. DeHaven J. I., Traynellis C., Riggs D. R., Ting E., Lamm D. L. Antibiotic and steroid therapy of massive systemic bacillus Calmette–Guérin toxicity. *Journal of Urology,* 147 (1992) 738–742. http://www.ncbi.nlm.nih.gov/pubmed/1538474 (accessed December 12, 2016).

29. Alexandroff A. B. Nicholson S., Patel P. M., Jackson A. M., Recent advances in bacillus Calmette–Guérin immunotherapy in bladder cancer. *Immunotherapy,* 2 (2010) 551–560, doi:10.2217/imt.10.32.

30. Gandhi N. M., Morales A., Lamm D. L. Bacillus Calmette–Guérin immunotherapy for genitourinary cancer. *BJU International,* 112 (2013) 288–297.

31. van Lingen A. V., Witjes J. A. Current intravesical therapy for non-muscle invasive bladder cancer. *Expert Opinion on Biological Therapy,* 13 (2013) 1371–1385, doi:10.1517/14712598.2013.824421.
32. Kamat A. M., Flaig T. W., Grossman H. B., Konety B., Lamm D. L., O'Donnell M. A., *et al.* Expert consensus document: Consensus statement on best practice management regarding the use of intravesical immunotherapy with BCG for bladder cancer. *Nature Reviews Urology,* 12 (2015) 1–11, doi:10.1038/nrurol.2015.58.
33. Um S.-J., Lee S.-K., Yang D.-K. Hypersensitivity pneumonitis following intravesical bacille Calmette–Guérin immunotherapy for superficial bladder cancer. *Journal of Investigational Allergology & Clinical Immunology* 19 (2009) 230–232. http://www.ncbi.nlm.nih.gov/pubmed/19610267 (accessed December 13, 2016).
34. Brausi M., Oddens J. R., Sylvester R. J., Bono A., Van De Beek C., Van Andel G., *et al.* Side effects of bacillus Calmette–Guérin (BCG) in the treatment of intermediate- and high-risk Ta, T1 papillary carcinoma of the bladder: Results of the EORTC genito-urinary cancers group randomised phase 3 study comparing one-third dose with full dose an. *European Urology,* 65 (2014) 69–76, doi:10.1016/j.eururo.2013.07.021.
35. Palou J. Factors related to side effects of intravesical bacillus Calmette–Guérin: Dose, maintenance treatment, and physicians? *European Urology,* 65 (2014) 77–78, doi:10.1016/j.eururo.2013.08.024.
36. Carrasco Hernández L., Castaño Núñez Á. L., Rodríguez Portal J. A. Hypersensitivity pneumonitis as a complication of intravesical BCG therapy for bladder cancer. *Archivos De Bronconeumologia* (English Ed.), 52 (2016) 445–446, doi:10.1016/j.arbr.2016.06.016.
37. Gonzalez O. Y., Musher D. M., Brar I., Furgeson S., Boktour M. R., Septimus E. J., *et al.* Spectrum of bacille Calmette–Guérin (BCG) infection after intravesical BCG immunotherapy. *Clinical Infectious Diseases,* 36 (2003) 140–148, doi:10.1086/344908.
38. Aljada I. S., Crane J. K., Corriere N., Wagle D. G., Amsterdam D. *Mycobacterium bovis* BCG causing vertebral osteomyelitis (Pott's disease) following intravesical BCG therapy. *Journal of Clinical Microbiology,* 37 (1999) 2106–2108. http://www.ncbi.nlm.nih.gov/pubmed/10325395 (accessed December 12, 2016).
39. Fouka E., Angelis N., Stefanopoulou P., Galanis N. BCG pneumonitis with a miliary radiological pattern complicating intravesical BCG immunotherapy. *Pneumonia,* 23 (2010) 384–387.

40. Álvarez-Múgica M., Gómez J. M. F., Vázquez V. B., Monzón A. J., Rodríguez J. M. F., Robles L. R., *et al.* Pancreatic and psoas abscesses as a late complication of intravesical administration of bacillus Calmette–Guérin for bladder cancer: a case report and review of the literature. *Journal of Medical Case Reports,* 3 (2009) 7323, doi:10.4076/1752-1947-3-7323.

41. Dammert P., Boujaoude Z., Rafferty W., Kass J. Fever of unknown origin and pancytopenia caused by culture-proven delayed onset disseminated bacillus Calmette–Guérin (BCG) infection after intravesical instillation. *Case Reports* 2013, bcr2013008949-bcr2013008949, doi:10.1136/bcr-2013-008949.

42. Fradet V., Gaudreau C., Perrotte P., Côté J., Paquin J.-M. Management of hepatic granulomatous tuberculosis complicating intravesical BCG for superficial bladder cancer. *Canadian Urological Association Journal,* 1 (2007) 269–272. http://www.ncbi.nlm.nih.gov/pubmed/18542802 (accessed December 12, 2016).

43. Gerbrandy S. J. F., Schreuders L. C., de Smet M. D. *Mycobacterium bovis* endophthalmitis from BCG immunotherapy for bladder cancer. *Ocular Immunology and Inflammation,* 16 (2008) 95–97, doi:10.1080/09273940802056273.

44. Golub V., Malhotra P., Patel S. Mycobacterial brain tuberculomas due to Bacille Calmette–Guérin intravesical chemotherapy for bladder cancer: A case report and literature review. *Canadian Journal of Infectious Diseases and Medical Microbiology,* 22 (2011) 104–106. http://www.ncbi.nlm.nih.gov/pubmed/22942888 (accessed December 12, 2016).

45. Gomez E., Chiang T., Louie T., Ponnapalli M., Eng R., Huang D. B. Prosthetic joint infection due to *Mycobacterium bovis* after intravesical instillation of bacillus Calmette–Guérin (BCG). *International Journal of Microbiology,* 2009 (2009) 527208, doi:10.1155/2009/527208.

46. Hakim S., Heaney J. A., Heinz T., Zwolak R. W. Psoas abscess following intravesical bacillus Calmette–Guérin for bladder cancer: A case report. *Journal of Urology,* 150 (1993) 188–189. http://www.ncbi.nlm.nih.gov/pubmed/8510250 (accessed December 12, 2016).

47. Nadasy K. A., Patel R. S., Emmett M., Murillo R. A., Tribble M. A., Black R. D., *et al.* Four cases of disseminated *Mycobacterium bovis* infection following intravesical BCG instillation for treatment of bladder carcinoma. *Southern Medical Journal,* 101 (2008) 91–95, doi:10.1097/SMJ.0b013e31815d4047.

48. Soylu A., Ince A. T., Polat H., Yasar N., Ciltas A., Ozkara S., *et al.* Peritoneal tuberculosis and granulomatous hepatitis secondary to treatment of bladder cancer with bacillus Calmette–Guérin. *Annals of Clinical Microbiology and Antimicrobials,* 8 (2009) 12, doi:10.1186/1476-0711-8-12.

49. Viallard J., Denis D., Texier-Maugein J., Parrens M., Faure I., Pellegrin J., *et al.* Disseminated infection after Bacille Calmette-Guérin instillation for treatment of bladder carcinoma. *Clinical Infectious Diseases,* 29 (1999) 451–452, doi:10.1086/520238.

50. Wolf Y. G., Wolf D. G., Higginbottom P. A., Dilley R. B. Infection of a ruptured aortic aneurysm and an aortic graft with Bacille Calmette–Guérin after intravesical administration for bladder cancer. *Journal of Vascular Surgery,* 22 (1995) 80–84. http://www.ncbi.nlm.nih.gov/pubmed/7602717 (accessed Decesmber 12, 2016).

51. Pommier J. D., Ben Lasfar N., Van Grunderbeeck N., Burdet C., Benchikh A., Nguyen S., *et al.* Complications following intravesical bacillus Calmette–Guérin treatment for bladder cancer: A case series of 22 patients. *Infectious Diseases* (Auckl), (2015) 1–7, doi:10.3109/23744235.2015.1055794.

52. Bowyer L., Hall R. R., Reading J., Marsh M. M. The persistence of Bacille Calmette–Guérin in the bladder after intravesical treatment for bladder cancer. *British Journal of Urology,* 75 (1995) 188–192, doi:10.1111/j.1464-410X.1995.tb07309.x.

53. Alvarez-Múgica M., Fernández J., Bulnes V., Jalón A., García J., Fernández J. M., *et al.* Fatal outcome due to sepsis by *Mycobacterium bovis* six years after BCG intravesical instillations. *Journal of Medical Cases,* 1 (2010) 81–83, doi:10.4021/jmc42w.

54. Lin I. Y. C., Van T. T. H., Smooker P. M. Live-attenuated bacterial vectors: Tools for vaccine and therapeutic agent delivery. *Vaccines,* 3 (2015) 940–972, doi:10.3390/vaccines3040940.

55. Lee C. H., Wu C. L., Shiau A. L. Endostatin gene therapy delivered by *Salmonella choleraesuis* in murine tumor models. *Journal of Gene Medicine,* 6 (2004) 1382–1393, doi:10.1002/jgm.626.

56. Domingos-Pereira S., Hojeij R., Reggi E., Derre L., Chevalier M. F., Romero P., *et al.* Local Salmonella immunostimulation recruits vaccine-specific CD8 T cells and increases regression of bladder tumor. *Oncoimmunology,* 4 (2015) e1016697, doi:http://dx.doi.org/10.1080/2162402X.2015.1016697.

57. Cummins C. S., Johnson J. L. *Corynebacterium parvum*: A Synonym for *Propionibacterium acnes*? *Journal of General Microbiology* (I974), 80 (1973) 433–442, doi:10.1099/00221287-80-2-433.

58. Kirschbau J. O., Kliman A. M. The pathogenic role of *Corynebacterium acnes* in acne vulgaris. *Archives of Dermatology*, 88 (1963) 832–833. http://www.ncbi.nlm.nih.gov/pubmed/14071457 (accessed November 22, 2016).

59. Neveu T., Branellec A., Biozzi G. Adjuvant properties of Corynebacterium parvum on antibody production and on the induction of delayed hypersensitivity toward conjugated proteins. *Annales de l'Institut Pasteur (Paris)*, 106 (1964) 771–777. http://www.ncbi.nlm.nih.gov/pubmed/14145260 (accessed November 22, 2016).

60. Halpern B. N., Brozzi G., Stiffel C., Mouton D., Biozzi G. Inhibition of tumour growth by administration of killed *Corynebacterium parvum*. *Nature*, 212 (1966) 853–854, doi:10.1038/212853a0.

61. deKernion J. B., Ramming K. P., Fraser K. A bladder tumor model response to immunotherapy. *National Cancer Institute Monograph*, (1978) 333. http://www.ncbi.nlm.nih.gov/pubmed/748789 (accessed November 21, 2016).

62. Purves E. C., Snell M., Cope W. A., Addison I. E., Copland R. F. P., Berenbaum M. C. Subcutaneous *Corynebacterium parvum* in bladder cancer: A controlled study of its immunological effects. *British Journal of Urology* 51 (1979) 278–282, doi:10.1111/j.1464-410X.1979.tb04709.x.

63. Lau B. H., Woolley J. L., Marsh C. L., Barker G. R., Koobs D. H., Torrey R. R. Superiority of intralesional immunotherapy with *Corynebacterium parvum* and *Allium sativum* in control of murine transitional cell carcinoma. *Journal of Urology*, 136 (1986) 701–705. http://www.ncbi.nlm.nih.gov/pubmed/3735559 (accessed November 21, 2016).

64. Woolley J. L., Lau B. H., Ruckle H. C., Torrey R. R. Phagocytic and natural killer cytotoxic responses of murine transitional cell carcinoma to postsurgical immunochemotherapy. *Journal of Urology* 140 (1988) 660–663. http://www.ncbi.nlm.nih.gov/pubmed/3411696 (accessed November 21, 2016).

65. Marsh C. L., Torrey R. R., Woolley J. L., Barker G. R., Lau B. H. Superiority of intravesical immunotherapy with *Corynebacterium parvum* and *Allium sativum* in control of murine bladder cancer. *Journal of Urology*, 137 (1987) 359–362. http://www.ncbi.nlm.nih.gov/pubmed/3806842 (accessed November 21, 2016).

66. Raica M., Ioart I., Gurtavenco A. Microscopic changes of the urinary bladder in patients with primary tumors locally treated with *Corynebacterium parvum*. *Morphologie Et Embryologie (Bucur)*, 35 (1989) 275–277. http://www.ncbi.nlm.nih.gov/pubmed/2533966 (accessed November 21, 2016).

67. Raica M. Effects of intravesical *Corynebacterium parvum* on recurrences of superficial tumors of the urinary bladder. *Anti-Cancer Drugs*, 3 (1992) 39–42. http://www.ncbi.nlm.nih.gov/pubmed/1623214 (accessed November 21, 2016).

68. Buhler J., Grignon Y., Gallon F. Breast cancer treated by antibiotherapy? Granulomatous mastitis with *Corynebacterium*. *Journal de Gynécologie Obstétrique et Biologie de la Reproduction* (Paris), 44 (2015) 679–682, doi:10.1016/j.jgyn.2015.01.011.

69. Kara Ö., Zarakolu P., Aşçioğlu S., Etgül S., Uz B., Büyükaşik Y., *et al.* Epidemiology and emerging resistance in bacterial bloodstream infections in patients with hematologic malignancies. *Infectious Diseases (Auckl)*, 47 (2015) 686–693, doi:10.3109/23744235.2015.1051105.

70. Biswal I., Mohapatra S., Deb M., Dawar R., Gaind R. Corynebacterium striatum: An emerging nosocomial pathogen in a case of laryngeal carcinoma. *Indian Journal of Medical Microbiology*, 32 (2014) 323–324, doi:10.4103/0255-0857.136589.

71. Ohashi Y., Nakai S., Tsukamoto T., Masumori N., Akaza H., Miyanaga N., *et al.* Habitual intake of lactic acid bacteria and risk reduction of bladder cancer. *Urologia Internationalis*, 68 (2002) 273–280, doi:10.1159/000058450.

72. Feyisetan O., Tracey C., Hellawell G. O. Probiotics, dendritic cells and bladder cancer. *BJU International*, 109 (2012) 1594–1597, doi:10.1111/j.1464-410X.2011.10749.x.

73. Kandasamy M., Bay B. H., Lee Y. K., Mahendran R. Lactobacilli secreting a tumor antigen and IL15 activates neutrophils and dendritic cells and generates cytotoxic T lymphocytes against cancer cells. *Cellular Immunology* 271 (2011) 89–96, doi:10.1016/j.cellimm.2011.06.004.

74. Cai S., Kandasamy M., Rahmat J. N., Tham S. M., Bay B. H., Lee Y. K., *et al.* *Lactobacillus rhamnosus* GG activation of dendritic cells and neutrophils depends on the dose and time of exposure. *Journal of Immunology Research*, 2016 (2016) 7402760, doi:10.1155/2016/7402760.

75. Seow S. W., Rahmat J. N., Mohamed A. A., Mahendran R., Lee Y. K., Bay B. H. *Lactobacillus* species is more cytotoxic to human bladder cancer cells than *Mycobacterium bovis* (bacillus Calmette–Guérin). *Journal of Urology*, 168 (2002) 2236–2239. http://www.ncbi.nlm.nih.gov/entrez/query.fcgi?cmd=Retrieve&db=PubMed&dopt=Citation&list_uids=12394766.

76. Seow S. W., Rahmat J. N., Bay B. H., Lee Y. K., Mahendran R. Expression of chemokine/cytokine genes and immune cell recruitment following the instillation of *Mycobacterium bovis*, bacillus Calmette-Guerin or *Lactobacillus rhamnosus* strain GG in the healthy murine bladder. *Immunology*, 124 (2008) 419–427, doi:10.1111/j.1365-2567.2007.02792.x.

77. Zaharoff D. A., Hoffman B. S., Hooper H. B., Benjamin C. J., Khurana K. K., Hance K. W., *et al.* Intravesical immunotherapy of superficial bladder cancer with chitosan/interleukin-12. *Cancer Research*, 69 (2009) 6192–6199, doi:10.1158/0008-5472.CAN-09-1114.

78. Biot C., Rentsch C. A., Gsponer J. R., Birkhäuser F. D., Jusforgues-Saklani H., Lemaître F., *et al.*, Preexisting BCG-specific T cells improve intravesical immunotherapy for bladder cancer. *Science Translational Medicine*, 4 (2012) 137ra72, doi:10.1126/scitranslmed.3003586.

79. Arnold J., de Boer E. C., O'Donnell M. A., Böhle A., Brandau S. Immunotherapy of experimental bladder cancer with recombinant BCG expressing interferon-gamma. *Journal of Immunotherapy*, 27 (2004) 116–123. http://www.ncbi.nlm.nih.gov/pubmed/14770083 (accessed July 4, 2015).

80. Asano M., Karasawa E., Takayama T. Antitumor activity of *Lactobacillus casei* (LC 9018) against experimental mouse bladder tumor (MBT-2). *Journal of Urology*, 136 (1986) 719–721.

81. Lim B.-K., Mahendran R., Lee Y.-K., Bay B.-H. Chemopreventive effect of *Lactobacillus rhamnosus* on growth of a subcutaneously implanted bladder cancer cell line in the mouse. *Japanese Journal of Cancer Research*, 93 (2002) 36–41. http://www.ncbi.nlm.nih.gov/pubmed/11802806 (accessed November 22, 2016).

82. Aso Y., Akazan H. Prophylactic effect of a *Lactobacillus casei* preparation on the recurrence of superficial bladder cancer. BLP Study Group. *Urologia* Internationalis, 49 (1992) 125–129. http://www.ncbi.nlm.nih.gov/pubmed/1466089 (accessed November 22, 2016).

83. Aso Y., Akaza H., Kotake T., Tsukamoto T., Imai K., Naito S. Preventive effect of a *Lactobacillus casei* preparation on the recurrence of superficial bladder cancer in a double-blind trial. The BLP Study Group. *European Urology* 27 (1995) 104–109. http://www.ncbi.nlm.nih.gov/pubmed/7744150 (accessed December 13, 2016).

84. Naito S., Koga H., Yamaguchi A., Fujimoto N., Hasui Y., Kuramoto H., *et al.* Prevention of recurrence with epirubicin and *Lactobacillus casei* after transurethral resection of bladder cancer. *Journal of Urology* 179 (2008) 485–490, doi:10.1016/j.juro.2007.09.031.

85. Yin X., Yu B., Tang Z., He B., Ren J., Xiao X., *et al. Bifidobacterium infantis*-mediated HSV-TK/GCV suicide gene therapy induces both extrinsic and intrinsic apoptosis in a rat model of bladder cancer. *Cancer Gene Therapy*, 20 (2013) 77–81, doi:10.1038/cgt.2012.86.

86. Reis L., Castilho M., Mobilon C., da Silveira W., Azevedo V., Fávaro W. *Lactococcus lactis* secreting attenuated recombinant staphylococcal enterotoxin B (RSEB) exceeds bacillus Calmette–Guérin (BCG) in the treatment of non-muscle invasive bladder cancer (NMIBC), *Journal of Urology*, 189 (2013) e217–e218, doi:10.1016/j.juro.2013.02.1925.

87. Lamm D. L., Reichert D. F., Harris S. C., Lucio R. M. Immunotherapy of murine transitional cell carcinoma. *Journal of Urology*, 128 (1982) 1104–1108. http://www.ncbi.nlm.nih.gov/pubmed/6757465 (accessed November 29, 2016).

88. Lee K., Ewing J. F., Sluss P. M. Effect of bacterial lipopolysaccharide on growth of murine bladder cancer, MBT-2. *Urological Research*, 17 (1989) 285–288. http://www.ncbi.nlm.nih.gov/pubmed/2510388 (accessed November 25, 2016).

89. Shih K.-S., Lin C.-C., Hung H.-F., Yang Y.-C., Wang C.-A., Jeng K.-C., *et al.* One-step chromatographic purification of *Helicobacter pylori* neutrophil-activating protein expressed in *Bacillus subtilis*. *PLOS One*, 8 (2013) e60786, doi:10.1371/journal.pone.0060786.

90. Codolo G., Fassan M., Munari F., Volpe A., Bassi P., Rugge M., *et al.* HP-NAP inhibits the growth of bladder cancer in mice by activating a cytotoxic Th1 response. *Cancer Immunology, Immunotherapy*, 61 (2012) 31–40, doi:10.1007/s00262-011-1087-2.

91. Codolo G., Munari F., Fassan M., de Bernard M. Evaluation of the efficacy of the *H. pylori* protein HP-NAP as a therapeutic tool for treatment of bladder cancer in an orthotopic murine model. *Journal of Visualized Experiments* (2015) e52743, doi:10.3791/52743.

92. Perabo F. G. E., Willert P. L., Wirger A., Schmidt D. H., Von Ruecker A., Mueller S. C. Superantigen-activated mononuclear cells induce apoptosis in transitional cell carcinoma. *Anticancer Research,* 25 (2005)3565–3573.http://www.ncbi.nlm.nih.gov/pubmed/16101181 (accessed November 21, 2016).

93. Reis L. O., Ferreira U., Billis A., Cagnon V. H. a, Fávaro W. J. Anti-angiogenic effects of the superantigen staphylococcal enterotoxin B and bacillus Calmette–Guérin immunotherapy for nonmuscle invasive bladder cancer. *Journal of Urology,* 187 (2012) 438–445, doi:10.1016/j.juro.2011.10.022.

94. Han C., Hao L., Chen M., Hu J., Shi Z., Zhang Z., *et al.* Target expression of staphylococcus enterotoxin A from an oncolytic adenovirus suppresses mouse bladder tumor growth and recruits CD3+ T cell. *Tumor Biology,* 34 (2013) 2863–2869, doi:10.1007/s13277-013-0847-3.

95. Gabig T. G., Waltzer W. C., Whyard T., Romanov V. *Clostridium perfringens* enterotoxin as a potential drug for intravesical treatment of bladder cancer. *Biochemical and Biophysical Research Communications,* 478 (2016) 887–892, doi:10.1016/j.bbrc.2016.08.046.

96. Heimbrook D. C., Stirdivant S. M., Ahern J. D., Balishin N. L., Patrick D. R., Edwards G. M., *et al.* Transforming growth factor alpha-Pseudomonas exotoxin fusion protein prolongs survival of nude mice bearing tumor xenografts. *Proceedings of the National Academy of Sciences of the United States of America,* 87 (1990) 4697–4701. http://www.ncbi.nlm.nih.gov/pubmed/2352944 (accessed November 29, 2016).

97. Goldberg M. R., Heimbrook D. C., Russo P., Sarosdy M. F., Greenberg R. E., Giantonio B. J., *et al.* Phase I clinical study of the recombinant oncotoxin TP40 in superficial bladder cancer. *Clinical Cancer Research,* 1 (1995) 57–61. http://www.ncbi.nlm.nih.gov/entrez/query.fcgi?cmd=Retrieve&db=PubMed&dopt=Citation&list_uids=9815887.

98. Keppler-Hafkemeyer A., Brinkmann U., Pastan I. Role of Caspases in immunotoxin-induced apoptosis of cancer cells. *Biochemistry,* 37 (1998) 16934–16942, doi:10.1021/bi980995m.

99. Kowalski M., Entwistle J., Cizeau J., Niforos D., Loewen S., Chapman W., *et al.* A phase i study of an intravesically administered immunotoxin targeting EpCAM for the treatment of nonmuscle-invasive bladder cancer in BCG-refractory and BCG-intolerant patients. *Drug Design, Development and Therapy,* 4 (2010) 313–320, doi:10.2147/DDDT.S14071.

100. Kowalski M., Guindon J., Brazas L., Moore C., Entwistle J., Cizeau J., *et al.* A phase II study of oportuzumab monatox: An immunotoxin therapy for patients with noninvasive urothelial carcinoma in situ previously Treated with Bacillus Calmette–Guérin. *Journal of Urology,* 188 (2012) 1712–1718, doi:10.1016/j.juro.2012.07.020.

101. Sakano S., Shimabukuro T., Ohmoto Y., Naito K. Cytokine-mediated antitumor effect of OK-432 on urinary bladder tumor cells in vitro. *Urological Research,* 25 (1997) 239–245. http://www.ncbi.nlm.nih.gov/pubmed/9286031 (accessed December 13, 2016).

102. Y.-Tian F., Tang K., Guan W., Yang T., Xu H., Zhuang Q.-Y., *et al.* OK-432 Suppresses proliferation and metastasis by tumor associated macrophages in bladder cancer. *Asian Pacific Journal of Cancer Prevention,* 16 (2015) 4537–4542. http://www.ncbi.nlm.nih.gov/pubmed/26107200 (accessed November 30, 2016).

103. Pfyffer G. E. Chapter 28: *Mycobacterium*: General characteristics, laboratory detection, and staining procedures, *Manual of Clinical Microbiology,* 11th Ed., American Society of Microbiology, (2015) pp. 536–569, doi:10.1128/9781555817381.ch30.

104. Tortoli E. Microbiological features and clinical relevance of new species of the genus *Mycobacterium. Clinical Microbiology Reviews,* 27 (2014) 727–752, doi:10.1128/CMR.00035-14.

105. Hoefsloot W., van Ingen J., Andrejak C., Ängeby K., Bauriaud R., Bemer P., *et al.* The geographic diversity of nontuberculous mycobacteria isolated from pulmonary samples: An NTM-NET collaborative study. *European Respiratory Journal,* 42 (2013) 1604–1613, doi:10.1183/09031936.00149212.

106. van der Werf M. J., Ködmön C., Katalinić-Janković V., Kummik T., Soini H., Richter E., *et al.* Inventory study of non-tuberculous mycobacteria in the European Union. *BMC Infectious Diseases,* 14 (2014) 62, doi:10.1186/1471-2334-14-62.

107. Griffith D. E., Aksamit T., Brown-Elliott B. A., Catanzaro A., Daley C., Gordin F., *et al.* An official ATS/IDSA statement: Diagnosis, treatment, and prevention of nontuberculous mycobacterial diseases. *American Journal of Respiratory and Critical Care Medicine* 175 (2007) 367–416, doi:10.1164/rccm.200604-571ST.

108. Johnson M. M., Odell J. A. Nontuberculous mycobacterial pulmonary infections. *Journal of Thoracic Disease,* 6 (2014) 210–220, doi:10.3978/j.issn.2072-1439.2013.12.24.

109. van Ingen J. Diagnosis of nontuberculous mycobacterial infections. *Seminars in Respiratory and Critical Care Medicine,* 34 (2013) 103–109, doi:10.1055/s-0033-1333569.

110. Daffé M. Chapter 1: The global architecture of the mycobacterial cell envelope, in: *The Mycobacterial Cell Envelope, American Society of Microbiology*, (2008) 3–11, doi:10.1128/9781555815783.ch1.

111. Secanella-Fandos S., Luquin M., Julián E. Connaught and Russian strains showed the highest direct antitumor effects of different bacillus Calmette–Guérin substrains. *Journal of Urology,* 189 (2013) 711–718, doi:10.1016/j.juro.2012.09.049.

112. Julián E., Roldán M., Sánchez-Chardi A., Astola O., Agustí G., Luquin M. Microscopic cords, a virulence-related characteristic of *Mycobacterium tuberculosis*, are also present in nonpathogenic mycobacteria. *Journal of Bacteriology*, 192 (2010) 1751–1760.

113. Krieg A. M. CpG motifs in bacterial DNA and their immune effects. *Annual Review of Immunology*, 20 (2002) 709–760, doi:10.1146/annurev.immunol.20.100301.064842.

114. Ishikawa E., Ishikawa T., Morita Y. S., Toyonaga K., Yamada H., Takeuchi O., *et al.* Direct recognition of the mycobacterial glycolipid, trehalose dimycolate, by C-type lectin Mincle. *Journal of Experimental Medicine,* 206 (2009) 2879–2888, doi:10.1084/jem.20091750.

115. Feinberg H., Rambaruth N. D. S., Jégouzo S. A. F., Jacobsen K. M., Djurhuus R., Poulsen T. B., *et al.* Binding sites for acylated trehalose analogs of glycolipid ligands on an extended carbohydrate recognition domain of the macrophage receptor Mincle. *Journal of Biological Chemistry*, 291 (2016) 21222–21233, doi:10.1074/jbc.M116.749515.

116. Jung S.-B., Yang C.-S., Lee J.-S., Shin A.-R., Jung S.-S., Son J. W., *et al.* The mycobacterial 38-kilodalton glycolipoprotein antigen activates the mitogen-activated protein kinase pathway and release of proinflammatory cytokines through toll-like receptors 2 and 4 in human monocytes. *Infection and Immunity*, 74 (2006) 2686–2696, doi:10.1128/IAI.74.5.2686-2696.2006.

117. Kadival G. V, Chaparas S. D., Hussong D. Characterization of serologic and cell-mediated reactivity of a 38-kDa antigen isolated from *Mycobacterium tuberculosis*. *Journal of Immunology*, 139 (1987) 2447–2451. http://www.ncbi.nlm.nih.gov/pubmed/2443566 (accessed December 14, 2016).

118. Harboe M., Wiker H. G. The 38-kDa protein of *Mycobacterium tuberculosis*: A review. *Journal of Infectious Diseases,* 166 (1992) 874–884. http://www.ncbi.nlm.nih.gov/pubmed/1527425 (accessed December 14, 2016).

119. Court N., Rose S., Bourigault M.-L., Front S., Martin O. R., Dowling J. K., *et al.* Mycobacterial PIMs inhibit host inflammatory responses through CD14-dependent and CD14-independent mechanisms. *PLOS One*, 6 (2011) e24631, doi:10.1371/journal.pone.0024631.

120. Chatterjee D., Khoo K. H. Mycobacterial lipoarabinomannan: An extraordinary lipoheteroglycan with profound physiological effects. *Glycobiology*, 8 (1998) 113–120, doi:10.1093/glycob/8.2.113.

121. Brennan P. J. Structure, function, and biogenesis of the cell wall of *Mycobacterium tuberculosis*. *Tuberculosis*, 83 (2003) 91–97, doi:10.1016/S1472-9792(02)00089-6.

122. Daffé M., Crick D. C., Jackson M. Genetics of capsular polysaccharides and cell envelope (Glyco) lipids. *Microbiology Spectrum*, 2 (2014) MGM2-0021-2013, doi:10.1128/microbiolspec.MGM2-0021-2013.f1.

123. Okamoto M., Sato M. Toll-like receptor signaling in anti-cancer immunity. *Journal of Medical Investigation*, 50 (2003) 9–24. http://www.ncbi.nlm.nih.gov/pubmed/12630564 (accessed December 13, 2016).

124. Higuchi T., Shimizu M., Owaki A., Takahashi M., Shinya E., Nishimura T., *et al.* A possible mechanism of intravesical BCG therapy for human bladder carcinoma: Involvement of innate effector cells for the inhibition of tumor growth. *Cancer Immunology, Immunotherapy*, 58 (2009) 1245–1255, doi:10.1007/s00262-008-0643-x.

125. LaRue H., Ayari C., Bergeron A., Fradet Y. Toll-like receptors in urothelial cells—targets for cancer immunotherapy. *Nature Reviews Urology*, 10 (2013) 537–545, doi:10.1038/nrurol.2013.153.

126. Kresowik T. P., Griffith T. S. Bacillus Calmette–Guérin immunotherapy for urothelial carcinoma of the bladder. *Immunotherapy*, 1 (2009) 281–288, doi:10.2217/1750743X.1.2.281.

127. Nigou J., Zelle-Rieser C., Gilleron M., Thurnher M., Puzo G. Mannosylated lipoarabinomannans inhibit IL-12 production by human dendritic cells: Evidence for a negative signal delivered through the mannose receptor. *Journal of Immunology*, 166 (2001) 7477–7485. http://www.ncbi.nlm.nih.gov/pubmed/11390501 (accessed December 13, 2016).

128. Nigou J., Gilleron M., Rojas M., García L. F., Thurnher M., Puzo G. Mycobacterial lipoarabinomannans: Modulators of dendritic cell function and the apoptotic response. *Microbes and Infection*, 4 (2002) 945–953. http://www.ncbi.nlm.nih.gov/pubmed/12106787 (accessed December 13, 2016).

129. Quesniaux V. J., Nicolle D. M., Torres D., Kremer L., Guérardel Y., Nigou J., *et al.* Toll-like receptor 2 (TLR2)-dependent-positive and TLR2-independent-negative regulation of proinflammatory cytokines by mycobacterial lipomannans. *Journal of Immunology*, 172 (2004) 4425–4434. http://www.ncbi.nlm.nih.gov/pubmed/15034058 (accessed December 13, 2016).

130. Torrelles J. B., Schlesinger L. S. Diversity in *Mycobacterium tuberculosis* mannosylated cell wall determinants impacts adaptation to the host. *Tuberculosis*, 90 (2010) 84–93, doi:10.1016/j.tube.2010.02.003.

131. Briken V., Porcelli S. A., Besra G. S., Kremer L. Mycobacterial lipoarabinomannan and related lipoglycans: From biogenesis to modulation of the immune response. *Molecular Microbiology*, 53 (2004) 391–403, doi:10.1111/j.1365-2958.2004.04183.x.

132. Hayashi D., Takii T., Fujiwara N., Fujita Y., Yano I., Yamamoto S., *et al.* Comparable studies of immunostimulating activities in vitro among *Mycobacterium b* bacillus Calmette–Guérin (BCG) substrains. *FEMS Immunology and Medical Microbiology*, 56 (2009) 116–128, doi:10.1111/j.1574-695X.2009.00559.x.

133. Dao D. N., Sweeney K., Hsu T., Gurcha S. S., Nascimento I. P., Roshevsky D., *et al.* Mycolic acid modification by the mmaA4 gene of M. tuberculosis modulates IL-12 production. *PLOS Pathogens*, 4 (2008) e1000081, doi:10.1371/journal.ppat.1000081.

134. Tran V., Ahn S. K., Ng M., Li M., Liu J. Loss of lipid virulence factors reduces the efficacy of the BCG vaccine. *Scientific Reports*, 6 (2016) 29076, doi:10.1038/srep29076.

135. Chen J. M., Islam S. T., Ren H., Liu J. Differential productions of lipid virulence factors among BCG vaccine strains and implications on BCG safety. *Vaccine*, 25 (2007) 8114–8122, doi:10.1016/j.vaccine.2007.09.041.

136. Kumar P., Tyagi R., Das G., Bhaskar S. *Mycobacterium indicus pranii* and *Mycobacterium bovis* BCG lead to differential macrophage activation in Toll-like receptor-dependent manner. *Immunology*, 143 (2014) 258–268, doi:10.1111/imm.12306.

137. Brambilla C., Llorens-Fons M., Julián E., Noguera-Ortega E., Tomàs-Martínez C., Pérez-Trujillo M., *et al.* Mycobacteria clumping increase their capacity to damage macrophages. *Frontiers in Microbiology*, 7 (2016) 1562, doi:10.3389/fmicb.2016.01562.

138. Mahairas G. G., Sabo P. J., Hickey M. J., Singh D. C., Stover C. K. Molecular analysis of genetic differences between *Mycobacterium bovis* BCG and virulent *M. bovis*. *Journal of Bacteriology*, 178 (1996) 1274–

1282. http://www.ncbi.nlm.nih.gov/pubmed/8631702 (accessed December 13, 2016).

139. Yu D. S., Lee C. F., Chang S. Y. Immunotherapy for orthotopic murine bladder cancer using bacillus Calmette–Guérin recombinant protein Mpt-64. *Journal of Urology*, 177 (2007) 738–742, doi:10.1016/j.juro.2006.09.074.

140. Sänger C., Busche A., Bentien G., Spallek R., Jonas F., Böhle A., *et al.* Immunodominant PstS1 antigen of *Mycobacterium tuberculosis* is a potent biological response modifier for the treatment of bladder cancer. *BMC Cancer*, 4 (2004) 86, doi:10.1186/1471-2407-4-86.

141. Tokunaga T., Yamamoto H., Shimada S., Abe H., Fukuda T., Fujisawa Y., *et al.* Antitumor activity of deoxyribonucleic acid fraction from *Mycobacterium bovis* BCG. Isolation I., physicochemical characterization, and antitumor activity. *Journal of the National Cancer Institute*, 72 (1984) 955–962. http://eutils.ncbi.nlm.nih.gov/entrez/eutils/elink.fcgi?dbfrom=pubmed&id=6200641&retmode=ref&cmd=prlinks\npapers2://publication/uuid/276FC7B9-EBD8-4C73-97FD-84B511F7A9F8.

142. Shimada S., Yano O., Tokunaga T. In vivo augmentation of natural killer cell activity with a deoxyribonucleic acid fraction of BCG. *Japanese Journal of Cancer Research*, 77 (1986) 808–816. http://www.ncbi.nlm.nih.gov/pubmed/2428798 (accessed November 29, 2016).

143. Shimada S., Yano O., Inoue H., Kuramoto E., Fukuda T., Yamamoto H., *et al.* Antitumor activity of the DNA fraction from *Mycobacterium bovis* BCG. II. Effects on various syngeneic mouse tumors. *Journal of the National Cancer Institute*, 74 (1985) 681–688. http://www.ncbi.nlm.nih.gov/pubmed/3856070 (accessed December 13, 2016).

144. Yamamoto S., Yamamoto T., Kataoka T., Kuramoto E., Yano O., Tokunaga T. Unique palindromic sequences in synthetic oligonucleotides are required to induce IFN and augment IFN-mediated natural killer activity. *Journal of Immunology*, 148 (1992) 4072–4076. http://www.ncbi.nlm.nih.gov/pubmed/1376349 (accessed November 29, 2016).

145. Kataoka T., Yamamoto S., Yamamoto T., Kuramoto E., Kimura Y., Yano O., *et al.* Antitumor activity of synthetic oligonucleotides with sequences from cDNA encoding proteins of *Mycobacterium bovis* BCG. *Japanese Journal of Cancer Research*, 83 (1992) 244–247. http://www.ncbi.nlm.nih.gov/pubmed/1582885 (accessed November 29, 2016).

146. Atkins H., Davies B. R., Kirby J. A., Kelly J. D. Polarisation of a T-helper cell immune response by activation of dendritic cells with CpG-

containing oligonucleotides: A potential therapeutic regime for bladder cancer immunotherapy. *British Journal of Cancer*, 89 (2003) 2312–2319, doi:10.1038/sj.bjc.6601474.

147. Hegele A., Dalpke A., Barth P., Varga Z., Heeg K., Hofmann R., *et al.* Antineoplastic effect of immunostimulatory DNA (CpG-ODN) in a murine C57-BL6/MB-49 transitional cell carcinoma model. *Anticancer Research*, 24 (2004) 2225–2230. http://www.ncbi.nlm.nih.gov/pubmed/15330165 (accessed November 30, 2016).

148. Ninalga C., Loskog A., Klevenfeldt M., Essand M., Totterman T. H. CpG oligonucleotide therapy cures subcutaneous and orthotopic tumors and evokes protective immunity in murine bladder cancer. *Journal of Immunotherapy*, 28 (2005) 20–27, doi:00002371-200501000-00003 [pii].

149. Mangsbo S. M., Ninalga C., Essand M., Loskog A., Tötterman T. H. CpG therapy is superior to BCG in an orthotopic bladder cancer model and generates CD4+ T-cell immunity *Journal of Immunotherapy*, 31 (2008) 34–42, doi:10.1097/CJI.0b013e3181587d29.

150. Mangsbo S. M., Sandin L. C., Anger K., Korman A. J., Loskog A., Tötterman T. H. Enhanced tumor eradication by combining CTLA-4 or PD-1 blockade with CpG therapy. *Journal of Immunotherapy*, 33 (2010) 225–235, doi:10.1097/CJI.0b013e3181c01fcb.

151. Filion M. C., Filion B., Reader S., Menard S., Phillips N. C. Modulation of interleukin-12 synthesis by DNA lacking the CpG motif and present in a mycobacterial cell wall complex. *Cancer Immunology, Immunotherapy*, 49 (2000) 325–334. http://www.ncbi.nlm.nih.gov/pubmed/10946815 (accessed November 30, 2016).

152. Filion M. C., Lépicier P., Morales A., Phillips N. C. *Mycobacterium phlei* cell wall complex directly induces apoptosis in human bladder cancer cells. *British Journal of Cancer*, 79 (1999) 229–235, doi:10.1038/sj.bjc.6690038.

153. Filion M. C., Phillips N. C. Therapeutic potential of mycobacterial cell wall-DNA complexes. *Expert Opinion on Investigational Drugs*, 10 (2001) 2157–2165, doi:10.1517/13543784.10.12.2157.

154. Kuromatsu I., Matsuo K., Takamura S., Kim G., Takebe Y., Kawamura J., *et al.* Induction of effective antitumor immune responses in a mouse bladder tumor model by using DNA of an alpha antigen from mycobacteria. *Cancer Gene Therapy*, 8 (2001) 483–490, doi:10.1038/sj.cgt.7700330.

155. Zhang P., Wang J., Wang D., Wang H., Shan F., Chen L., *et al.* Dendritic cell vaccine modified by Ag85A gene enhances anti-tumor immunity

against bladder cancer. *International Immunopharmacology*, 14 (2012) 252–260, doi:10.1016/j.intimp.2012.07.014.

156. Zlotta A. R., Van Vooren J. P., Denis O., Drowart A., Daffé M., Lefèvre P., *et al.* What are the immunologically active components of bacille Calmette–Guérin in therapy of superficial bladder cancer? *International Journal of Cancer*, 87 (2000) 844–852.

157. Yarkoni E., Rapp H. J. Immunotherapy of experimental cancer by intralesional injection of emulsified nonliving mycobacteria: Comparison of *Mycobacterium bovis* (BCG), *Mycobacterium phlei*, and *Mycobacterium smegmatis*. *Infection and Immunity*, 28 (1980) 887–892.

158. Ribi E. E., Milner K. C., Granger D. L., Kelly M. T., Yamamoto K., Brehmer W., *et al.* Immunotherapy with nonviable microbial components. *Annals of the New York Academy of Sciences*, 277 (1976) 228–238. http://www.ncbi.nlm.nih.gov/pubmed/187099 (accessed April 15, 2015).

159. Gray G. R., Ribi E. E., Granger D., Parker R., Azuma I., Yamamoto K. Immunotherapy of cancer: Tumor suppression and regression by cell walls of *Mycobacterium phlei* attached to oil droplets. *Journal of the National Cancer Institute*, 55 (1975) 727–730.

160. Yarkoni E., Rapp H. J., Zbar B. Immunotherapy of a guinea pig hepatoma with ultrasonically prepared mycobacterial vaccines. *Cancer Immunology, Immunotherapy*, 2 (1977) 143–146, doi:10.1007/BF00200061.

161. Akaza H., Iwasaki A., Ohtani M., Ikeda N., Niijima K., Toida I., *et al.* Expression of antitumor response. Role of attachment and viability of Bacillus Calmette–Guérin to bladder cancer cells. *Cancer*, 72 (1993) 558–563. http://www.ncbi.nlm.nih.gov/pubmed/8319187 (accessed December 13, 2016).

162. Hwang T.-L., Fang C.-L., Chen C.-H., Fang J.-Y. Permeation enhancer-containing water-in-oil nanoemulsions as carriers for intravesical cisplatin delivery. *Pharmaceutical Research* 26 (2009) 2314–2323.

163. Noguera-Ortega E., Blanco-Cabra N., Rabanal R. M., Sánchez-Chardi A., Roldán M., Guallar-Garrido S., *et al.* Mycobacteria emulsified in olive oil-in-water trigger a robust immune response in bladder cancer treatment. *Scientific Reports*, 6 (2016) 27232, doi:10.1038/srep27232.

164. Homhuan A., Kogure K., Akaza H., Futaki S., Naka T., Fujita Y., *et al.* New packaging method of mycobacterial cell wall using octaarginine-

modified liposomes: Enhanced uptake by and immunostimulatory activity of dendritic cells. *Journal of Controlled Release*, 120 (2007) 60–69, doi:10.1016/j.jconrel.2007.03.017.

165. Nakamura T., Fukiage M., Higuchi M., Nakaya A., Yano I., Miyazaki J., *et al.* Nanoparticulation of BCG-CWS for application to bladder cancer therapy. *Journal of Controlled Release*, 176 (2014) 44–53, doi:10.1016/j.jconrel.2013.12.027.

166. Nakamura T., Fukiage M., Suzuki Y., Yano I., Miyazaki J., Nishiyama H., *et al.* Mechanism responsible for the antitumor effect of BCG-CWS using the LEEL method in a mouse bladder cancer model. *Journal of Controlled Release*, 196 (2014) 161–167, doi:10.1016/j.jconrel.2014.10.007.

167. Kato T., Bilim V., Yuuki K., Naito S., Yamanobe T., Nagaoka A., *et al.* Bacillus Calmette–Guérin and BCG cell wall skeleton suppressed viability of bladder cancer cells in vitro. *Anticancer Research*, 30 (2010) 4089–4096. http://www.ncbi.nlm.nih.gov/pubmed/21036724.

168. Uenishi Y., Takii T., Yano I., Sunagawa M. Separation and molecular characterization of mycolic acid from the cell wall skeleton of *Mycobacterium bovis* BCG Tokyo 172 (SMP-105) and BCG substrains by normal-phase high performance liquid chromatography and liquid chromatography/mass spectrometry. *Journal of Microbiological Methods*, 77 (2009) 320–322, doi:10.1016/j.mimet.2009.03.006.

169. Uenishi Y., Kusunose N., Yano I., Sunagawa M. Isolation and identification of arabinose mycolates of Cell Wall Skeleton (CWS) derived from *Mycobacterium bovis* BCG Tokyo 172 (SMP-105). *Journal of Microbiological Methods*, 80 (2010) 302–305, doi:10.1016/j.mimet.2010.01.003.

170. Joraku A., Homhuan A., Kawai K., Yamamoto T., Miyazaki J., Kogure K., *et al.* Immunoprotection against murine bladder carcinoma by octaarginine-modified liposomes incorporating cell wall of *Mycobacterium bovis* bacillus Calmette–Guérin. *BJU International*, 103 (2009) 686–693, doi:10.1111/j.1464-410X.2008.08235.x.

171. Miyazaki J., Kawai K., Kojima T., Oikawa T., Joraku A., Shimazui T., *et al.* The liposome-incorporating cell wall skeleton of *Mycobacterium bovis* bacillus Calmette–Guérin can directly enhance the susceptibility of cancer cells to lymphokine-activated killer cells through up-regulation of natural-killer group 2, member D ligands. *BJU International*, 108 (2011) 1520–1526, doi:10.1111/j.1464-410X.2010.10056.x.

172. Chin J. L., Kadhim S. A., Batislam E., Karlik S. J., Garcia B. M., Nickel J. C., *et al.* Mycobacterium cell wall: An alternative to intravesical bacillus

Calmette Guerin (BCG) therapy in orthotopic murine bladder cancer. *Journal of Urology,* 156 (1996) 1189–1193. http://www.ncbi.nlm.nih.gov/pubmed/8709344 (accessed December 13, 2016).

173. Vézina S. A., Archambault D. Modulatory effect of mycobacterium cell wall extract (Regressin) on lymphocyte blastogenic activity and macrophage cytokine gene transcription in swine. *Clinical and Diagnostic Laboratory Immunology,* 4 (1997) 314–320. http://www.ncbi.nlm.nih.gov/pubmed/9144370 (accessed December 13, 2016).

174. Morales A., Chin J. L., Ramsey E. W. Mycobacterial cell wall extract for treatment of carcinoma in situ of the bladder. *Journal of Urology,* 166 (2001) 1633–1638.

175. Morales A., Phadke K., Steinberg G. D. Intravesical mycobacterial cell Wall-DNA complex in the treatment of carcinoma in situ of the bladder after standard intravesical therapy has failed. *Journal of Urology,* 181 (2009) 1040–1045, doi:10.1016/j.juro.2008.11.019.

176. Morales A., Herr H., Steinberg G., Given R., Cohen Z., Amrhein J., *et al.* Efficacy and safety of MCNA in patients with nonmuscle invasive bladder cancer at high risk for recurrence and progression after failed treatment with bacillus Calmette–Guérin. *Journal of Urology,* 193 (2015) 1135–1143, doi:10.1016/j.juro.2014.09.109.

177. Morales A., Cohen Z. *Mycobacterium phlei* cell wall-nucleic acid complex in the treatment of nonmuscle invasive bladder cancer unresponsive to bacillus Calmette–Guérin. *Expert Opinion on Biological Therapy,* 16 (2016) 273–283, doi:10.1517/14712598.2016.1134483.

178. Kelley D. R., Ratliff T. L., Catalona W. J., Shapiro A., Lage J. M., Bauer W. C., *et al.* Intravesical bacillus Calmette–Guérin therapy for superficial bladder cancer: effect of bacillus Calmette–Guérin viability on treatment results. *The Journal of Urology,* 134 (1985) 48–53. https://doi.org/10.1016/S0022-5347(17)46976-X.

179. Secanella-Fandos S., Noguera-Ortega E., Olivares F., Luquin M., Julián E. Killed but metabolically active *Mycobacterium bovis* bacillus Calmette–Guérin retains the antitumor ability of live bacillus Calmette–Guérin. *Journal of Urology,* 191 (2014) 1422–1428, doi:10.1016/j.juro.2013.12.002.

180. Murata M. Activation of Toll-like receptor 2 by a novel preparation of cell wall skeleton from *Mycobacterium bovis* BCG Tokyo (SMP-105) sufficiently enhances immune responses against tumors. *Cancer Science,* 99 (2008) 1435–1440.

181. Jackson A., Alexandroff A., Fleming D., Prescott S., Chisholm G., James K. Bacillus- Calmette–Guérin (BCG) organisms directly alter the growth of bladder-tumor cells. *International Journal of Oncology*, 5 (1994) 697–703. http://www.ncbi.nlm.nih.gov/pubmed/21559633 (accessed December 14, 2016).

182. Shah G., Zhang G., Chen F., Cao Y., Kalyanaraman B., See W. Loss of bacillus Calmette–Guérin viability adversely affects the direct response of urothelial carcinoma cells to bacillus Calmette–Guérin exposure. *Journal of Urology*, 191 (2014) 823–829, doi:10.1016/j.juro.2013.09.012.

183. Zhang Y., Khoo H. E., Esuvaranathan K. Effects of Bacillus Calmette-Guèrin and interferon alpha-2B on cytokine production in human bladder cancer cell lines. *Journal of Urology*, 161 (1999) 977–983.http://www.ncbi.nlm.nih.gov/pubmed/10022737(accessed September 22, 2015).

184. Kemp T. J., Ludwig A. T., Earel J. K., Moore J. M., VanOosten R. L., Moses B., *et al.* Neutrophil stimulation with *Mycobacterium bovis* bacillus Calmette–Guérin (BCG) results in the release of functional soluble TRAIL/Apo-2L. *Blood*, 106 (2005) 3474–3482, doi:10.1182/blood-2005-03-1327.

185. Yamada H., Kuroda E., Matsumoto S., Matsumoto T., Yamada T., Yamashita U. Prostaglandin E2 down-regulates viable bacille Calmette–Guérin-induced macrophage cytotoxicity against murine bladder cancer cell MBT-2 in vitro. *Clinical and Experimental Immunology*, 128 (2002) 52–58. http://www.pubmedcentral.nih.gov/articlerender.fcgi?artid=1906368&tool=pmcentrez&rendertype=abstract (accessed September 26, 2015).

186. Secanella-Fandos S. *Funcionalitat dels micobacteris ambientals de creixement ràpid com a agents antitumorals*, Universitat Autònoma de Barcelona, 2012. http://www.tdx.cat/handle/10803/117614 (accessed September 22, 2015).

187. Ikeda N., Toida I., Iwasaki A., Kawai K., Akaza H. Surface antigen expression on bladder tumor cells induced by bacillus Calmette-Guérin (BCG): A role of BCG internalization into tumor cells. *International Journal of Urology*, 9 (2002) 29–35, doi:10.1046/j.1442-2042.2002.00415.x.

188. Tsuji S., Matsumoto M., Takeuchi O., Akira S., Azuma I., Hayashi A., *et al.* Maturation of human dendritic cells by cell wall skeleton of *Mycobacterium bovis* bacillus Calmette–Guérin: Involvement of toll-like receptors. *Infection and Immunity*, 68 (2000) 6883–6890. http://

www.pubmedcentral.nih.gov/articlerender.fcgi?artid=97794&tool=pmcentrez&rendertype=abstract (accessed May 14, 2015).

189. Shapiro A., Ratliff T. L., Oakley D. M., Catalona W. J. Reduction of bladder tumor growth in mice treated with intravesical bacillus Calmette–Guérin and its correlation with bacillus Calmette–Guérin viability and natural killer cell activity. *Cancer Research*, 43 (1983) 1611–1615. http://www.ncbi.nlm.nih.gov/pubmed/6339040.

190. Günther J. H., Frambach M., Deinert I., Brandau S., Jocham D., Böhle A. Effects of acetylic salicylic acid and pentoxifylline on the efficacy of intravesical BCG therapy in orthotopic murine bladder cancer (MB49). *Journal of Urology*, 161 (1999) 1702–1706. http://www.ncbi.nlm.nih.gov/pubmed/10210443 (accessed December 14, 2016).

191. de Boer E. C., Rooijakkers S. J., Schamhart D. H. J., Kurth K. H. Cytokine gene expression in a mouse model: The first instillations with viable bacillus Calmette–Guérin determine the succeeding Th1 response. *Journal of Urology*, 170 (2003) 2004–2008, doi:10.1097/01.ju.0000091826.83705.79.

192. Lamm D. L., Iverson T., Wangler V. 1785 Clinical experience with heat-inactivated bacillus Calmette–Guérin (BCG) immunotherapy. *Journal of Urology*, 189 (2013) e733–e734, doi:10.1016/j.juro.2013.02.2875.

193. Noguera-Ortega E., Secanella-Fandos S., Eraña H., Gasión J., Rabanal R. M., Luquin M., *et al.* Nonpathogenic *Mycobacterium brumae* inhibits bladder cancer growth in vitro, ex vivo, and in vivo. *European Urology Focus*, 2 (2016) 67–76, doi:10.1016/j.euf.2015.03.003.

194. Chaudhuri P., Mukhopadhyay S. Bladder preserving approach for muscle invasive bladder cancer—role of mycobacterium w. *Journal of the Indian Medical Association*, 101 (2003) 559–560. http://www.ncbi.nlm.nih.gov/pubmed/15168998 (accessed April 15, 2015).

195. Yates D. R., Brausi M. A., Catto J. W. F., Dalbagni G., Rouprêt M., Shariat S. F., *et al.* Treatment options available for bacillus Calmette–Guérin failure in non-muscle-invasive bladder cancer. *European Urology*, 62 (2012) 1088–1096, doi:10.1016/j.eururo.2012.08.055.

196. Subramaniam M., In L. L., Kumar A., Ahmed N., Nagoor N. H. Cytotoxic and apoptotic effects of heat killed *Mycobacterium indicus pranii* (MIP) on various human cancer cell lines. *Scientific Reports*, 6 (2016) 19833, doi:10.1038/srep19833.

197. Kreider J. W., Bartlett G. L., Purnell D. M. Immunotherapeutic effectiveness of BCG inactivated by various modalities. *Cancer*, 46 (1980) 480–487.

198. Thanhäuser A., Böhle A., Flad H. D., Ernst M., Mattern T., Ulmer A. J. Induction of bacillus-Calmette–Guérin-activated killer cells from human peripheral blood mononuclear cells against human bladder carcinoma cell lines in vitro. *Cancer Immunology, Immunotherapy,* 37 (1993) 105–111.

199. Noguera-Ortega E., Rabanal R. M., Secanella-Fandos S., Torrents E., Luquin M., Julián E. γ irradiated mycobacteria enhance survival in bladder tumor bearing mice although less efficaciously than live mycobacteria. *Journal of Urology,* 195 (2016) 198–205, doi:10.1016/j.juro.2015.07.011.

200. Baran J., Baj-Krzyworzeka M., W glarczyk K., Ruggiero I., Zembala M. Modulation of monocyte-tumour cell interactions by *Mycobacterium vaccae. Cancer Immunology, Immunotherapy,* 53 (2004) 1127–1134, doi:10.1007/s00262-004-0552-6.

201. Rodríguez-Güell E., Agustí G., Corominas M., Cardona P.-J., Casals I., Parella T., *et al.* The production of a new extracellular putative long-chain saturated polyester by smooth variants of *Mycobacterium vaccae* interferes with Th1-cytokine production. *Antonie Van Leeuwenhoek,* 90 (2006) 93–108, doi:10.1007/s10482-006-9062-1.

202. Hachem R., Raad I., Rolston K. V., Whimbey E., Katz R., Tarrand J., *et al.* Cutaneous and pulmonary infections caused by *Mycobacterium vaccae. Clinical Infectious Diseases,* 23 (1996) 173–175.

203. Skiest D. J., Levi M. E. Catheter-related bacteremia due to *Mycobacterium smegmatis. Southern Medical Journal,* 91 (1998) 36–37. http://www.ncbi.nlm.nih.gov/pubmed/9438400 (accessed December 13, 2016).

204. Pennekamp A., Pfyffer G. E., Wüest J., George C. A., Ruef C. *Mycobacterium smegmatis* infection in a healthy woman following a facelift: Case report and review of the literature. *Annals of Plastic Surgery,* 39 (1997) 80–83. http://www.ncbi.nlm.nih.gov/pubmed/9229098 (accessed December 13, 2016).

205. Wallace R. J., Nash D. R., Tsukamura M., Blacklock Z. M., Silcox V. A. Human disease due to *Mycobacterium smegmatis. Journal of Infectious Diseases,* 158 (1988) 52–59. http://www.ncbi.nlm.nih.gov/pubmed/3392420 (accessed December 13, 2016).

206. Kumar K. J., Chandra J., Mandal R. N., Dutta R., Jain N. K. Fatal pulmonary infection caused by *Mycobacterium smegmatis* in an infant. *Indian Journal of Pediatrics,* 62 (1995) 619–621. http://www.ncbi.nlm.nih.gov/pubmed/10829933 (accessed December 13, 2016).

207. Young S. L., Murphy M., Zhu X. W., Harnden P., O'Donnell M. A., James K., *et al.* Cytokine-modified *Mycobacterium smegmatis* as a novel

anticancer immunotherapy. *International Journal of Cancer,* 112 (2004) 653–660, doi:10.1002/ijc.20442.

208. Hudson M. A., Ritchey J. K., Catalona W. J., Brown E. J., Ratliff T. L. Comparison of the fibronectin-binding ability and antitumor efficacy of various mycobacteria. *Cancer Research,* 50 (1990) 3843–3847.

209. Blanc P., Dutronc H., Peuchant O., Dauchy F.-A., Cazanave C., Neau D., *et al.* Nontuberculous mycobacterial infections in a French hospital: A 12-year retrospective study. *PLOS One,* 11 (2016) e0168290, doi:10.1371/journal.pone.0168290.

210. Luquin M., Ausina V., Vincent-Levy-Frebault V., Laneelle M. A., Belda F., Garcia-Barcelo M., *et al. Mycobacterium brumae sp. nov.,* a rapidly growing, nonphotochromogenic mycobacterium. *International Journal of Systematic Bacteriology,* 43 (1993) 405–413, doi:10.1099/00207713-43-3-405.

211. Rodriguez-Guell E., Agusti G., Corominas M., Luquin M., Julian E. Impaired gamma interferon response to *Mycobacterium vaccae* antigens in patients with cavitary pulmonary tuberculosis. *Clinical and Vaccine Immunology,* 15 (2008) 1485–1488, doi:10.1128/CVI.00131-08.

212. Lee S. A., Raad I. I., Adachi J. A., Han X. Y. Catheter-related bloodstream infection caused by *Mycobacterium brumae. Journal of Clinical Microbiology,* 42 (2004) 5429–5431, doi:10.1128/JCM.42.11.5429-5431.2004.

213. Jiménez M. S., Julián E., Luquin M. Misdiagnosis of *Mycobacterium brumae* infection. *Journal of Clinical Microbiology,* 49 (2011) 1190-1-2, doi:10.1128/JCM.01540-10.

214. Zlotta A. R., Drowart A., Van Vooren J. P., De Cock M., Pirson M., Palfliet K., *et al.* Evolution and clinical significance of the T cell proliferative and cytokine response directed against the fibronectin binding antigen 85 complex of bacillus Calmette–Guérin during intravesical treatment of superficial bladder cancer. *Journal of Urology,* 157 (1997) 492–498, doi:10.1016/S0022-5347(01)65185-1.

215. Jackson A. M., Alexandroff A. B., Kelly R. W., Skibinska A., Esuvaranathan K., Prescott S., *et al.* Changes in urinary cytokines and soluble intercellular adhesion molecule-1 (ICAM-1) in bladder cancer patients after bacillus Calmette–Guérin (BCG) immunotherapy. *Clinical and Experimental Immunology,* 99 (1995) 369–375. http://www.ncbi.nlm.nih.gov/pubmed/7882559 (accessed December 13, 2016).

216. Douglass L., Schoenberg M. The future of intravesical drug delivery for non-muscle invasive bladder cancer. *Bladder Cancer,* 2 (2016) 285–292, doi:10.3233/BLC-160056.

217. Velasco-Velázquez M. A., Barrera D., González-Arenas A., Rosales C., Agramonte-Hevia J. Macrophage–*Mycobacterium tuberculosis* interactions: Role of complement receptor 3. *Microbial Pathogenesis*, 35 (2003) 125–131. http://www.ncbi.nlm.nih.gov/pubmed/12927520 (accessed December 15, 2016).

218. Muñoz M., Lanéelle M. A., Luquin M., Torrelles J., Julián E., Ausina V., *et al.* Occurrence of an antigenic triacyl trehalose in clinical isolates and reference strains of *Mycobacterium tuberculosis*. *FEMS Microbiology Letters*, 157 (1997) 251–259. http://www.ncbi.nlm.nih.gov/pubmed/9435105 (accessed December 14, 2016).

219. Muñoz M., Luquin M., García-Barcelo M., Julián E., Ausina V., Lanéelle M. A. Distribution of surface-exposed antigenic glycolipids in recent clinical isolates of *Mycobacterium tuberculosis*. *Research in Microbiology*, 148 (1997) 405–412, doi:10.1016/S0923-2508(97)83871-5.

220. Neyrolles O., Guilhot C. Recent advances in deciphering the contribution of *Mycobacterium tuberculosis* lipids to pathogenesis. *Tuberculosis*, 91 (2011) 187–195, doi:10.1016/j.tube.2011.01.002.

221. Bafica A., Scanga C. A., Feng C. G., Leifer C., Cheever A., Sher A. TLR9 regulates Th1 responses and cooperates with TLR2 in mediating optimal resistance to *Mycobacterium tuberculosis*. *Journal of Experimental Medicine*, 202 (2005) 1715–1724, doi:10.1084/jem.20051782.

222. Tima H. G., Al Dulayymi J. R., Denis O., Lehebel P., Baols K. S., Mohammed M. O., *et al.* Inflammatory properties and adjuvant potential of synthetic glycolipids homologous to mycolate esters of the cell wall of *Mycobacterium tuberculosis*. *Journal of Innate Immunity*, (2016), doi:10.1159/000450955.

223. Morita D., Hattori Y., Nakamura T., Igarashi T., Harashima H., Sugita M. Major T cell response to a mycolyl glycolipid is mediated by CD1c molecules in rhesus macaques. *Infection and Immunity*, 81 (2013) 311–316, doi:10.1128/IAI.00871-12.

224. Kasmar A. G., van Rhijn I., Cheng T.-Y., Turner M., Seshadri C., Schiefner A., *et al.* CD1b tetramers bind $\alpha\beta$ T cell receptors to identify a mycobacterial glycolipid-reactive T cell repertoire in humans. *Journal of Experimental Medicine*, 208 (2011) 1741–1747, doi:10.1084/jem.20110665.

225. Moody D. B., Reinhold B. B., Guy M. R., Beckman E. M., Frederique D. E., Furlong S. T., *et al.* Structural requirements for glycolipid antigen recognition by CD1b-restricted T cells. *Science*, 278 (1997) 283–286.

http://www.ncbi.nlm.nih.gov/pubmed/9323206 (accessed December 15, 2016).

226. Sweet L., Zhang W., Torres-Fewell H., Serianni A., Boggess W., Schorey J. *Mycobacterium avium* glycopeptidolipids require specific acetylation and methylation patterns for signaling through toll-like receptor 2. *Journal of Biological Chemistry*, 283 (2008) 33221–33231, doi:10.1074/jbc.M805539200.

227. Fujiwara N., Naka T., Ogawa M., Yamamoto R., Ogura H., Taniguchi H. Characteristics of *Mycobacterium smegmatis* J15cs strain lipids. *Tuberculosis*, 92 (2012) 187–192, doi:10.1016/j.tube.2011.10.001.

228. Layre E., Collmann A., Bastian M., Mariotti S., Czaplicki J., Prandi J., *et al.* Mycolic acids constitute a scaffold for mycobacterial lipid antigens stimulating CD1-Restricted T Cells. *Chemical Biology*, 16 (2009) 82–92, doi:10.1016/j.chembiol.2008.11.008.

229. Hattori Y., Morita D., Fujiwara N., Mori D., Nakamura T., Harashima H., *et al.* Glycerol monomycolate is a novel ligand for the human, but not mouse macrophage inducible C-type lectin, Mincle. *Journal of Biological Chemistry*, 289 (2014) 15405–15412, doi:10.1074/jbc.M114.566489.

230. Yonekawa A., Saijo S., Hoshino Y., Miyake Y., Ishikawa E., Suzukawa M., *et al.* Dectin-2 is a direct receptor for mannose-capped lipoarabinomannan of mycobacteria. *Immunity*, 41 (2014) 402–413, doi:10.1016/j.immuni.2014.08.005.

231. Killick K. E., Ní Cheallaigh C., O'Farrelly C., Hokamp K., MacHugh D. E., Harris J. Receptor-mediated recognition of mycobacterial pathogens. *Cellular Microbiology*, 15 (2013) 1484–1495, doi:10.1111/cmi.12161.

232. Mishra A. K., Alves J. E., Krumbach K., Nigou J., Castro A. G., Geurtsen J., *et al.* Differential arabinan capping of lipoarabinomannan modulates innate immune responses and impacts T helper cell differentiation. *Journal of Biological Chemistry*, 287 (2012) 44173–44183, doi:10.1074/jbc.M112.402396.

233. Sieling P., Chatterjee D., Porcelli S., Prigozy T., Mazzaccaro R., Soriano T., *et al.* CD1-restricted T cell recognition of microbial lipoglycan antigens. *Science* 269 (1995) 227–230.

234. Brightbill H. D., Libraty D. H., Krutzik S. R., Yang R. B., Belisle J. T., Bleharski J. R., *et al.* Host defense mechanisms triggered by microbial lipoproteins through toll-like receptors. *Science*, 285 (1999) 732–736. http://www.ncbi.nlm.nih.gov/pubmed/10426995 (accessed December 15, 2016).

235. Means T. K., Wang S., Lien E., Yoshimura A., Golenbock D. T., Fenton M. J. Human toll-like receptors mediate cellular activation by *Mycobacterium tuberculosis*. *Journal of Immunology*, 163 (1999) 3920–3927. http://www.ncbi.nlm.nih.gov/pubmed/10490993 (accessed December 15, 2016).

236. Minnikin D. E., Kremer L., Dover L. G., Besra G. S. The methyl-branched fortifications of *Mycobacterium tuberculosis*. *Chemical Biology*, 9 (2002) 545–553. http://www.ncbi.nlm.nih.gov/pubmed/12031661 (accessed December 14, 2016).

237. Stamm C. E., Collins A. C., Shiloh M. U. Sensing of *Mycobacterium tuberculosis* and consequences to both host and bacillus. *Immunological Reviews*, 264 (2015) 204–219, doi:10.1111/imr.12263.

238. Muñoz M., Raynaud C., Lanéelle M. A., Julián E., López Marín L. M., Silve G., *et al.* Seroreactive species-specific lipooligosaccharides of *Mycobacterium mucogenicum sp. nov.* (formerly *Mycobacterium chelonae*-like organisms): Identification and chemical characterization. *Microbiology*, 144 (1998) 137–148, doi:10.1099/00221287-144-1-137.

239. Li H., Ulstrup J. C., Jonassen T. O., Melby K., Nagai S., Harboe M. Evidence for absence of the MPB64 gene in some substrains of *Mycobacterium bovis* BCG, *Infection and Immunity*, 61 (1993) 1730–1734. http://www.ncbi.nlm.nih.gov/pubmed/8478061 (accessed December 15, 2016).

240. Toyonaga K., Torigoe S., Motomura Y., Kamichi T., Hayashi J. M., Morita Y. S., *et al.* C-type lectin receptor DCAR recognizes mycobacterial phosphatidyl-inositol mannosides to promote a Th1 response during infection. *Immunity*, (2016), doi:10.1016/j.immuni.2016.10.012.

241. Hossain M. M., Norazmi M.-N. Pattern recognition receptors and cytokines in *Mycobacterium tuberculosis* infection—the double-edged sword? *BioMed Research International*, 2013 (2013) 1–18, doi:10.1155/2013/179174.

242. Bowdish D. M. E., Sakamoto K., Kim M.-J., Kroos M., Mukhopadhyay S., Leifer C. A., *et al.* MARCO, TLR2, and CD14 are required for macrophage cytokine responses to mycobacterial trehalose dimycolate and *Mycobacterium tuberculosis*. *PLOS Pathogens*, 5 (2009) e1000474, doi:10.1371/journal.ppat.1000474.

243. Ishikawa E., Ishikawa T., Morita Y. S., Toyonaga K., Yamada H., Takeuchi O., *et al.* Direct recognition of the mycobacterial glycolipid,

trehalose dimycolate, by C-type lectin Mincle. *Journal of Experimental Medicine,* 206 (2009) 2879–2888, doi:10.1084/jem.20091750.

244. Miyake Y., Oh-hora M., Yamasaki S. C-Type lectin receptor MCL facilitates Mincle expression and signaling through complex formation. *Journal of Immunology,* 194 (2015) 5366–5374, doi:10.4049/jimmunol.1402429.

245. Dey B., Dey R. J., Cheung L. S., Pokkali S., Guo H., Lee J.-H., *et al.* A bacterial cyclic dinucleotide activates the cytosolic surveillance pathway and mediates innate resistance to tuberculosis. *Nature Medicine,* 21 (2015) 401–406, doi:10.1038/nm.3813.

246. Yang Y., Yin C., Pandey A., Abbott D., Sassetti C., Kelliher M. A. NOD2 Pathway activation by MDP or *Mycobacterium tuberculosis* infection involves the stable polyubiquitination of Rip2. *Journal of Biological Chemistry,* 282 (2007) 36223–36229, doi:10.1074/jbc.M703079200.

Chapter 5

Genetically Modified *Salmonella* as Cancer Therapeutics: Mechanisms, Advances, and Challenges

Xiaoxin Zhang[a] **and Zi-Chun Hua**[a,b,c]

[a]*School of Life Sciences, Nanjing University, 163 Xianlin Dadao, Nanjing 210023, Jiangsu, China*
[b]*Changzhou High-Tech Research Institute of Nanjing University and Jiangsu Target Pharma Laboratories, Inc., Changzhou 213164, China*
[c]*Shenzhen Research Institute of Nanjing University, Shenzhen 518057, China*

huazc@nju.edu.cn

Bacteria-mediated cancer therapy is an emerging concept as it possesses some unique properties that make it unachievable through traditional methods. Bacteria can not only inhibit tumor growth and prolong mice survival time but also deliver therapeutic agents. *Salmonella* is one of the most extensively studied bacteria over the past decades. Although understanding of the anticancer function of *Salmonella* has grown tremendously and a variety of *Salmonella* mutants with higher potency have been developed, the phase I clinical trials using *Salmonella* mutants were disappointing. Thus, studies toward the ultimate goal are required. This chapter summarizes the recent developments in *Salmonella*-mediated cancer therapy and highlight the challenges that lie ahead.

Microbial Infections and Cancer Therapy: Recent Advances
Edited by Ananda M. Chakrabarty and Arsénio M. Fialho

ISBN 978-981-4774-86-4 (Hardcover), 978-1-351-04190-4 (eBook)
www.panstanford.com

5.1 Introduction

As long as three hundred years ago, there were reports that tumors regressed after patients got infected with bacteria [1]. Then, more case reports were published. In the late 19th century, William Coley, a New York physician, combined heat-killed gram-positive *Streptococcus* and gram-negative *Serratia marcescens* to treat his patients, which was widely used for sarcomas patients until 1963 [2, 3]. His work laid the pioneer foundation for bacterial tumor therapy.

Up to now, many genera of bacteria have been developed to treat tumors in animal models or human clinical trials [4–9]. Among them, *Salmonella* is the most extensively studied for bacterial tumor therapy. *Salmonella enterica* serovar Typhimurium is a rod-shaped gram-negative bacteria. It can preferentially accumulate in tumor, reaching ratios of 1000:1 to 10,000:1 as tumors versus normal tissues. In addition, *Salmonella* can inhibit tumor growth in a broad range of human and mouse tumors. However, poor tumor targeting and no therapeutic effects were observed during the phase I clinical trials using *Salmonella* to control tumor growth (Table 5.1). Thus, more studies of the mechanisms responsible for its tumor targeting and anticancer capacity and optimization of its delivery system are required in order to engineer the perfect *Salmonella* vectors. The following chapter presents a recent overview of *Salmonella*-mediated cancer therapy.

Table 5.1 Preclinical examples of *Salmonella*-mediated cancer therapy

Species	Identifier	Tumor (sample size)	Results	Refs.
VNP20009	NCT00004216	Metastatic melanoma (24)	Focal tumor colonization in 3 patients No tumor shrinkage	[10]
	NCT00004988	Metastatic melanoma (4)	Tumor biopsy culture positive in 1 patient No tumor shrinkage	[11]
	NCT00006254	Squamous cell carcinoma (3)	Tumor colonization in 2 patients No tumor shrinkage	[12]

χ4550	NCT01099631	Hepatocellular carcinoma (22)	Terminated—reasons not disclosed	
VXM01	NCT01486329	Pancreatic cancer (72)	Reduction in tumor perfusion after vaccination. Fate of tumors not disclosed	[13]

5.2 Mechanisms of Tumor Suppression

5.2.1 Host Immunity and *Salmonella*

5.2.1.1 Innate immunity and *Salmonella*

Salmonella has an indirect killing impact on tumor cells, which is aided by cooperation with the host's immune system through recruitment of inflammatory immune cells and cytokines. Lee *et al.* compared the anticancer activities of *Salmonella* in wild-type mice and toll-like receptor 4 (TLR4)-deficient mice and found that TLR4 played an important role in *Salmonella*-induced tumor inhibition [14]. This was later confirmed by Kaimala and colleagues' work demonstrating that the anticancer capacity of *Salmonella* relied mostly on the induction of innate immune responses through the TLR-MyD88 signaling pathway [15]. The activation of TLR serves as a priming signal required for the activation of NLRP3 inflammasome. Phan and colleagues reported that *Salmonella* activated inflammasome pathways, resulting in a marked increase of IL-β in a *Salmonella*-colonized tumor [16]. Interleukin-1 beta (IL-1β), produced by the infiltrated dendritic cells, played an important role in *Salmonella*-mediated cancer therapy [17]. Depletion of IL-1β using neutralizing antibodies abrogated the anticancer effects of *Salmonella*. A similar result was also observed in our study. Three VNP20009 mutants with unchanged tumor targeting ability induced far less IL-1β in tumors and displayed reduced anticancer capacities [18].

Interestingly, as a large number of neutrophils immigrated into tumors, they formed a rim and restricted *Salmonella* from replicating in necrotic and hypoxic regions [19]. Depletion of host neutrophils led more bacteria to accumulate in the tumor. However, the infiltrated neutrophils exerted their antitumor effects through secretion of tumor necrosis factor alpha (TNF-α), which disrupted the tumor vessels and led to a bacteria flux into the tumor, along with blood [20, 21]. In addition, Kim *et al.* and Guo *et al.* identified macrophages as another main producer of TNF-α, and coadministration of TNF-α enhanced the anticancer effects of *Salmonella* [17, 22]. Taken together, *Salmonella* treatments make intratumoral myeloid cells less suppressive.

5.2.1.2 Adaptive immunity and *Salmonella*

When *Salmonella* was administrated to tumor-bearing mice, both anti-*Salmonella*-specific and tumor antigen–specific T cells were recruited into tumors [23]. Lee *et al.* compared the anticancer activities of *Salmonella* in wild-type CD4 T cell–deficient and CD8 T cell–deficient mice to study the role of T cells in *Salmonella*-mediated cancer therapy [24]. While *Salmonella* inhibited tumor growth by 50% in wild-type mice, only 34%–42% tumor growth was observed in CD4-deficient mice and macrophages and neutrophils were also significantly decreased, demonstrating that T cells are indispensable for the efficacy of *Salmonella* against tumors. In addition, *Salmonella* promoted an antitumor Th1-type response characterized by increased frequencies of IFN-γ-secreting CD4+ T and CD8+ T cells and a reduction of regulatory T cells [20, 25]. To overcome a tumor-induced immunosuppressive environment, *Salmonella* reduced the expression of tumor indoleamine 2,3-dioxygenase 1 and induced connexin 43 (Cx43) expression [26, 27]. By upregulation of Cx43, functional gap junctions between tumor cells and dendritic cells were established to transfer tumor antigenic peptides to dendritic cells, thereby activating cytotoxic T cells against tumor antigens. In addition, B cells played an important role in the antitumor activity mediated by *Salmonella*. As bacterial loads in B cell–deficient mice were higher than in wild-type mice, B cells were found to inhibit the dissemination of *Salmonella* to other healthy organs [28].

5.2.2 The Traits of *Salmonella* Required for Cancer Therapy

With rapid developments in the genetic modification of *Salmonella*, more and more researchers began to study *Salmonella* factors affecting tumor colonization and anticancer capacity. *Salmonella* pathogenicity island (SPI)-2 was the first identified genetic system required for the anticancer capacity of *Salmonella* [29]. This was more deeply investigated by our lab. The knockout of the genes required for intramacrophage survival demonstrated that the genes were not required for tumor colonization but essential for anticancer capacity of *Salmonella*. What's more important, our results indicated that the anticancer capacity of VNP20009 didn't correlate to its tumor targeting ability [18].

However, only a limited number of genes were deleted in these studies. To identify the genes responsible for tumor colonization, a high throughput screen of a single gene deletion was performed by Valenzuela *et al.* and Arrach *et al.*, and a group of genes affecting tumor colonization was identified [30, 31]. Among these genes, there was a motility gene *motAB*, which was consistent with the previous finding that stated motility was critical for effective distribution and accumulation of bacteria in tumor tissue [32, 33]. In addition, motile *Salmonella* bacteria contain various chemotaxis proteins, which directs the bacteria to different regions within the tumor [34–37]. Kasinskas and Forbes changed bacterial localization within tumors by deleting specific receptors in *Salmonella*, thereby improving the anticancer capacity of *Salmonella* [34]. However, a recent study reported that *Salmonella* lost wide-type motility and flagella during long-term tumor colonization, probably as a strategy to minimize energy consumption and maximize proliferation [38]. Besides this, the complete genome sequence revealed that VNP20009 had additional mutations in chemotaxis and motility [39, 40]. It remains to be elucidated whether these mutations are harmful or beneficial to the anticancer capacity of VNP20009.

5.3 Optimization of *Salmonella*-Mediated Delivery Systems

As *Salmonella* colonizes both in well-oxygenated regions and necrotic regions, which enables it to target primary tumors as well as metastases, these bacteria are promising gene therapy vectors. To maximize the potency of bacteria-mediated cancer gene therapy, five parameters of the systems are needed to be carefully optimized.

5.3.1 Optimization of Bacterial Vectors

5.3.1.1 Attenuation of *Salmonella* vectors

As *Salmonella* specifically targets tumors, it is widely used as a tumor targeting shuttle of therapeutic molecules. However, wild-type *Salmonella* is a pathogen and can cause severe infections in humans. Thus, safety is one of the major concerns of bacterial vectors and multiple avirulent *Salmonella* were developed for bacterial cancer therapy (Table 5.2). To attenuate the virulent vectors, Low *et al.* generated VNP20009 by disrupting *msbB* and deleting *purI* [41, 42]. The disruption of *msbB*, which is required for LPS biosynthesis, reduced TNF-α induction and increased the LD_{50} 10,000-fold. VNP20009 displayed an anticancer phenotype in animal models and proved safe in the phase I clinical trials [11, 43]. In addition, A1-R is metabolically deficient in arginine and leucine and can effectively eradicate primary and metastatic tumors in nude mouse models of various tumors [44–49].

However, the mutants were randomly introduced and other genes in the strain might be affected coincidentally. Katherine and colleagues found that VNP20009 bred additional deletions, which might impair its antitumor capacity *in vivo* [40]. For example, there is a single nucleotide polymorphism in the chemotaxis gene *cheY* of VNP20009. VNP20009 is therefore impaired in flagella synthesis and becomes nonchemotactic. With the availability of entire bacterial genome sequences and rapid development of technics, *Salmonella* can now easily be manipulated at genetic levels. Our lab engineered a *Salmonella* mutant by deleting *phoP* and *phoQ* by the RED recombinase method to enable the mutant to release a shRNA-expressing plasmid [50]. The mutant exhibited a better safety profile than VNP20009. In addition, *Salmonella* deleting znuABC or *aroA* also displayed promising anticancer effects [51].

Table 5.2 *Salmonella* mutants tested in experimental tumors

Name	Species	Model	Result	Refs.
VNP20009	*S. typhimurium* (Δ*msbB*Δ*purI*)	Melanoma, breast, lung, and colorectal cancer	Tumor growth reduced	[41, 52, 53]
A1R	*S. typhimurium* (Δ*leu*Δ*arg*)	Prostate, breast, ovarian, pancreatic, sarcoma, and glioma cancer	Tumor growth reduced	[44, 45, 49, 54–58]
LH430	*S. typhimurium* (Δ*phoP*Δ*phoQ*)	Laryngeal, cervical, prostate, and melanoma cancer	Tumor growth reduced	[59–62]
SL7207	*S. typhimurium* (Δ*sifA*)	Glioma, colon, and neuroblastoma cancer	Tumor growth reduced	[5, 19, 21, 63]
BRD509	*S. typhimurium* (Δ*aroA*Δ*aroD*)	Melanoma cancer	Tumor growth reduced	[64]
SL3261	*S. typhimurium* (Δ*aroA*)	Melanoma and colorectal cancer	Tumor growth reduced	[64, 65]

5.3.1.2 Screen of tumor-specific *Salmonella*

Necrotic/hypoxic areas in tumors provide a unique environment suitable for bacteria. To screen for the mutants that can specifically target a tumor, Arrach *et al.* generated 41,000 *Salmonella* mutants by transposon insertion and identified a class of mutants that showed reduced fitness in normal organs and unchanged fitness in tumors [31]. In addition to this, Yu *et al.* engineered a *Salmonella* strain that exclusively survived in anaerobic conditions to improve its safety profile [66]. By exploiting the reprogrammed glucose metabolism in tumor, our lab created metabolic engineered mutants with knockout glycolysis and oxidative phosphorylation and screened for the mutants that altered the tumor metabolism microenvironment and exhibited a better anticancer capacity.

Motility and a homogeneous localization of bacteria are other important elements of engineering bacteria [35, 36]. It was reported that the further the bacteria penetrated, the better were the therapeutic outcomes that could be achieved [33, 67]. Zhang and Forbes recently found that trg-deficient *Salmonella* penetrated deeper into tumors, which resulted in a more homogeneous treatment than its parental strains [68]. Thus, trg-deficient *Salmonella* is a promising therapeutic agent for the delivery of therapeutic agents.

5.3.1.3 Attenuation versus immunogenicity

However, it should be noted that the balance between attenuation and immune stimulation is important for therapeutic success. For example, the rfaD-deficient *Salmonella* displayed reduced antitumor effects as the strain was overattenuated. In addition, our study found that although deleting the genes *slyA*, *STM3120*, and *htrA* made the mutants less virulent, their antitumor capacities were significantly impaired [18]. Thus, it would be interesting to design a conditionally modified strain. It was reported that aroA-deficient mutants induced increased levels of proinflammatory cytokines and improved tumor therapeutic activity [69]. In addition to this, Frahm *et al.* recently developed a delayed attenuation system, where they put the complementing gene under the control of an inducible promoter to make the bacteria attenuated after a few rounds of replication *in vivo* [70]. The infected mice were only transiently affected but displayed better therapeutic outcomes.

5.3.2 Genetic Stability of Expression of Heterologous Genes

For bacterial delivery of cytotoxic compounds, genetic stability and a controllable high expression of heterologous genes are critical to ensure long-term release of therapeutic proteins. The heterologous genes can be either integrated into the bacterial chromosome or expressed on a plasmid. Replacement of specific sequences of chromosome with a therapeutic gene cassette allows the maximum genetic stability, as chromosomal DNA rarely undergoes mutation or deletion. Green fluorescent protein (GFP), cytosine deaminase (CDase) gene, and LIGHT have been successfully integrated into chromosome [12, 71, 72]. However, as only one copy of the heterologous gene is integrated into the chromosome, limited heterologous proteins are expressed and therapeutic outcomes are restricted.

Another approach is to carry heterologous proteins on plasmids. Therefore, plasmid stability is the top priority for delivering cargo proteins into a tumor mass. Danino *et al.* recently studied the dynamics of plasmid instability *in vivo*, which showed that the rate of plasmid-carrying bacteria dropped from roughly 50% at 12 h to 10% at 24 h post intravenous injection into the tumor-bearing mice [73]. The plasmid loss results from an uneven bacterial replication as plasmid-free *Salmonella* replicate faster than plasmid-bearing *Salmonella* [74]. Thus, different methods were used to enhance plasmid retention, (i) toxin/antitoxin-based systems and (ii) conditional lethal systems.

The hok/sok locus is of the toxin/antitoxin-based system, where the hok gene encodes a cell killing protein and the sok gene transcripts an unstable antisense RNA complementary to the hok mRNA [74]. In newly born plasmid-free cells, sok-RNA is rapidly degraded, whereas the stable toxin hok mRNA is still available and encodes hok protein, thus ensuring a rapid and selective killing of these cells. The system has been utilized by Din *et al.* to minimize the extent of plasmid loss in the absence of antibiotic selection *in vivo* [75].

Another strategy to prevent plasmid loss is the conditional lethal system. In this system, an essential anabolism gene is inactivated and a copy of the intact gene is inserted into a plasmid to complement the mutation in the chromosome and ensure the presence of the plasmid. Yu and colleagues constructed a *Salmonella* mutant lacking the *asd* gene, which encodes an enzyme required for synthesis of diaminopimelic acid (DAP), an essential component of the cell wall [66]. Mutants without a plasmid-borne *asd* or cells grown in the absence of DAP lysed. Similarly, Kim *et al.* also constructed a balanced-lethal system based on the deletion of the *glmS* gene, which encodes an essential enzyme for cell wall synthesis [76]. Both systems have been successfully used in bacterial cancer therapy.

5.3.3 Regulation of Therapeutic Protein Expression

Another important aspect of using *Salmonella* as a delivery vector is to select an appropriate promoter to control protein expression. There are three categories of promoters used in *Salmonella*-mediated cancer therapy: constitutive promoters, inducible promoters, and microenvironment-sensing promoters. Compared with the other promoters, the constitutive promoter always produces therapeutic cargos, which may get distributed systemically and cause off-target side effects.

In contrast, the inducible promoters, which respond to chemical compounds or γ-irradiation, have been employed to control protein expression. Frahm *et al.* and Loessner *et al.* successfully employed the tightly regulated pBAD system, which was activated by L-arabinose to induce heterologous gene expression *in vivo* [70, 77]. The salicylate system is also tightly regulated and both intraperitoneal and intravenous administration of salicylate acid–induced gene expression *in vivo* [78, 79]. Although L-arabinose and salicylate are nontoxic and can amplify gene expression, they are limited to passive diffusion and inadequate tumor penetration. Another approach for using γ-irradiation to trigger gene expression can overcome these limitations. γ-Irradiation can easily penetrate a tumor and only treat cancerous regions. The RecA promoter was thus used to control TNF-related apoptosis-inducing ligand (TRAIL) and TNF-α expression [80, 81]. When irradiation caused double strand breaks in the bacterial genome, the RecA and its promoter were activated to induce therapeutic gene expression. However, this system produces high basal gene expression. To reduce the basal expression and increase radiation responsiveness, an extra Cheo box was incorporated into the RecA promoter to reduce basal expression and make the promoter more specific to radiation-induced activation [82].

Another strategy to strictly control protein expression is the quorum sensing system, which regulates protein expression based on population density. The system consists of two genes: *luxI* and *luxR*. *luxI* synthesizes the autoinducers, which freely cross the bacterial membrane and activate the transcriptional regulator protein LuxR. The autoinducer and LuxR complex binds to the *luxI* promoter and activates its transcription. Therefore, when the bacterial population density reaches a threshold and there are enough autoinducers, the gene under the control of the *luxI* promoter is expressed. The system has been used in previous research to trigger protein expression in tumors [75, 83]. Besides this, this system has been employed to amplify the expression of the desired protein induced with small molecules (e.g., L-arabinose) that diffuse poorly within the tumor mass [84]. Dai *et al.* showed that this system improved bacterial cell sensitivity to chemical signaling and bacterial protein production 350-fold in tumor tissue [84].

As *Salmonella* can sense and adapt to its microenvironment by regulating gene transcription, an alternative way to control gene expression is the microenvironment-sensing promoter. To identify the promoters that exclusively express genes in tumors, Arrach *et al.*, Leschner *et al.*, Flentie *et al.*, and our lab used high throughput methods to screen and identify tumor microenvironment-induced promoters [71, 85–87]. In their findings, different promoters that were specially activated in a tumor microenvironment were found and the pH and hypoxia were determined as the main stimulus for upregulation of gene expression. Thus, more hypoxia-sensitive promoters were identified. For example, hypoxia-sensitive promoters nirB, pepT, FF+20*, and adhE were used in *Salmonella*-mediated cancer therapy to confine the expression of therapeutic proteins to the anoxic region of tumors [71, 88–90]. However, these hypoxia promoters only regulated gene expression at indicated oxygen concentrations. Previous studies have shown that oxygen concentrations within tumors were highly heterogeneous and oxygen levels varied between different types of tumors [91]. To precisely control therapeutic gene expression in tumors with various oxygen levels, our lab is working on the identification of the promoters responsive to different oxygen levels for the precise expression of therapeutic genes under different tumor environments.

5.3.4 Compartmentalization of Therapeutic Agents

When *Salmonella* enters phagocytes, it is restricted to *Salmonella*-containing vaculos (SCVs) and isolated from the cytosol of the host cell. Localization within SCVs hampers the delivery of therapeutic particles into the cytosol of the host cell, especially when it is used for vaccines. Several strategies were exploited, including (i) direct surface display, (ii) the export of antigen to the extracellular space, and (iii) bacterial lysis.

5.3.4.1 Direct surface display

The display of proteins on bacteria is an attractive way to enhance bacterial tumor targeting efficiency and present heterologous proteins to the host immune system. The heterologous genes were fused into the gene encoding bacterial outer membrane proteins OmpA [92–94]. In addition, LamB and flagellin can be utilized to present heterologous proteins or peptides on the bacterial outer membrane. Anticarcinoembryonic antigen (scFV), anti-CD20 peptide, and RGD peptide were reported to be displayed on attenuated *Salmonella* and resulted in increased tumor targeting efficiency and therapeutic effects. Anti-CD20 antibody was displayed on attenuated *Salmonella* delivering a prodrug-converting enzyme to treat human lymphoma [94]. Park *et al.* showed that the display of the RGD peptide sequence on the outer membrane of *Salmonella* resulted in increased tumor targeting efficiency and therapeutic effects [93]. It has been assumed that the display of heterologous antigen has the potential to elicit potent humoral immunity. However, no successful evidence or example has been reported yet.

5.3.4.2 The export of heterologous proteins to extracellular space

The second approach is to export heterologous proteins to extracellular space. To export the protein, the *Salmonella* type three secretion system (TTSS) is employed. TTSS, which consists of structural proteins and effectors, is a needle-like structure expressed on bacterial cell surface to deliver bacterial protein into eukaryotic host cells. This translocation is mediated by the N-terminal amino acid sequence of effectors and changes in the C-terminal region of effectors do not interfere with translocation. Nishikawa *et al.* and Zhu *et al.* reported that tumor antigens secreted through SopE on SP-1 could efficiently elicit specific tumor responses [62, 95]. Compared with TTSS on SP-1, which is mainly assembled during bacterial invasion of host cell, TTSS on

SP-2 is mainly assembled when bacteria reside within the vaculos of host cells, thereby ensuring the necessary communication between bacteria and host cells. Furthermore, Manuel *et al.* systematically compared a serious of genes on SP-2 and found that the TAA fused to sseJ exhibited maximal potency for antigen translocation [96]. Consequently, complete tumor regression was observed. Thus, the delivery of tumor-associated antigens via TTSS is a prerequisite for active delivery as it can overcome major histocompatibility complex (MHC) class I–restricted immune responses. However, it should be taken into account that there are proteins or protein motifs that are not amenable to secretion through this pathway, for example, the proteins that cannot be unfolded. Therefore, if such a domain is present in the heterologous protein, it would hamper heterologous protein delivery via the type III secretion pathway.

5.3.4.3 The cell lysis system

Another strategy is the programmed cell lysis system. The system not only avoids potential risks posed by unintentional release of the genetically modified organisms into the environment but also readily passes through a bacterial membrane, thus further enhancing the immune responses to the expressed antigen. Jeong *et al.* and Camacho *et al.* placed the lysis genes of *Salmonella* phage Ieps5 under the control of an inducible promoter to release a therapeutic compound at a specified time [76, 79]. Another means with which to achieve programmed cell lysis is to employ *Salmonella* with deletions in asdA and murA, which results in complete lysis [97]. The expression of the complementing genes is controlled by an inducible promoter, such as pBAD. While the method releases the heterologous agents, it kills the bacteria and does not allow for continuous expression. In addition, the inducer employed to trigger bacterial lysis is limited by passive diffusion and may not reach the bacteria. To overcome these limitations, Din *et al.* designed a *Salmonella* strain that lysed in synchronized cycles [75]. The lytic system (φX174 gene E) was controlled by bacterial density. When the bacteria reached a threshold population, they lysed to release the therapeutic agents. After quorum lysed, the remaining survival bacteria began to grow, resulting in a pulsatile delivery system. Thus, the programmed cell lysis system shows a promising future for active delivery.

5.3.5 Expression of Anticancer Agents and Modulation of the Tumor Microenvironment

Various genes have been exploited and developed for *Salmonella*-mediated bacterial cancer therapy. On the basis of the mode of their functions, the genes can be divided into three categories (Table 5.3). The toxins that directly kill cancer cells are one of major therapeutic compounds that are delivered by *Salmonella*. Some of them are native bacterial toxins and function by forming pores in mammalian cell membranes and inducing apoptosis, such as hlyE [88]. Others are proapoptotic proteins that target eukaryotic cell signaling. For example, our lab engineered *Salmonella* to deliver a C-terminally truncated Fas-associated protein with death domain (FADD), which is more cytotoxic to murine melanoma cells [98]. Compared with bacterial toxins, which are effective anticancer agents as they are native to bacterial physiology, the proapoptotic proteins are more selectively cytotoxic to tumor cells.

Table 5.3 The therapeutic agents delivered by *Salmonella*

Therapeutic approach	Therapeutic gene	Refs.
Cytotoxic agents	*hlyE*	[88]
	Pseudomonas exotoxin A	[111]
	HPV16 E7 fusion protein,	[112]
	Cytotoxic protein cytolysin A (clyA)	[113]
	Cp53	[79]
	FalL	[114]
	TRAIL	[80, 89]
	Flt3L	[115]
	TNF-α	[101]
Cytokines	LIGHT	[72]
	IL-2	[99, 100, 116, 117]

	IL12	[118, 119]
	IL18	[120]
	CCL21	[121]
Antigens and antibodies	Prostate antigen + cholera toxin subunit B	[122]
	HSP70+taa	[95]
	RAF	[123]
	VEGF receptor	[118, 124]
Prodrug system	Prodrug-activating enzyme carboxypeptidase G2 Herpes simplex virus thymidine kinase Prodrug-converting enzyme	[94, 125]
	Purine nucleoside phosphorylase	[126]
	Mouse a-fetoprotein (AFP) gene	[127]
Vascular	Cytosine deaminase gene	[12, 128, 129]
	Thrombospondin-1 (TSP-1)	[130]

As a tumor creates an environment where immune surveillance fails to work, an alternative method for bacterial cancer therapy is to boost the immune system to fight against cancer. *Salmonella* has been exploited to carry a number of different cytokines or tumor-associated antigens to enhance its anticancer activity. Cytokines exert their antitumor capacities by inducing and activating immune cells. *Salmonella* can selectively release cytokines into the tumor without causing severe side effects, and promising results were obtained from *Salmonella*-carried immunostimulatory molecules, such as IL-2, TNF-α, and LIGHT [72, 99–101]. The delivery of a tumor-associated antigen is another approach that is used in bacterial-mediated cancer immunotherapy. By fusing the proteins that were upregulated in tumors to secretion signals described above, these bacterial therapies can effectively prevent or treat tumors [102–104]. To create a more effective immune response to tumor, various adjuvants were also added. The addition of adjuvants not only helps cross the mucosal barrier but also facilitates cross presentation of exogenous antigens [105].

Salmonella were also utilized to deliver shRNA to selectively silence the overexpressed proteins in tumors. Up to now, many genes have been silenced using this system [106–108]. For example, as *Salmonella* could predominantly target and kill cancer stem cells (CSCs), which were reported to correlate with tumor progression, metastatic potential, and poor prognosis, our lab silenced the expression of ATP binding cassette bump 5 (ABCB5), a CSC marker of melanoma cells [107, 109, 110]. VNP-shABCB5 made cancer cells more vulnerable to chemotherapy, and promising therapeutic effects were obtained. In addition, our lab engineered a VNP(*PhoP*/Q−) mutant that exhibited a better safety level and released a shRNA-expressing plasmid into the cytoplasm of host cells [50].

5.4 Combined Therapy

5.4.1 Combined with Chemotherapy

In the past decades, chemotherapy was widely used to fight cancer. However, drug resistance is one of major obstacles that hinder greater success of chemotherapy. To overcome this limitation, engineered *Salmonella* was combined with chemotherapeutic drugs and some promising results were obtained. Previous studies showed that *Salmonella* plus cyclophosphamide, trastuzumab, or cisplatin acted additively to retard tumor growth and extensively prolonged the mice survival time [107, 131, 132]. Most recently, Mercado-Lubo *et al.* identified the *Salmonella* type III secreted effector SipA as the key virulence factor responsible for modulating the multidrug resistance transporter P-glycoprotein (P-gp) [133]. This finding may explain the enhanced anticancer activity of the combined therapy. In addition, Yano and colleagues showed that the *Salmonella* A1-R strain made quiescent cancer cells sensitive to cytotoxic chemotherapy by decoying cancer cells cycle from G0/G1 to S/G2/M [134]. Therefore, the combination of *Salmonella* and cisplatinum or paclitaxel exhibited better anticancer activity compared with treatment alone. As CSCs in tumors tend to be resistant to chemotherapy, our group targeted ABCB5, which conferred drug resistance in CSC by small short interfering RNA delivered by VNP20009 [107].

The combined treatment of VNP20009 carrying shABCB5 with CTX efficiently reduced tumor growth and prolonged survival time by reducing ABCB5 expression and inhibiting chemotherapy resistance.

Another problem of conventional cancer chemotherapy is lack of tumor specificity. *Salmonella*-mediated enzyme prodrug therapy, which converts nontoxic chemical compounds into cytotoxic drugs, decreases the side effects from the treatment. Several prodrug converting enzymes have been attempted in *Salmonella*. Expression of CDase in *Salmonella* has been reported to convert 5-fuorocytosine into 5-fuorouracil and inhibit colon tumor growth. This system was also tested in a small clinical trial with three patients [12]. Although CDase expressing *Salmonella* colonized in the tumors of two of the three patients and converted 5-FC to 5-FU, no significant tumor regression was observed. This failure might result from poor tumor colonization of VNP20009, similar to the problem that VNP20009 faced in the phase I clinical trial. The uneven biodistribution of *Salmonella* in a tumor might also lead to this failure. As *Salmonella* mainly accumulated in hypoxic regions where prodrugs hardly reached, further genetic modification is required to optimize the targeting of *Salmonella*.

5.4.2 Combined with Other Treatments

Combining with radiotherapy is another promising strategy that *Salmonella* utilizes to enhance its anticancer capacity. Avogadri and colleagues demonstrated that *Salmonella*-based therapy coupled with low-dose radiotherapy enhanced the anticancer capacity of *Salmonella* by dampening tumor immune escape mechanisms [135]. Similarly, Yoon *et al.* also reported using *Salmonella* with γ-radiation to potently suppress tumor growth [136].

In addition, therapeutic effects of *Salmonella* could be enhanced by combining it with purified proteins. The antiangiogenic agents, including endostatin, vascular endothelial growth factor (VEGF), and endostatin-derivated peptide HM-3, have been successfully administrated in combination with *Salmonella*, and all showed promising clinical potentials [137–139].

Most recently, researchers have started to develop a novel strategy of combing *Salmonella* with nanoparticles. By coating *Salmonella* with synthetic nanoparticles, Hu *et al.* engineered a coating of live bacteria to deliver DNA vaccines to the tumor [140]. It was shown that the protective nanoparticle coating layer not only helped the bacteria to escape the phagosomes but also enhanced the acid tolerance of *Salmonella* in the stomach and intestines after oral administration and successful inhibition of tumor growth was achieved. Another approach used by Mercado-Lubo *et al.* was to combine *Salmonella* proteins with gold nanoparticles to mimic the ability of *Salmonella* to reverse multidrug resistance [133]. Although it circumvented the safety concern of using *Salmonella*, the application of nanoparticles also discarded all the benefits that *Salmonella* owns as a vehicle. For example, nanoparticles distribute nonspecifically and inadequately accumulate in a tumor. In addition, it is a one-point release system and does not allow for continuous expression of therapeutic drugs.

5.5 Conclusion

As *Salmonella* possesses unique properties to make it specially colonize in tumors and inhibit tumor growth, it is a promising anticancer agent. Despite proven safe, clinical trials using *Salmonella* to control tumors were disappointing. Thus, tremendous efforts have been devoted to enhance its anticancer capacity. These improvements will definitely promote *Salmonella*-based cancer therapy potential and improve its clinical outcome.

Acknowledgment

This study was supported by grants from the Doctoral Station Science Foundation of the Chinese Ministry of Education (20130091130003), the Chinese National Natural Sciences Foundation (81630092, 81573338, 81421091), the National Key Research Program by Ministry of Science and Technology (2014CB744501, 2016YFC0902700), the Shenzhen Science and Technology Innovation Committee (JCYJ20160331152141936), and the Shenzhen Peacock Plan (KQTD20140630165057031).

References

1. Wei M. Q., Mengesha A., Good D., Anne J. Bacterial targeted tumour therapy—dawn of a new era. *Cancer Letters*, 259(1) (2008) 16–27.
2. HoptionCann S. A., van Netten J. P., van Netten C. Dr William Coley and tumour regression: A place in history or in the future. *Postgraduate Medical Journal*, 79(938) (2003) 672–680.
3. Coley W. B. The treatment of inoperable sarcoma by bacterial toxins (the mixed toxins of the *Streptococcus erysipelas* and the *Bacillus prodigiosus*). *Proceedings of the Royal Society of Medicine*, 3 (Surg Sect) (1910) 1–48.
4. Forbes N. S. Engineering the perfect (bacterial) cancer therapy. *Nature Reviews, Cancer*, 10(11) (2010) 785–794.
5. Yu Y. A., Shabahang S., Timiryasova T. M., Zhang Q., Beltz R., Gentschev I., *et al.* Visualization of tumors and metastases in live animals with bacteria and vaccinia virus encoding light-emitting proteins. *Nature Biotechnology*, 22(3) (2004) 313–320.
6. Pan Z. K., Weiskirch L. M., Paterson Y. Regression of established B16F10 melanoma with a recombinant *Listeria monocytogenes* vaccine. *Cancer Research*, 59(20) (1999) 5264–5269.
7. Arakawa M., Sugiura K., Reilly H. C., Stock C. C. Oncolytic effect of *Proteus mirabilis* upon tumor-bearing animals. II. Effect on transplantable mouse and rat tumors. *GANN*, 59(2) (1968) 117–122.
8. Bhatnagar P. K., Awasthi A., Nomellini J. F., Smit J., Suresh M. R. Anti-tumor effects of the bacterium *Caulobacter crescentus* in murine tumor models. *Cancer Biology & Therapy*, 5(5) (2006) 485–491.
9. Kohwi Y., Imai K., Tamura Z., Hashimoto Y. Antitumor effect of *Bifidobacterium infantis* in mice. *GANN*, 69(5) (1978) 613–618.
10. Toso J. F., Gill V. J., Hwu P., Marincola F. M., Restifo N. P., Schwartzentruber D. J., *et al.* Phase I study of the intravenous administration of attenuated *Salmonella typhimurium* to patients with metastatic melanoma. *Journal of Clinical Oncology*, 20(1) (2002) 142–152.
11. Heimann D. M., Rosenberg S. A. Continuous intravenous administration of live genetically modified *Salmonella typhimurium* in patients with metastatic melanoma. *Journal of Immunotherapy (Hagerstown, Md.: 1997)*, 26(2) (2003) 179–180.
12. Nemunaitis J., Cunningham C., Senzer N., Kuhn J., Cramm J., Litz C., *et al.* Pilot trial of genetically modified, attenuated *Salmonella*

expressing the *E. Coli* cytosine deaminase gene in refractory cancer patients. *Cancer Gene Therapy*, 10(10) (2003) 737–744.

13. Schmitz-Winnenthal F. H., Hohmann N., Niethammer A. G., Friedrich T., Lubenau H., Springer M., *et al.* Anti-angiogenic activity of VXM01, an oral T-cell vaccine against VEGF receptor 2, in patients with advanced pancreatic cancer: A randomized, placebo-controlled, phase 1 trial. *Oncoimmunology*, 4(4) (2015) e1001217.
14. Lee C. H., Wu C. L., Shiau A. L. Toll-like receptor 4 mediates an antitumor host response induced by *Salmonella choleraesuis*. *Clinical Cancer Research*, 14(6) (2008) 1905–1912.
15. Kaimala S., Mohamed Y. A., Nader N., Issac J., Elkord E., Chouaib S., *et al. Salmonella*-mediated tumor regression involves targeting of tumor myeloid suppressor cells causing a shift to m1-like phenotype and reduction in suppressive capacity. *Cancer Immunology, Immunotherapy: CII*, 63(6) (2014) 587–599.
16. Phan T. X., Nguyen V. H., Duong M. T., Hong Y., Choy H. E., Min J. J. Activation of inflammasome by attenuated *Salmonella typhimurium* in bacteria-mediated cancer therapy. *Microbiology and Immunology*, 59(11) (2015) 664–675.
17. Kim J. E., Phan T. X., Nguyen V. H., Dinh-Vu H. V., Zheng J. H., Yun M., *et al. Salmonella typhimurium* suppresses tumor growth via the pro-inflammatory cytokine interleukin-1β. *Theranostics*, 5(12) (2015) 1328–1342.
18. Zhang X., Xu Q., Yang L., Lai Y., Zhang Z., Han C., *et al.* The genes slyA, STM3120 and htrA are required for the anticancer ability of VNP20009. *Oncotarget*, 7 (2016) 81187–81196, doi: 10.18632/oncotarget.13217.
19. Westphal K., Leschner S., Jablonska J., Loessner H., Weiss S. Containment of tumor-colonizing bacteria by host neutrophils. *Cancer Research*, 68(8) (2008) 2952–2960.
20. Lee C. H., Wu C. L., Chen S. H., Shiau A. L. Humoral immune responses inhibit the antitumor activities mediated by *Salmonella enterica* serovar Choleraesuis. *Journal of Immunotherapy (Hagerstown, Md.: 1997)*, 32(4) (2009) 376–388.
21. Leschner S., Westphal K., Dietrich N., Viegas N., Jablonska J., Lyszkiewicz M., *et al.* Tumor invasion of *Salmonella enterica* serovar Typhimurium is accompanied by strong hemorrhage promoted by TNF-α. *PLOS One*, 4(8) (2009) e6692.

22. Guo Z. L., Yu B., Ning B. T., Chan S., Lin Q. B., Li J. C., *et al.* Genetically modified "obligate" anaerobic *Salmonella typhimurium* as a therapeutic strategy for neuroblastoma. *Journal of Hematology & Oncology*, 8 (2015) 99.

23. Avogadri F., Martinoli C., Petrovska L., Chiodoni C., Transidico P., Bronte V., *et al.* Cancer immunotherapy based on killing of *Salmonella*-infected tumor cells. *Cancer Research*, 65(9) (2005) 3920–3927.

24. Lee C. H., Hsieh J. L., Wu C. L., Hsu P. Y., Shiau A. L. T cell augments the antitumor activity of tumor-targeting *Salmonella*. *Applied Microbiology and Biotechnology*, 90(4) (2011) 1381–1388.

25. Liu T., Chopra A. K. An enteric pathogen *Salmonella enterica* serovar Typhimurium suppresses tumor growth by down regulating $CD44^{high}$ and CD4T regulatory (T_{reg}) cell expression in mice: The critical role of lipopolysaccharide and braun lipoprotein in modulating tumor growth. *Cancer Gene Therapy*, 17(2) (2010) 97–108.

26. Kuan Y. D., Lee C. H. *Salmonella* overcomes tumor immune tolerance by inhibition of tumor indoleamine 2,3-dioxygenase 1 expression. *Oncotarget*, 7(1) (2016) 374–385.

27. Saccheri F., Pozzi C., Avogadri F., Barozzi S., Faretta M., Fusi P., *et al.* Bacteria-induced gap junctions in tumors favor antigen cross-presentation and antitumor immunity. *Science Translational Medicine*, 2(44) (2010) 44ra57.

28. Lee C. H., Hsieh J. L., Wu C. L., Hsu H. C., Shiau A. L. B cells are required for tumor-targeting *Salmonella* in host. *Applied Microbiology and Biotechnology*, 92(6) (2011) 1251–1260.

29. Pawelek J. M., Sodi S., Chakraborty A. K., Platt J. T., Miller S., Holden D. W., *et al.* *Salmonella* pathogenicity island-2 and anticancer activity in mice. *Cancer Gene Therapy*, 9(10) (2002) 813–818.

30. Silva-Valenzuela C. A., Desai P. T., Molina-Quiroz R. C., Pezoa D., Zhang Y., *et al.* Solid tumors provide niche-specific conditions that lead to preferential growth of *Salmonella*. *Oncotarget*, 7(23) (2016) 35169–35180.

31. Arrach N., Cheng P., Zhao M., Santiviago C. A., Hoffman R. M., McClelland M. High-throughput screening for *Salmonella* avirulent mutants that retain targeting of solid tumors. *Cancer Research*, 70(6) (2010) 2165–2170.

32. Toley B. J., Forbes N. S. Motility is critical for effective distribution and accumulation of bacteria in tumor tissue. *Integrative Biology: Quantitative Biosciences From Nano To Macro*, 4(2) (2012) 165–176.

33. Ganai S., Arenas R. B., Sauer J. P., Bentley B., Forbes N. S. In tumors *Salmonella* migrate away from vasculature toward the transition zone and induce apoptosis. *Cancer Gene Therapy*, 18(7) (2011) 457–466.

34. Kasinskas R. W., Forbes N. S. *Salmonella typhimurium* lacking ribose chemoreceptors localize in tumor quiescence and induce apoptosis. *Cancer Research*, 67(7) (2007) 3201–3209.

35. Kasinskas R. W., Forbes N. S. *Salmonella typhimurium* specifically chemotax and proliferate in heterogeneous tumor tissue in vitro. *Biotechnology and Bioengineering*, 94(4) (2006) 710–721.

36. Forbes N. S., Munn L. L., Fukumura D., Jain R. K. Sparse initial entrapment of systemically injected *Salmonella typhimurium* leads to heterogeneous accumulation within tumors. *Cancer Research*, 63(17) (2003) 5188–5193.

37. Panteli J. T., Forbes N. S. Engineered bacteria detect spatial profiles in glucose concentration within solid tumor cell masses. *Biotechnology and Bioengineering*, 113(11) (2016) 2474–2484.

38. Choe E., Kazmierczak R. A., Eisenstark A. Phenotypic evolution of therapeutic *Salmonella enterica* serovar Typhimurium after invasion of tramp mouse prostate tumor. *mBio*, 5(4) (2014) e01182–e01114.

39. Broadway K. M., Modise T., Jensen R. V., Scharf B. E. Complete genome sequence of *Salmonella enterica* serovar Typhimurium VNP20009, a strain engineered for tumor targeting. *Journal of Biotechnology*, 192(Pt A) (2014) 177–178.

40. Broadway K. M., Denson E. A., Jensen R. V., Scharf B. E. Rescuing chemotaxis of the anticancer agent *Salmonella enterica* serovar Typhimurium VNP20009. *Journal of Biotechnology*, 211 (2015) 117–120.

41. Low K. B., Ittensohn M., Le T., Platt J., Sodi S., Amoss M., *et al.* Lipid a mutant *Salmonella* with suppressed virulence and TNF alpha induction retain tumor-targeting in vivo. *Nature Biotechnology*, 17(1) (1999) 37–41.

42. Low K. B., Ittensohn M., Luo X., Zheng L. M., King I., Pawelek J. M., *et al.* Construction of VNP20009: A novel, genetically stable antibiotic-sensitive strain of tumor-targeting *Salmonella* for

parenteral administration in humans. *Methods in Molecular Medicine*, 90 (2004) 47–60.

43. Toso J. F., Gill V. J., Hwu P., Marincola F. M., Restifo N. P., *et al.* Phase i study of the intravenous administration of attenuated *Salmonella typhimurium* to patients with metastatic melanoma. *Journal of Clinical Oncology*, 20(1) (2002) 142–152.
44. Zhao M., Geller J., Ma H., Yang M., Penman S., Hoffman R. M. Monotherapy with a tumor-targeting mutant of *Salmonella typhimurium* cures orthotopic metastatic mouse models of human prostate cancer. *Proceedings of the National Academy of Sciences of the United States of America*, 104(24) (2007) 10170–10174.
45. Zhao M., Yang M., Ma H., Li X., Tan X., Li S., *et al.* Targeted therapy with a *Salmonella typhimurium* leucine–arginine auxotroph cures orthotopic human breast tumors in nude mice. *Cancer Research*, 66(15) (2006) 7647–7652.
46. Zhang Y., Miwa S., Zhang N., Hoffman R. M., Zhao M. Tumor-targeting *Salmonella typhimurium* A1-R arrests growth of breast-cancer brain metastasis. *Oncotarget*, 6(5) (2015) 2615–2622.
47. Matsumoto Y., Miwa S., Zhang Y., Zhao M., Yano S., Uehara F., *et al.* Intraperitoneal administration of tumor-targeting *Salmonella typhimurium* A1-R inhibits disseminated human ovarian cancer and extends survival in nude mice. *Oncotarget*, 6(13) (2015) 11369–11377.
48. Toneri M., Miwa S., Zhang Y., Hu C., Yano S., Matsumoto Y., *et al.* Tumor-targeting *Salmonella typhimurium* A1-R inhibits human prostate cancer experimental bone metastasis in mouse models. *Oncotarget*, 6(31) (2015) 31335–31343.
49. Nagakura C., Hayashi K., Zhao M., Yamauchi K., Yamamoto N., Tsuchiya H., *et al.* Efficacy of a genetically-modified *Salmonella typhimurium* in an orthotopic human pancreatic cancer in nude mice. *AntiCancer Research*, 29(6) (2009) 1873–1878.
50. Cheng X., Zhang X., Zhou Y., Zhang C., Hua Z. C. A *Salmonella typhimurium* mutant strain capable of RNAi delivery: Higher tumor-targeting and lower toxicity. *Cancer Biology & Therapy*, 15(8) (2014) 1068–1076.
51. Chirullo B., Ammendola S., Leonardi L., Falcini R., Petrucci P., Pistoia C., *et al.* Attenuated mutant strain of *Salmonella typhimurium* lacking the ZnuABC transporter contrasts tumor growth promoting anti-cancer immune response. *Oncotarget*, 6(19) (2015) 17648–17660.

52. Yu B., Yang M., Shi L., Yao Y. D., Jiang Q. Q., Li X. F., *et al.* Explicit hypoxia targeting with tumor suppression by creating an "obligate" anaerobic *Salmonella typhimurium* strain. *Scientific Reports*, 2 (2012) 436.
53. Zhang Y., Zhang N., Zhao M., Hoffman R. M. Comparison of the selective targeting efficacy of *Salmonella typhimurium* A1-R and VNP20009 on the Lewis lung carcinoma in nude mice. *Oncotarget*, 6(16) (2015) 14625–14631.
54. Hayashi K., Zhao M., Yamauchi K., Yamamoto N., Tsuchiya H., Tomita K., *et al.* Systemic targeting of primary bone tumor and lung metastasis of high-grade osteosarcoma in nude mice with a tumor-selective strain of *Salmonella typhimurium*. *Cell Cycle* (Georgetown, Tex.), 8(6) (2009) 870–875.
55. Yam C., Zhao M., Hayashi K., Ma H., Kishimoto H., McElroy M., *et al.* Monotherapy with a tumor-targeting mutant of *S. typhimurium* inhibits liver metastasis in a mouse model of pancreatic cancer. *The Journal of Surgical Research*, 164(2) (2010) 248–255.
56. Kimura H., Zhang L., Zhao M., Hayashi K., Tsuchiya H., Tomita K., *et al.* Targeted therapy of spinal cord glioma with a genetically modified *Salmonella typhimurium*. *Cell Proliferation*, 43(1) (2010) 41–48.
57. Matsumoto Y., Miwa S., Zhang Y., Hiroshima Y., Yano S., Uehara F., *et al.* Efficacy of tumor-targeting *Salmonella typhimurium* A1-R on nude mouse models of metastatic and disseminated human ovarian cancer. *Journal of Cellular Biochemistry*, 115(11) (2014) 1996–2003.
58. Momiyama M., Zhao M., Kimura H., Tran B., Chishima T., Bouvet M., *et al.* Inhibition and eradication of human glioma with tumor-targeting *Salmonella typhimurium* in an orthotopic nude-mouse model. *Cell Cycle* (Georgetown, Tex.), 11(3) (2012) 628–632.
59. Zhang L., Gao L., Zhao L., Guo B., Ji K., Tian Y., *et al.* Intratumoral delivery and suppression of prostate tumor growth by attenuated *Salmonella enterica* serovar Typhimurium carrying plasmid-based small interfering RNAs. *Cancer Research*, 67(12) (2007) 5859–5864.
60. Guan G. F., Zhao M., Liu L. M., Jin C. S., Sun K., Zhang D. J., *et al.* *Salmonella typhimurium* mediated delivery of apoptin in human laryngeal cancer. *International Journal of Medical Sciences*, 10(12) (2013) 1639–1648.

61. Li X., Li Y., Hu J., Wang B., Zhao L., Ji K., *et al.* Plasmid-based E6-specific siRNA and co-expression of wild-type p53 suppresses the growth of cervical cancer in vitro and in vivo. *Cancer Letters*, 335(1) (2013) 242–250.

62. Nishikawa H., Sato E., Briones G., Chen L. M., Matsuo M., Nagata Y., *et al.* In vivo antigen delivery by a *Salmonella typhimurium* type III secretion system for therapeutic cancer vaccines. *The Journal of Clinical Investigation*, 116(7) (2006) 1946–1954.

63. Berger E., Soldati R., Huebener N., Hohn O., Stermann A., Durmus T., *et al. Salmonella* SL7207 application is the most effective DNA vaccine delivery method for successful tumor eradication in a murine model for neuroblastoma. *Cancer Letters*, 331(2) (2013) 167–173.

64. al-Ramadi B. K., Fernandez-Cabezudo M. J., El-Hasasna H., Al-Salam S., Bashir G., Chouaib S. Potent anti-tumor activity of systemically administered IL2-expressing *Salmonella* correlates with decreased angiogenesis and enhanced tumor apoptosis. *Clinical Immunology* (Orlando, Fla.), 130(1) (2009) 89–97.

65. Yang N., Zhu X., Chen L., Li S., Ren D. Oral administration of attenuated *S. typhimurium* carrying shRNA-expressing vectors as a cancer therapeutic. *Cancer Biology & Therapy*, 7(1) (2008) 145–151.

66. Yu B., Yang M., Shi L., Yao Y., Jiang Q., Li X., *et al.* Explicit hypoxia targeting with tumor suppression by creating an "obligate" anaerobic *Salmonella typhimurium* strain. *Scientific Reports*, 2 (2012) 436.

67. Thornlow D. N., Brackett E. L., Gigas J. M., Van Dessel N., Forbes N. S. Persistent enhancement of bacterial motility increases tumor penetration. *Biotechnology and Bioengineering*, 112(11) (2015) 2397–2405.

68. Zhang M., Forbes N. S. Trg-deficient *Salmonella* colonize quiescent tumor regions by exclusively penetrating or proliferating. *Journal of Controlled Release*, 199 (2015) 180–189.

69. Felgner S., Frahm M., Kocijancic D., Rohde M., Eckweiler D., Bielecka A., *et al.* aroA-deficient *Salmonella enterica* serovar Typhimurium is more than a metabolically attenuated mutant. *mBio*, 7(5) (2016) pii: e01220-16.

70. Frahm M., Felgner S., Kocijancic D., Rohde M., Hensel M., Curtiss R. 3rd, *et al.* Efficiency of conditionally attenuated *Salmonella enterica* serovar Typhimurium in bacterium-mediated tumor therapy. *mBio*, 6(2) (2015) pii: e00254-15.

71. Chen J., Wei D., Zhuang H., Qiao Y., Tang B., Zhang X., *et al.* Proteomic screening of anaerobically regulated promoters from *Salmonella* and its antitumor applications. *Molecular & Cellular Proteomics*, 10(6) (2011) M111.009399.

72. Loeffler M., Le'Negrate G., Krajewska M., Reed J. C. Attenuated *Salmonella* engineered to produce human cytokine light inhibit tumor growth. *Proceedings of the National Academy of Sciences of the United States of America*, 104(31) (2007) 12879–12883.

73. Danino T., Lo J., Prindle A., Hasty J., Bhatia S. N. In vivo gene expression dynamics of tumor-targeted bacteria. *ACS Synthetic Biology*, 1(10) (2012) 465–470.

74. Kroll J., Klinter S., Schneider C., Voss I., Steinbuchel A. Plasmid addiction systems: Perspectives and applications in biotechnology. *Microbial Biotechnology*, 3(6) (2010) 634–657.

75. Din M. O., Danino T., Prindle A., Skalak M., Selimkhanov J., Allen K., *et al.* Synchronized cycles of bacterial lysis for in vivo delivery. *Nature*, 536(7614) (2016) 81–85.

76. Kim K., Jeong J. H., Lim D., Hong Y., Yun M., Min J. J., *et al.* A novel balanced-lethal host-vector system based on *glmS*. *PLOS One*, 8(3) (2013) e60511.

77. Loessner H., Endmann A., Leschner S., Westphal K., Rohde M., Miloud T., *et al.* Remote control of tumour-targeted *Salmonella enterica* serovar Typhimurium by the use of L-arabinose as inducer of bacterial gene expression in vivo. *Cellular Microbiology*, 9(6) (2007) 1529–1537.

78. Royo J. L., Becker P. D., Camacho E. M., Cebolla A., Link C., Santero E., *et al.* In vivo gene regulation in *Salmonella* spp. by a salicylate-dependent control circuit. *Nature Methods*, 4(11) (2007) 937–942.

79. Camacho E. M., Mesa-Pereira B., Medina C., Flores A., Santero E. Engineering *Salmonella* as intracellular factory for effective killing of tumour cells. *Scientific Reports*, 6 (2016) 30591.

80. Ganai S., Arenas R. B., Forbes N. S. Tumour-targeted delivery of trail using *Salmonella typhimurium* enhances breast cancer survival in mice. *British Journal of Cancer*, 101(10) (2009) 1683–1691.

81. Nuyts S., Van Mellaert L., Theys J., Landuyt W., Bosmans E., Anne J., *et al.* Radio-responsive recA promoter significantly increases TNF-alpha production in recombinant clostridia after 2 Gy irradiation. *Gene Therapy*, 8(15) (2001) 1197–1201.

82. Nuyts S., Van Mellaert L., Barbe S., Lammertyn E., Theys J., Landuyt W., *et al.* Insertion or deletion of the Cheo box modifies radiation

inducibility of *Clostridium* promoters. *Applied and Environmental Microbiology*, 67(10) (2001) 4464–4470.

83. Swofford C. A., Van Dessel N., Forbes N. S. Quorum-sensing *Salmonella* selectively trigger protein expression within tumors. *Proceedings of the National Academy of Sciences of the United States of America*, 112(11) (2015) 3457–3462.

84. Dai Y., Toley B. J., Swofford C. A., Forbes N. S. Construction of an inducible cell-communication system that amplifies *Salmonella* gene expression in tumor tissue. *Biotechnology and Bioengineering*, 110(6) (2013) 1769–1781.

85. Flentie K., Kocher B., Gammon S. T., Novack D. V., McKinney J. S., Piwnica-Worms D. A bioluminescent transposon reporter-trap identifies tumor-specific microenvironment-induced promoters in *Salmonella* for conditional bacterial-based tumor therapy. *Cancer Discovery*, 2(7) (2012) 624–637.

86. Leschner S., Deyneko I. V., Lienenklaus S., Wolf K., Bloecker H., Bumann D., *et al.* Identification of tumor-specific *Salmonella typhimurium* promoters and their regulatory logic. *Nucleic Acids Research*, 40(7) (2012) 2984–2994.

87. Arrach N., Zhao M., Porwollik S., Hoffman R. M., McClelland M. *Salmonella* promoters preferentially activated inside tumors. *Cancer Research*, 68(12) (2008) 4827–4832.

88. Ryan R. M., Green J., Williams P. J., Tazzyman S., Hunt S., Harmey J. H., *et al.* Bacterial delivery of a novel cytolysin to hypoxic areas of solid tumors. *Gene Therapy*, 16(3) (2009) 329–339.

89. Chen J., Yang B., Cheng X., Qiao Y., Tang B., Chen G., *et al. Salmonella*-mediated tumor-targeting trail gene therapy significantly suppresses melanoma growth in mouse model. *Cancer Science*, 103(2) (2012) 325–333.

90. Cheng X., Zhang X., Cheng W., Chen J., Ma C., Yang B., *et al.* Tumor-specific delivery of histidine-rich glycoprotein suppresses tumor growth and metastasis by anti-angiogenesis and vessel normalization. *Current Gene Therapy*, 14(2) (2014) 75–85.

91. Brown J. M., Wilson W. R. Exploiting tumour hypoxia in cancer treatment. *Nature reviews. Cancer*, 4(6) (2004) 437–447.

92. Bereta M., Hayhurst A., Gajda M., Chorobik P., Targosz M., Marcinkiewicz J., *et al.* Improving tumor targeting and therapeutic potential of *Salmonella* VNP20009 by displaying cell surface CEA-specific antibodies. *Vaccine*, 25(21) (2007) 4183–4192.

93. Park S. H., Zheng J. H., Nguyen V. H., Jiang S. N., Kim D. Y., Szardenings M., *et al.* RGD peptide cell-surface display enhances the targeting and therapeutic efficacy of attenuated *Salmonella*-mediated cancer therapy. *Theranostics*, 6(10) (2016) 1672–1682.

94. Massa P. E., Paniccia A., Monegal A., de Marco A., Rescigno M. *Salmonella* engineered to express CD20-targeting antibodies and a drug-converting enzyme can eradicate human lymphomas. *Blood*, 122(5) (2013) 705–714.

95. Zhu X., Zhou P., Cai J., Yang G., Liang S., Ren D. Tumor antigen delivered by *Salmonella* III secretion protein fused with heat shock protein 70 induces protection and eradication against murine melanoma. *Cancer Science*, 101(12) (2010) 2621–2628.

96. Xu X., Hegazy W. A., Guo L., Gao X., Courtney A. N., Kurbanov S., *et al.* Effective cancer vaccine platform based on attenuated *Salmonella* and a type III secretion system. *Cancer Research*, 74(21) (2014) 6260–6270.

97. Kong W., Wanda S. Y., Zhang X., Bollen W., Tinge S. A., Roland K. L., *et al.* Regulated programmed lysis of recombinant *Salmonella* in host tissues to release protective antigens and confer biological containment. *Proceedings of the National Academy of Sciences of the United States of America*, 105(27) (2008) 9361–9366.

98. Yang Y. W., Zhang C. M., Huang X. J., Zhang X. X., Zhang L. K., Li J. H., *et al.* Tumor-targeted delivery of a C-terminally truncated FADD (N-FADD) significantly suppresses the B16F10 melanoma via enhancing apoptosis. *Scientific Reports*, 6 (2016) 34178.

99. Ha X. Q., Yin Q., Zhao H. B., Hui L., Wang M. L., Peng J. H., *et al.* Inhibitory effects of the attenuated *Salmonella typhimurium* containing the IL-2 gene on hepatic tumors in mice. *Journal of Biomedicine & Biotechnology*, 2012 (2012) 946139.

100. Sorenson B. S., Banton K. L., Frykman N. L., Leonard A. S., Saltzman D. A. Attenuated *Salmonella typhimurium* with IL-2 gene reduces pulmonary metastases in murine osteosarcoma. *Clinical Orthopaedics and Related Research*, 466(6) (2008) 1285–1291.

101. Yoon W. S., Chae Y. S., Hong J., Park Y. K. Antitumor therapeutic effects of a genetically engineered *Salmonella typhimurium* harboring TNF-α in mice. *Applied Microbiology and Biotechnology*, 89(6) (2011) 1807–1819.

102. Xiong G., Husseiny M. I., Song L., Erdreich-Epstein A., Shackleford G. M., Seeger R. C., *et al.* Novel cancer vaccine based on genes of *Salmonella* pathogenicity island 2. *International Journal of Cancer*, 126(11) (2010) 2622–2634.

103. Wang Y. J., Hou Y., Huang H., Liu G. R., White A. P., Liu S. L. Two oral HBx vaccines delivered by live attenuated *Salmonella*: Both eliciting effective anti-tumor immunity. *Cancer Letters*, 263(1) (2008) 67–76.

104. Stark F. C., Sad S., Krishnan L. Intracellular bacterial vectors that induce CD8(+) T cells with similar cytolytic abilities but disparate memory phenotypes provide contrasting tumor protection. *Cancer Research*, 69(10) (2009) 4327–4334.

105. Lin I. Y., Van T. T., Smooker P. M. Live-attenuated bacterial vectors: Tools for vaccine and therapeutic agent delivery. *Vaccines*, 3(4) (2015) 940–972.

106. Blache C. A., Manuel E. R., Kaltcheva T. I., Wong A. N., Ellenhorn J. D., Blazar B. R., *et al.* Systemic delivery of *Salmonella typhimurium* transformed with IDO shRNA enhances intratumoral vector colonization and suppresses tumor growth. *Cancer Research*, 72(24) (2012) 6447–6456.

107. Zhang X., Cheng X., Lai Y., Zhou Y., Cao W., Hua Z. C. *Salmonella* VNP20009-mediated RNA interference of ABCB5 moderated chemoresistance of melanoma stem cell and suppressed tumor growth more potently. *Oncotarget*, 7(12) (2016) 14940–14950.

108. Manuel E. R., Blache C. A., Paquette R., Kaltcheva T. I., Ishizaki H., Ellenhorn J. D., *et al.* Enhancement of cancer vaccine therapy by systemic delivery of a tumor-targeting *Salmonella*-based STAT3 shRNA suppresses the growth of established melanoma tumors. *Cancer Research*, 71(12) (2011) 4183–4191.

109. Chang W. W., Kuan Y. D., Chen M. C., Lin S. T., Lee C. H. Tracking of mouse breast cancer stem-like cells with *Salmonella*. *Experimental Biology and Medicine*, 237(10) (2012) 1189–1196.

110. Hiroshima Y., Zhao M., Zhang Y., Maawy A., Hassanein M. K., Uehara F., *et al.* Comparison of efficacy of *Salmonella typhimurium* A1-R and chemotherapy on stem-like and non-stem human pancreatic cancer cells. *Cell Cycle*, 12(17) (2013) 2774–2780.

111. Quintero D., Carrafa J., Vincent L., Bermudes D. EGFR-targeted chimeras of pseudomonas toxA released into the extracellular milieu by attenuated *Salmonella* selectively kill tumor cells. *Biotechnology and Bioengineering*, 113(12) (2016) 2698–2711.

112. Yoon W., Choi J. H., Kim S., Park Y. K. Engineered *Salmonella typhimurium* expressing E7 fusion protein, derived from human papillomavirus, inhibits tumor growth in cervical tumor-bearing mice. *Biotechnology Letters*, 36(2) (2014) 349–356.

113. Nguyen V. H., Kim H. S., Ha J. M., Hong Y., Choy H. E., Min J. J. Genetically engineered *Salmonella typhimurium* as an imageable therapeutic probe for cancer. *Cancer Research*, 70(1) (2010) 18–23.

114. Loeffler M., Le'Negrate G., Krajewska M., Reed J. C. Inhibition of tumor growth using *Salmonella* expressing Fas ligand. *Journal of the National Cancer Institute*, 100(15) (2008) 1113–1116.

115. Yoon W. S., Choi W. C., Sin J. I., Park Y. K. Antitumor therapeutic effects of *Salmonella typhimurium* containing Flt3 ligand expression plasmids in melanoma-bearing mouse. *Biotechnology Letters*, 29(4) (2007) 511–516.

116. Barnett S. J., Soto L. J. 3rd, Sorenson B. S., Nelson B. W., Leonard A. S., Saltzman D. A. Attenuated *Salmonella typhimurium* invades and decreases tumor burden in neuroblastoma. *Journal of Pediatric Surgery*, 40(6) (2005) 993–997, discussion 997–998.

117. Sorenson B. S., Banton K. L., Frykman N. L., Leonard A. S., Saltzman D. A. Attenuated *Salmonella typhimurium* with interleukin 2 gene prevents the establishment of pulmonary metastases in a model of osteosarcoma. *Journal of Pediatric Surgery*, 43(6) (2008) 1153–1158.

118. Keke F., Hongyang Z., Hui Q., Jixiao L., Jian C. A combination of flk1-based DNA vaccine and an immunomodulatory gene (IL-12) in the treatment of murine cancer. *Cancer Biotherapy & Radiopharmaceuticals*, 19(5) (2004) 649–657.

119. Jang M. J., Kim J. E., Chung Y. H., Lee W. B., Shin Y. K., Lee J. S., *et al.* Dendritic cells stimulated with outer membrane protein A (OmpA) of *Salmonella typhimurium* generate effective anti-tumor immunity. *Vaccine*, 29(13) (2011) 2400–2410.

120. Loeffler M., Le'Negrate G., Krajewska M., Reed J. C. IL-18-producing *Salmonella* inhibit tumor growth. *Cancer Gene Therapy*, 15(12) (2008) 787–794.

121. Loeffler M., Le'Negrate G., Krajewska M., Reed J. C. *Salmonella typhimurium* engineered to produce CCL21 inhibit tumor growth. *Cancer Immunology, Immunotherapy*, 58(5) (2009) 769–775.

122. Fensterle J., Bergmann B., Yone C. L., Hotz C., Meyer S. R., Spreng S., *et al.* Cancer immunotherapy based on recombinant *Salmonella enterica* serovar Typhimurium aroA strains secreting prostate-specific antigen and cholera toxin subunit B. *Cancer Gene Therapy*, 15(2) (2008) 85–93.

123. Gentschev I., Fensterle J., Schmidt A., Potapenko T., Troppmair J., Goebel W., *et al.* Use of a recombinant *Salmonella enterica* serovar

Typhimurium strain expressing c-RAF for protection against c-RAF induced lung adenoma in mice. *BMC Cancer*, 5 (2005) 15.

124. Lu X. L., Jiang X. B., Liu R. E., Zhang S. M. The enhanced anti-angiogenic and antitumor effects of combining flk1-based DNA vaccine and IP-10. *Vaccine*, 26(42) (2008) 5352–5357.

125. Friedlos F., Lehouritis P., Ogilvie L., Hedley D., Davies L., Bermudes D., *et al.* Attenuated *Salmonella* targets prodrug activating enzyme carboxypeptidase G2 to mouse melanoma and human breast and colon carcinomas for effective suicide gene therapy. *Clinical Cancer Research*, 14(13) (2008) 4259–4266.

126. Fu W., Lan H., Liang S., Gao T., Ren D. Suicide gene/prodrug therapy using *Salmonella*-mediated delivery of *Escherichia coli* purine nucleoside phosphorylase gene and 6-methoxypurine 2′-deoxyriboside in murine mammary carcinoma 4T1 model. *Cancer Science*, 99(6) (2008) 1172–1179.

127. Chou C. K., Hung J. Y., Liu J. C., Chen C. T., Hung M. C. An attenuated *Salmonella* oral DNA vaccine prevents the growth of hepatocellular carcinoma and colon cancer that express alpha-fetoprotein. *Cancer Gene Therapy*, 13(8) (2006) 746–752.

128. Jazowiecka-Rakus J., Szala S. Antitumour activity of *Salmonella typhimurium* VNP20047 in B16(F10) murine melanoma model. *Acta Biochimica Polonica*, 51(3) (2004) 851–856.

129. Mesa-Pereira B., Medina C., Camacho E. M., Flores A., Santero E. Improved cytotoxic effects of *Salmonella*-producing cytosine deaminase in tumour cells. *Microbial Biotechnology*, 8(1) (2015) 169–176.

130. Lee C. H., Wu C. L., Shiau A. L. Systemic administration of attenuated *Salmonella choleraesuis* carrying thrombospondin-1 gene leads to tumor-specific transgene expression, delayed tumor growth and prolonged survival in the murine melanoma model. *Cancer Gene Therapy*, 12(2) (2005) 175–184.

131. Hiroshima Y., Zhang Y., Zhao M., Zhang N., Murakami T., Maawy A., *et al.* Tumor-targeting *Salmonella typhimurium* A1-R in combination with trastuzumab eradicates HER-2-positive cervical cancer cells in patient-derived mouse models. *PLOS One*, 10(6) (2015) e0120358.

132. Lee C. H., Wu C. L., Tai Y. S., Shiau A. L. Systemic administration of attenuated *Salmonella choleraesuis* in combination with cisplatin for cancer therapy. *Molecular Therapy*, 11(5) (2005) 707–716.

133. Mercado-Lubo R., Zhang Y., Zhao L., Rossi K., Wu X., Zou Y., *et al.* A *Salmonella* nanoparticle mimic overcomes multidrug resistance in tumours. *Nature Communications*, 7 (2016) 12225.

134. Yano S., Zhang Y., Zhao M., Hiroshima Y., Miwa S., Uehara F., *et al.* Tumor-targeting *Salmonella typhimurium* A1-R decoys quiescent cancer cells to cycle as visualized by FUCCI imaging and become sensitive to chemotherapy. *Cell Cycle* (Georgetown, Tex.), 13(24) (2014) 3958–3963.

135. Avogadri F., Mittal D., Saccheri F., Sarrafiore M., Ciocca M., Larghi P., *et al.* Intra-tumoral *Salmonella typhimurium* induces a systemic anti-tumor immune response that is directed by low-dose radiation to treat distal disease. *European Journal of Immunology*, 38(7) (2008) 1937–1947.

136. Yoon W. S., Kim S., Seo S., Park Y. *Salmonella typhimurium* with gamma-radiation induced H2AX phosphorylation and apoptosis in melanoma. *Bioscience, Biotechnology, and Biochemistry*, 78(6) (2014) 1082–1085.

137. Jia L. J., Xu H. M., Ma D. Y., Hu Q. G., Huang X. F., Jiang W. H., *et al.* Enhanced therapeutic effect by combination of tumor-targeting *Salmonella* and endostatin in murine melanoma model. *Cancer Biology & Therapy*, 4(8) (2005) 840–845.

138. Hiroshima Y., Zhang Y., Murakami T., Maawy A., Miwa S., Yamamoto M., *et al.* Efficacy of tumor-targeting *Salmonella typhimurium* A1-R in combination with anti-angiogenesis therapy on a pancreatic cancer patient-derived orthotopic xenograft (PDOX) and cell line mouse models. *Oncotarget*, 5(23) (2014) 12346–12357.

139. Zhao C., He J., Cheng H., Zhu Z., Xu H. Enhanced therapeutic effect of an antiangiogenesis peptide on lung cancer in vivo combined with *Salmonella* VNP20009 carrying a Sox2 shRNA construct. *Journal of Experimental & Clinical Cancer Research*, 35(1) (2016) 107.

140. Hu Q., Wu M., Fang C., Cheng C., Zhao M., Fang W., *et al.* Engineering nanoparticle-coated bacteria as oral DNA vaccines for cancer immunotherapy. *Nano Letters*, 15(4) (2015) 2732–2739.

Chapter 6

Genetically Engineered Oncolytic *Salmonella typhimurium*

Jin Hai Zheng[a] **and Jung-Joon Min**[a,b]

[a]*Laboratory of In Vivo Molecular Imaging, Institute for Molecular Imaging and Theranostics, 264 Seoyangro, Hwasun, Jeonnam 58128, Republic of Korea*
[b]*Department of Nuclear Medicine, Chonnam National University Medical School, 5 Hak 1 dong, Dong-gu, Gwangju 61469, Republic of Korea*

jjmin@jnu.ac.kr

Attenuated strains of *Salmonella typhimurium* specifically colonize and proliferate in cancer tissues, resulting in marked tumor reduction or even complete eradication. This chapter focuses on *S. typhimurium* defective in ppGpp synthesis (ΔppGpp). This strain was found to have a median lethal dose (LD_{50}) 100,000 to 1,000,000 times higher than that of the wild type, with specific targeting of various tumor types in mice and good safety profiles. To improve the efficacy of bacteria-mediated cancer therapy, the bacteria were genetically engineered to deliver and overexpress anticancer proteins under the control of inducible promoters. In addition, the attenuated bacteria can be engineered to express reporter genes for noninvasive imaging *in vivo*.

Microbial Infections and Cancer Therapy: Recent Advances
Edited by Ananda M. Chakrabarty and Arsénio M. Fialho

ISBN 978-981-4774-86-4 (Hardcover), 978-1-351-04190-4 (eBook)
www.panstanford.com

6.1 Introduction

6.1.1 Bacterial Cancer Therapy

Bacteria-mediated cancer therapy was first introduced at the end of the 19th century, when the American bone surgeon Dr. William B. Coley tried to treat inoperable sarcoma patients with *Streptococcus pyogenes*. Over the next 40 years, over 1000 cancer patients were treated with Coley's toxin, a mixture of heat-inactivated *Streptococcus pyogenes* and *Serratia marcescens*, with cures observed in more than 25% of the sarcoma patients and in some patients with other types of cancer [1]. Because these results were rarely reproducible, Coley's toxin gradually disappeared from medical practice after the advent of radiotherapy and chemotherapy. Advances in immunology and biotechnology, however, have clarified the mechanism underlying the effects of Coley's toxin, leading to renascent research on bacterial cancer therapy.

Tumor microenvironments are characterized by hypoxia, the release of small molecular nutrients from dying cancer cells, and protection from immune surveillance, all of which favor the specific growth of anaerobic bacteria in tumor tissues. Over the past two decades, several obligatory and facultative anaerobic bacteria, including *Bifidobacterium* [2], *Clostridium* [3], *Salmonella* [4–6], and *Escherichia coli* [7, 8], have been tested in mouse cancer models and in phase I clinical trials in human cancer patients. Attenuated strains of *S. typhimurium* have shown excellent tumor targeting and induction of robust anticancer activity, and several genetically engineered attenuated strains of *S. typhimurium* have been tested in tumor models [9]. One example is the VNP20009 strain, with mutations in *purI* and *msbB*, which showed a 10-fold reduction in tumor necrosis factor alpha (TNF-α)-induced shock compared with wild-type *S. typhimurium* [2]. Tumor biopsies taken after administration of this strain to patients with metastatic melanoma and renal carcinoma showed substantial tumor colonization [2]. Another attenuated *S. typhimurium* strain, A1-R, which is defective in leucine and arginine synthesis, was found to inhibit tumor growth in various mouse models [5, 10].

6.1.2 ΔppGpp *S. typhimurium* Strain and Cancer Therapy

The ΔppGpp *S. typhimurium* strain, which is defective in guanosine 5′-diphosphate-3′-diphosphate synthesis, has shown anticancer effects in animals without notable toxicity [11, 12]. This strain was constructed from wild-type *S. typhimurium* strain 14028s by double depletion of *relA* and *spoT*, strongly attenuating its infectiveness in mice and its invasiveness *in vitro* due to the lack of the key intermediate molecule ppGpp. The LD_{50} of live ΔppGpp *Salmonella* administered orally or intraperitoneally to female Balb/c mice was about 10^5-fold higher than that of wild-type *S. typhimurium* [13]. Following its intravenous injection, tumor tissues were found to accumulate concentrations of ΔppGpp *S. typhimurium* as high as 10^{10} colony-forming units (CFU)/g, or about 10,000-fold higher than its concentration in the liver [6].

Systemic administration of avirulent ppGpp *S. typhimurium* to mice was found to activate host immune responses. Pattern recognition receptors (PRRs) on immune cells, such as toll-like receptors (TLRs), broadly recognize molecules shared by pathogens, but not host cells or tissues. Among the molecules recognized by TLRs are specifically conserved components on bacteria, called pathogen-associated molecular patterns (PAMPs). These bacterial PAMPs, such as lipopolysaccharide (LPS), flagellin, and CpG sites, bind to TLRs and activate TLR signaling pathways to induce innate and adaptive immune responses. Colonization of tumor tissues by ΔppGpp *S. typhimurium* was found to increase the production of proinflammatory cytokines, including TNF-α, interleukin (IL)-1β, and IL-18 [14, 15]; to activate the inflammasome pathway [15]; and to polarize tumor-associated macrophages (TAMs) into M1-like macrophages [6, 16].

6.1.3 Strategies for Enhanced Bacterial Cancer Therapy

To increase bacterial anticancer activity, engineered strains of ΔppGpp *S. typhimurium* have been used as delivery and expression vectors to send payloads specifically to tumor tissues. For example, attenuated *S. typhimurium* has been engineered to express the cytolytic protein cytolysin A (ClyA) [11, 17], the immune stimulatory ligand *Vibrio vulnificus* flagellin B (FlaB) [6], the mitochondrial target domain (Noxa) [18], the apoptotic cell death inducer L-asparaginase (L-ASNase) [19], and the immunotoxin (TNF-α-PE38) [20], with these strains showing greatly enhanced tumor suppression compared with ΔppGpp *S. typhimurium* in various mouse tumor models. Moreover, bacterial distribution *in vivo* has been monitored by engineering the attenuated *S. typhimurium* to express bacterial, firefly, or renilla luciferase [11, 17], allowing these bacteria to be easily tracked using optical imaging devices.

6.2 Generation of Attenuated Strains and Molecular Imaging Strategies

6.2.1 Engineering of *S. typhimurium* Strains for Virulence Attenuation

Wild-type *S. typhimurium* is extremely toxic when administered directly to animals, but very low doses are usually insufficient to induce notable anticancer effects. Thus, these bacteria must be attenuated by genetic engineering before their application to cancer research. Several approaches have been used to generate attenuated *S. typhimurium* strains with decreased toxicity and increased tumor targeting.

- Bacterial components can be modified to reduce inflammatory stimulation of the host immune system. For example, the LPS mutant strain VNP20009, with deletions of *purI* and *msbB* from the bacterial chromosome, showed a 10,000-fold increase in LD_{50} in animals [4].
- Nutrient auxotrophs can be generated by depleting certain genes, such as leucine, arginine, and aromatic acid synthetases [10, 21], making the growth of these strains dependent on the extracellular nutrient supply. However, in the tumor microenvironment, small molecular nutrients released from apoptotic/necrotic cancer cells may enhance the ability of these attenuated *S. typhimurium* strains to colonize and proliferate in tumor tissues.
- The expression of toxic genes can be inactivated or down-regulated. Deletions of *relA* and *spoT* suppressed the synthesis of ppGpp, markedly down-regulating the expression

of various virulence genes, including those encoded on *Salmonella* pathogenicity island 1 (SPI1) that are required for the invasion of host cells and induction of macrophage apoptosis [22].

- Advantage can be taken of the tumor microenvironment, with hypoxia utilized to express essential bacterial genes, such as *asd*, which encode the enzyme aspartate-semialdehyde dehydrogenase and are under the control of hypoxia-inducible promoter (HIP)-1. Thus, these bacteria can survive only under hypoxic conditions, greatly reducing their cytotoxicity to normal tissues and increasing their tumor-specific proliferation [23].

6.2.2 Expression of Reporter Genes for Noninvasive Imaging

To monitor bacterial distribution *in vivo*, attenuated strains have been engineered to express reporter genes for noninvasive imaging. Administration of attenuated *S. typhimurium* expressing fluorescence proteins, such as green fluorescence protein (GFP), followed by noninvasive optical fluorescence molecular imaging, can detect bacteria both *in vitro* and *in vivo* [5]. Limitations, however, include autofluorescence and limited depth of penetration. Bioluminescence imaging is widely used in preclinical molecular imaging as it has some advantages over other imaging modalities, including excellent sensitivity, multiplexing capabilities, and lack of endogenous bioluminescence. The bacterial luciferase (Lux) operon consists of the *lux A, B, C, D,* and *E* genes. The *lux A* and *B* genes encode the α and β subunits of luciferase, which catalyze light emission, whereas the *lux C, D,* and *E* genes encode enzymes responsible for aldehyde synthesis of $FMNH_2$, which is readily provided by the electron transport chain present in all bacteria. Introduction of the Lux operon into the bacterial chromosome, along with P22HT *int* transduction, results in continuous robust expression of the luminescence gene, with no additional exogenous substrate required [17]. Administration of engineered light-emitting ΔppGpp *S. typhimurium* to various mouse cancer models showed specific signals in tumors (Fig. 6.1). In addition to bacterial luciferase, firefly luciferase, which requires the substrate D-luciferin, and renilla luciferase, which reacts with the substrate coelenterazine and its analogs, have been utilized as reporters for *in vivo* imaging to monitor bacterial colonization or anticancer gene expression [11]. Moreover, attenuated *S. typhimurium* expressing herpes simplex virus *thymidine kinase* (HSV1-*tk*) selectively colonized tumor xenografts and effectively sequestered a radiolabeled nucleoside analog, 2′-fluoro-1-β-D-arabino-furanosyl-5-iodouracil (FIAU), allowing detection by positron emission tomography (PET) [24].

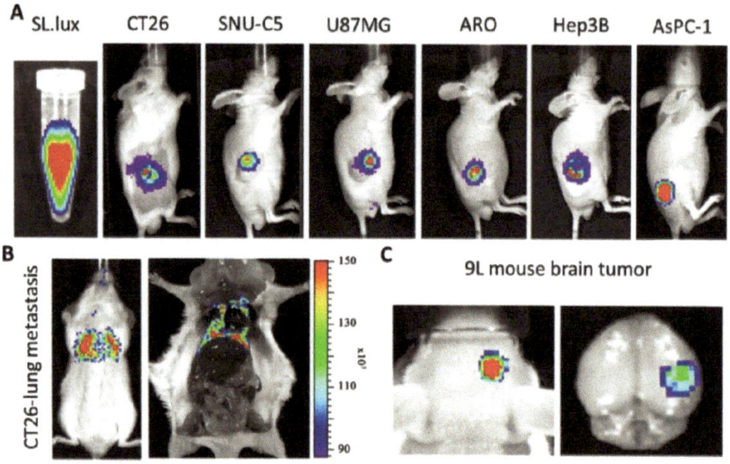

Figure 6.1 Bacterial targeting in several kinds of cancer models. Attenuated ΔppGpp *S. typhimurium* transduced with the bacterial *lux* operon for noninvasive imaging. (A) Bacterial bioluminescence imaging in several kinds of subcutaneous cancer models. (B) Bacterial targeting in a CT26 lung metastasis model, involving intravenous injection of cancer cells. (C) Attenuated *S. typhimurium* colonization of a 9L orthotopic mouse brain tumor. CT26, murine colon adenocarcinoma; SNU-C5, human gastric carcinoma; U87MG, human glioblastoma; ARO, human thyroid cancer; Hep3B, human hepatocellular carcinoma; AsPC-1, human pancreatic cancer.

6.3 Surface Engineering for Enhanced Tumor Targeting

The abilities of attenuated *S. typhimurium* to colonize and proliferate in tumors and to suppress tumor growth have been found to be specific to cancer types. The targeting efficiency of attenuated *S. typhimurium* in some cancer models was found to be lower, reducing bacterially mediated antitumor activity. Various strategies involving the display of cancer-specific binding domains have therefore been developed to enhance tumor-specific bacterial colonization. For example, the protein alpha V beta 3 ($\alpha_V\beta_3$) integrin is highly expressed on activated endothelial cells, newly generated blood vessels, and some tumor cells and is regarded essential for cancer angiogenesis [25]. The arginine-glycine-aspartate (RGD) specifically binds to $\alpha_V\beta_3$ integrin with high affinity and has been utilized in cancer diagnostic imaging after conjugation with certain imaging probes (e.g., fluorochromes for optical imaging, radionuclides for PET imaging, and magnetic compounds for magnetic resonance imaging). In addition, conjugation of RGD with chemotherapeutic agents, such as doxorubicin, chlorambucil, and camptothecin, can greatly increase the anticancer specificity of these agents and reduce their toxicity to normal tissues [26, 27]. Engineered *S. typhimurium* displaying RGD on its surface showed strongly increased tumor targeting in $\alpha_V\beta_3$-overexpressing cancer xenografts, inhibiting tumor development and improving animal survival [12]. In addition, the presence of an anti-CD20 single-domain antibody on the surface of attenuated *S. typhimurium* and expression of a prodrug-converting enzyme further suppressed the growth of human lymphoma xenografts in mouse models [28].

Current biotechnology techniques, including phage display, yeast display, gene sequencing, and biosynthesis, will enable the identification of additional cancer-specific markers, including tumor-specific antigens and cancer-related overexpression of surface receptors, as well as cancer-binding domains. This may result in additional engineering of attenuated *S. typhimurium*, further improving the targeting and delivery of bacteria-mediated treatment of certain types of cancers.

6.4 Engineering of *Salmonella* for Payload Expression

6.4.1 Inducible Expression System

Delivery and expression of cancer therapeutic genes using engineered attenuated *S. typhimurium* were found to drastically suppress tumor growth. Following systemic administration to tumor-bearing mice via the tail vein, however, genetically engineered *S. typhimurium* became initially and transiently localized to reticuloendothelial organs. Constitutive expression of anticancer drugs during the early phase of infection, before these bacteria specifically colonized tumor tissue, could induce unwanted damage in normal organs, such as the liver and spleen. To avoid systemic toxicity, different inducible promoters have been applied to bacterial drug delivery systems. The expression of therapeutic genes is usually induced three to four days after bacterial infection, when these bacteria have specifically colonized tumor tissues [6, 11, 17], thus minimizing toxicity to normal organs. Toxicity was analyzed by measuring serum or plasma concentrations of aspartate aminotransferase (AST), alanine aminotransferase (ALT), blood urea nitrogen (BUN), creatinine, C-reactive protein (CRP), and procalcitonin (PCT) after infection with ΔppGpp *S. typhimurium* harboring different plasmid structures. All of these parameters were within normal ranges, with no systemic toxicity observed, when therapeutic gene expression was induced after the bacteria specifically colonized tumor tissues; by contrast, ALT and AST concentrations were specifically increased, indicating liver damage, when gene expression was induced soon after infection [6, 11, 12]. Among the strategies utilized to trigger gene expression during *S. typhimurium*-mediated cancer therapy are external trigger systems involving an L-arabinose-inducible pBAD promoter [6, 17, 29], a tetracycline- or doxycycline-inducible pTet promoter [11], and a γ-irradiation-inducible pRecA promoter [30]; environmental sensing systems involving hypoxia-inducible fumarate and a nitrate reduction regulator [31]; and quorum sensing systems, in which target gene expression is triggered at the high bacterial densities usually observed in tumor tissues [32]. This section will describe the tetracycline/doxycycline-inducible pTet promoter and the L-arabinose-inducible pBAD promoter in more detail.

6.4.1.1 Tetracycline/doxycycline-inducible pTet promoter

Tetracycline and doxycycline, an analog of tetracycline, exhibit properties of ideal inducers, including the effective induction of gene expression at very low concentrations (nmol/l range); good bioavailability, in that they can penetrate both bacterial and animal cells; nontoxicity at therapeutic concentrations, with approval for human clinical use; and stability, allowing long-term therapeutic activity. Repressor-regulated tetracycline efflux systems contain two genes, *tetA* and *tetR*, separated by an intergenic region. This intergenic region contains two promoters, one that drives the expression of *tetR*, which encodes the TetR repressor to suppress gene transcription, and one that drives the expression of *tetA*, which encodes the TetA efflux pump. The intergenic region also contains two *tetO* operators that regulate gene expression. In the absence of tetracycline/doxycycline, TetR is bound to *tetO*, which prevents the expression of TetA and TetR. In the presence of tetracycline, TetR binds to tetracycline and undergoes a conformational change that results in the dissociation of TetR from the *tetO* operators and expression of TetA and TetR. Because of the divergent nature of *tetR* and *tetA* transcription, replacing *tetA* with a gene of interest and placing a second gene of interest downstream of the repressor gene (*tetR*) would enable bilateral dual gene expression in a tetracycline-inducible system. Expression of target genes carried by a dual-expression vector showed excellent correlation between the *tetA* and *tetR* promoters, with the former considered more powerful for gene transcription. Bacterial cancer therapy with a dual-expression vector carrying a therapeutic gene under the control of the *tetA* promoter and a reporter gene under the control of the *tetR* promoter would therefore enable noninvasive monitoring of bacterial distribution and anticancer gene expression *in vivo* [11]. This type of vector would therefore result in effective anticancer therapy and imaging simultaneously or expression of synergistic anticancer molecules, further enhancing its therapeutic efficacy.

6.4.1.2 L-arabinose-inducible pBAD promoter

Gene expression under the control of a pBAD promoter is tightly regulated by a nontoxic sugar, L-arabinose. The pBAD promoter originates from the *E. coli* arabinose operon. The pC promoter, which constitutively controls the transcription of *araC* in the opposite direction, is adjacent to the pBAD promoter. Constitutively expressed AraC positively and negatively regulates gene transcription by binding to the pBAD promoter. In the absence of L-arabinose, AraC dimerizes the O_2 and I_1 operator sites, forming a DNA loop. This looping prevents transcription of pBAD and pC by inhibiting the binding of cyclic AMP receptor protein (CAP) and RNA polymerase. In the presence of L-arabinose, arabinose bound to AraC dimerizes the I_1 and I_2 operators, allowing CAP and RNA polymerase to bind to linear DNA, activating the transcription of the pBAD and pC promoters. The pBAD promoter has been found to be an excellent promoter, with gene expression tightly regulated by L-arabinose, thus allowing the precise expression of target genes *in vivo* by remote control [6, 17, 29].

6.4.1.3 Strategy to enhance pBAD promoter performance with Ara mutant

The specific delivery and expression of anticancer drugs in tumor tissues under the control of the pBAD promoter was found to enhance the therapeutic effect of ΔppGpp *S. typhimurium*. L-arabinose, however, cannot accumulate in bacteria, as it is metabolized to D-xylulose-5-P by enzymes encoded by the *ara* operon in *Salmonella*. Thus, sustained high concentration of L-arabinose should enhance protein expression. Protein expression was enhanced by deleting the *ara* operon from ΔppGpp *S. typhimurium* using λ red recombination [33]. The *ara* operon was replaced with a linear DNA carrying an antibiotic-resistant gene with homology to its adjacent regions. Proteins expression by a plasmid encoding renilla luciferase variant 8 (rluc8) and cytolysin A (ClyA) was evaluated in the *ara* mutant and parental strains. *In vitro* luciferase assays demonstrated that, following L-arabinose induction, rluc8 expression was 49-fold higher in the *ara* mutant than in the parental strain. Similar findings were observed by noninvasive *in vivo* imaging, with the *ara* operon–deleted strain showing comparable signal intensity in tumors following intraperitoneal injection of 12 mg/mouse as the parental strain following injection of 120 mg/mouse. At the higher L-arabinose concentration (120 mg/mouse), the *ara* mutant strain showed a 30-fold stronger rluc8 signal and a greater expression of the oncolytic protein ClyA than the parental strain. Moreover, the mutant strain had higher anticancer activity in a subcutaneous CT26 mouse colon cancer model [33]. These findings suggest that this strategy can further improve the performance of the pBAD promoter and enable more efficient cancer killing.

6.4.2 Strategy to Enhance Plasmid Maintenance in Bacteria

The attenuated ΔppGpp *S. typhimurium* strain showed specific tumor colonization and served as an ideal vector for the delivery of anticancer genes encoded by genetically constructed plasmids. However, plasmid stability is critical for the successful delivery of payloads into tumor tissues, and the use of antibiotic-resistant genes as a selective determinant for plasmid maintenance is impractical *in vivo*. This problem was first addressed by the construction of a balanced-lethal system, involving a plasmid bearing the *asd* gene of *Streptococcus mutans* that complements a mutated *asd* gene in the chromosome of the *Salmonella* strain. The *asd* gene encodes an enzyme required for the synthesis of diaminopimeic acid (DAP), an essential component of cell wall peptidoglycans of gram-negative bacteria. Bacteria with *asd* mutants lacking DAP quickly undergo lysis. Because DAP is not present in mammalian tissues, this balanced-lethal system ensures that all surviving *asd* mutant *Salmonella* carry the recombinant *Asd*$^+$ plasmid [34]. This concept was also used to develop another balanced-lethal host system, involving an enzyme essential for peptidoglycan synthesis in *E. coli* and *S. typhimurium*. Mutants with a defective *glmS* gene are strictly dependent on the presence of exogenous D-glucosamine (GlcN) and N-acetyl-D-glucosamine (GlcNAc). Because these compounds are not found in mammalian tissues, this balanced lethal system requires that *Salmonella* carry a recombinant *GlmS*$^+$ plasmid for survival. A *glmS* mutant strain of *S. typhimurium* carrying a *GlmS*$^+$ plasmid showed very strict maintenance of the recombinant plasmid *in vivo*, enabling the efficient delivery of a therapeutic gene to tumor tissues [35].

6.4.3 Payloads for *Salmonella*-Mediated Cancer Therapy

Because the ΔppGpp *S. typhimurium* strain is highly attenuated and is unable to invade mammalian cells, bacterial toxicity should be limited to cancer cells. This attenuated strain showed selective colonization of various tumor types, with a concentration in tumors as high as 10^{10} CFU/g after systemic infection. Genetically engineered ΔppGpp *S. typhimurium* may therefore constitute a novel delivery and expression vector for cancer therapy (Table 6.1).

Table 6.1 Attenuated ΔppGpp *S. typhimurium* for cancer therapy

Strain	Promoter	Cargos	Cancer models	Description	Refs
ΔppGpp			CT26 and MC38	Activation of inflammasome	[14, 15]
	pBAD	ClyA	CT26 and Hep3B	Delivery of oncolytic protein	[17]
	pTet	ClyA, rluc8	CT26 and Hep3B[a]	Dual expression for cancer theranostics	[11]
	pBAD	FlaB	MC38 and orthotopic [b]HCT116 cancer	Stimulation of host anticancer activity	[9]
	pBAD	Noxa	CT26	Mitochondrial targeting domain inducing apoptosis	[18]
	pBAD	L-asparaginase	4T1,[c] MC38,[d] and AsPC-1[e]	Induction of cell apoptosis	[19]
	pBAD	TGFα-PE38	CT26,[f] 4T1, MC38, and SW620[g]	Immunotoxin	[20]
	pBAD	RGD	Human breast cancer and melanoma	Surface engineering with enhanced targeting	[12]
ΔppGpp, Δara	pBAD	ClyA	CT26	Enhance protein expression with *ara* mutant	[33]

[a]Hep3B: Human hepatocellular carcinoma
[b]HCT116: Human colorectal carcinoma
[c]4T1: Mouse mammary cancer
[d]MC38 and [f]CT26: Mouse colon carcinoma
[e]AsPC-1: Human pancreatic cancer
[g]SW620: Human colorectal adenocarcinoma

6.4.3.1 Cytotoxic protein: ClyA

ClyA (or haemolysin E, HlyE) is a pore-forming protein hemolytic protein expressed by *E. coli* and the *Salmonella enterica* serovars Typhi and Paratyphi A [36]. Outer-membrane vesicles (OMVs) released from bacteria contain ClyA protein, and ClyA is toxic to mammalian cells in a contact-dependent manner. Because ClyA kills mammalian cells in a nonspecific manner, constitutive expression of this protein would induce tissue damage in normal reticuloendothelial organs, such as the liver and spleen, which usually show high bacterial colonization during the initial stages of bacterial infection. Because tight control of ClyA expression *in vivo* is required for cancer treatment, we utilized inducible promoters to deliver ClyA to mouse tumors, thereby minimizing its nonspecific toxicity. Both L-arabinose-inducible pBAD promoter and tetracycline/doxycycline-inducible pTet promoter systems showed good expression of ClyA, with no evidence of toxicity, after bacteria specifically colonized tumor tissues. Treatment with ΔppGpp *S. typhimurium* secreting ClyA resulted in tumor regression of mouse colon cancer, human hepatocellular carcinoma, and lung metastasis, with prolonged animal survival [11, 17]. The nonspecific mammalian cell killing by ClyA-secreting *S. typhimurium* may have some advantages over other cancer-targeted chemotherapy regimens, as the former can also destroy cancer stromal cells in "cold" tumors such as pancreatic cancer, which are usually resistant to T cell infiltration and to therapeutic agents [37].

6.4.3.2 Immunomodulator: FlaB

Bacterial flagellin from both gram-positive and gram-negative bacteria is the natural ligand of toll-like receptor 5 (TLR5), and activation of the TLR5 signaling pathway mobilizes nuclear factor (NF)-κB and induces the production of TNF-α. Activation of TLR5 by purified flagellin results in the regression of TLR5-positive breast and colon cancers [38, 39]. However, this strategy is restricted to TLR5-positive cancer models and multiple injections are required. We recently used an engineered *S. typhimurium* to overexpress heterologous flagellin, enhancing cancer immunotherapy [6]. Because high concentrations of bacteria accumulate in tumors, and these bacteria continuously secrete abundant amounts of flagellin after induction, their anticancer effects are markedly enhanced. Flagellins in *V. vulnificus* flagellum are encoded by six flagellin structural genes (*flaA*, *flaB*, *flaF*, *flaC*, *flaD*, and *flaE*), with FlaB being the most crucial building block [40]. FlaB has been applied as an adjuvant in combination with human papillomavirus (HPV) E6/E7 antigens to treat both subcutaneous and orthotopic genital cancer models, inducing robust anticancer immunity and suggesting that FlaB is an excellent adjuvant for cancer immunotherapy [41, 42]. FlaB has high binding affinity to TLR5 and was more potent in stimulating TLR5 signaling than *Salmonella* flagellin FliC [40].

Colonization of tumor tissues by attenuated *S. typhimurium* tissues resulted in acute inflammation and the recruitment of immune cells, such as monocytes, macrophages, and neutrophils [6, 14]. Infection-mediated immune cell infiltration was associated with the interaction between bacterial LPS and the host toll-like receptor 4 (TLR4) signaling pathway [6]. LPS activation of TLR4 led to the production of chemokines, such as macrophage-inflammatory protein-2 (MIP-2) and KC, promoting the recruitment of neutrophils, macrophages, and immature dendritic cells (DCs) [43, 44]. Bacterial infection of TLR4 knockout mice failed to recruit immune cells, including monocytes/macrophages and neutrophils, whereas infection of TLR5$^{-/-}$ mice recruited as many immune cells as wild-type mice, indicating that TLR4, but not TLR5, is required for immune cell recruitment (Fig. 6.2). This study involved tumor models with low surface TLR5 expression, including the MC38 murine colon adenocarcinoma and HCT116 human colorectal carcinoma models, suggesting that the anticancer effect of FlaB is mediated through host TLR5. Treatment with FlaB-secreting *S. typhimurium* effectively suppressed tumor growth and metastasis in mouse cancer models, while prolonging animal survival [6]. Anticancer activities were completely abrogated in TLR4$^{-/-}$ and MyD88$^{-/-}$ knockout mice but only partly in TLR5$^{-/-}$ knockout mice, suggesting that TLR4 signaling and immune cell infiltration are necessary for FlaB-expressing bacteria-mediated cancer therapy (Fig. 6.3). FlaB subsequently secreted by colonizing *S. typhimurium* further activated recruited immune cells, resulting in the phenotypic and functional activation of TAMs, with polarization into M1-like macrophages and a reciprocal reduction in M2-like suppressive activities [6]. Because flagellin monomers bind to TLR5, endogenous flagellin assembled into the flagellum structure of *Salmonella* would be less likely to trigger the TLR5 signaling pathway. Indeed, this may be considered a new approach for cancer immunotherapy, with genetically engineered avirulent bacteria releasing multiple TLR ligands.

Table 6.2 Comparison of chemotherapy and bacterial cancer therapy

	Chemotherapy	Bacterial therapy
Tumor targeting	Relatively low	High specificity
Pharmacokinetics	Rapid clearance with a short half-life	Sustained high concentration
Tissue penetration	Limited	Deep penetration to distal cancer tissues
Toxicity	Toxic to normal tissues	Minimized tissue toxicity
Immune stimulation	Mild or low	Robust
Programmability	Low	High, gene engineering and remote control
Costs	Relatively high	Inexpensive

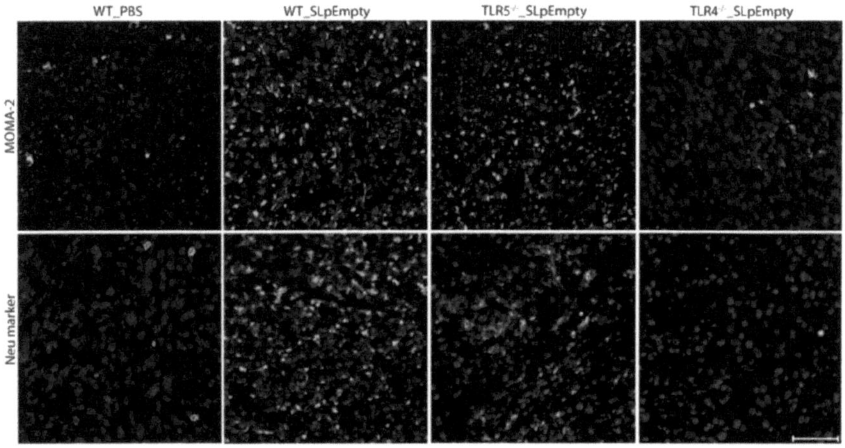

Figure 6.2 Immune cells infiltration in WT and knockout mice after *Salmonella* treatment. Immunofluorescence staining was performed to assess immune cell infiltration into tumors in WT, TLR5$^{-/-}$, and TLR4$^{-/-}$ mice subcutaneously implanted with MC38 mouse colon cancer cells three days after bacterial infection. MOMA-2, monoclonal antibody against monocytes and macrophages; Neu marker, monoclonal antibody against neutrophils. Representative images from three independent experiments are shown. Scale bar = 50 μm. Reprinted from Ref. [6], with permission from AAAS.

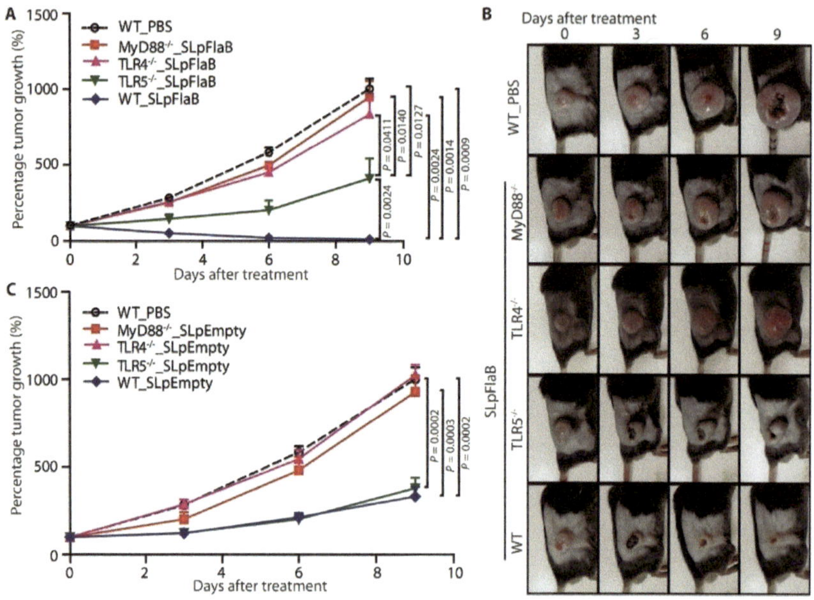

Figure 6.3 Effect of engineered FlaB-secreting *Salmonella* on tumor growth in knockout mice. C57BL/6 mice (WT, $TLR4^{-/-}$, $TLR5^{-/-}$, and $MyD88^{-/-}$; n = 8 per group) subcutaneously bearing MC38 tumors. When the tumors reached a volume of approximately 120 mm^3, the mice received SLpFlaB (1×10^7 CFU) or PBS via intravenous (i.v.) injection, followed by daily administration of 0.12 g L-arabinose beginning on 3 dpi. (A) Percent tumor growth after treatment with FlaB-expressing bacteria. *P* (WT_PBS vs. $MyD88^{-/-}$_SLpFlaB) = 1.000; *P* (WT_PBS vs. $TLR4^{-/-}$_SLpFlaB) = 0.3450. (B) Photographs of subcutaneous tumors in representative mice. (C) Percent tumor growth after treatment with *Salmonella* carrying an empty vector (SLpEmpty). *P* (WT_PBS vs. $MyD88^{-/-}$_SLpEmpty) = 0.7758; *P* (WT_PBS vs. $TLR4^{-/-}$_SLpEmpty) = 0.6943; *P* (WT_ SLpEmpty vs. $TLR5^{-/-}$_SLpEmpty) = 0.5054. Reprinted from Ref. [6], with permission from AAAS.

6.4.3.3 Mitochondrial target domain: Noxa

A dysfunction in cell apoptosis usually results in tumor cell development, proliferation, and resistance to treatment. Targeted cancer therapy to induce cell apoptosis would therefore eliminate the proliferation of abnormal cancer cells. In mammalian cells, the mitochondria-mediated apoptotic pathway is greatly regulated by the Bcl-2 family of proteins, each of which contains at least one of four conserved motifs known as Bcl-2 homology domains (BH1 to 4). These domains have been divided into three subfamilies. Noxa belongs to the BH3 subfamily and exhibits sequence homology only to the BH3 domain. Noxa has two functional domains, the BH3 domain and a mitochondrial targeting domain (MTD), the latter being a prodeath domain that induces calcium release from mitochondria by increasing their permeability [45]. To increase MTD penetration into cancer cells, MDT was fused with a cell-penetrating peptide (DS4.3) derived from a voltage-gated potassium channel. A phage-derived bacterial lysis system was utilized to release MTD from *S. typhimurium*, with both the DS4.3-MTD fused sequence and the phage lysis gene under the control of a pBAD promoter [18]. Targeted delivery of MTD with ΔppGpp *S. typhimurium* greatly enhanced cancer cell apoptosis under both *in vitro* and *in vivo* conditions following induction with L-arabinose [18].

6.4.3.4 Apoptotic cell death inducer: L-asparaginase

L-asparaginase (L-ASNase) from *E. coli* is a universal anticancer protein used to treat patients with acute lymphoblastic leukemia [46]. L-ASNase catalyzes the deamination of asparagine into aspartate and, to a lesser extent, the deamination of glutamine to glutamate. Both of these activities may be required for its therapeutic efficacy against malignancies. Asparagine depletion leads to the inhibition of global protein synthesis, inducing apoptotic cell death. The glutaminase activity of L-ASNase also promotes apoptosis, both by suppressing protein synthesis and by augmenting the effects of asparagine deficiency. To test the anticancer activity of L-ASNase delivered by engineered bacteria, genetically engineered ΔppGpp *S. typhimurium* were transformed with an L-ASNase encoding plasmid under the control of an L-arabinose-inducible pBAD promoter [19]. L-ASNase secreted by these bacteria induced apoptotic cell death under both *in vitro* and *in vivo* conditions. Administration of a single dose of L-ASNase-expressing *S. typhimurium* to nude mice implanted with murine colon cancer, breast cancer, or human pancreatic cancer greatly inhibited tumor growth and prolonged animal survival [19].

6.4.3.5 Immunotoxin: TGFα-PE38

Chimeric immunotoxins contain a cancer-binding domain that delivers a toxin to cancer cells, with the toxin entering and killing these cancer cells. Several recombinant immunotoxins targeting malignant tumors have been developed and are now undergoing clinical trials. TGFα-PE38 is an immunotoxin consisting of transforming growth factor alpha (TGFα), a natural ligand of epidermal growth factor receptor (EGFR), and a modified *Pseudomonas* exotoxin A (PE38) lacking an intrinsic cell-binding domain, a highly potent cytotoxic protein moiety. Cancer cells expressing high levels of EGFR undergo apoptosis upon treatment with TGFα-PE38. However, several limitations hamper the development of immunotoxin-based cancer therapy. For example, systemic administration of TGFα-PE38 at levels high enough to show therapeutic activity resulted in dose-limiting hepatotoxicity [47]. Although intratumoral administration of TGFα-PE38 prevented the hepatotoxicity and solved the problem of its short half-life, this agent showed limited efficacy in a clinical trial of human patients with recurrent malignant brain tumors, mainly due to inconsistent drug delivery [48]. However, genetically engineered attenuated *S. typhimurium* may overcome these limitations. Following bacterial colonization of tumor tissues, an external inducer can turn on continuous gene (*TGFα-PE38*) expression, resulting in high local drug concentration in tumor tissues, inducing the death of tumor cells without notable toxicity to normal organs. Indeed, genetically engineered TGFα-PE38-secreting *S. typhimurium* showed specific tumor killing in cancer models with high EGFR expression, as well as extended animal survival [20].

6.5 Stimulation of Host Immunity

6.5.1 Activation of the Inflammasome Pathway

The accumulation of attenuated *S. typhimurium* in tumor tissues activates the inflammasome pathway [14, 15]. During the process of bacterial infection, exposed bacterial compounds (PAMPs) bind to a group of PRRs on host cells, activating the host's innate immune response. NOD-like receptors (NLRs) are the cytosolic sensors of PAMPs that enter the cell via phagocytosis or invasion and of damage-associated molecular patterns (DAMPs) associated with cell stress. Three subfamilies of NLRs have been identified: NLRP1, NLRP3, and NLRC4 (also known as IPAF). IPAF inflammasomes are activated by bacterial flagellin associated with bacterial types 3 and 4 secretion systems [49]. NLRP3 inflammasomes are triggered by endogenous DAMPs or PAMPs, which induce K^+ efflux [50]. Caspase-1 activation is required for the production of mature proinflammatory cytokines, including IL-1β and IL-18. Caspase-1 is activated by the binding of TNF-α or TLR ligands to cell receptors, leading to the activation and translocation of NF-κB into the nucleus, in which pro-IL-1β and NLRP3 are expressed. Alternatively, activation of the inflammasome leads to the assembly of NLRP3 protein complexes and the cleavage of pro-caspase-1 to its active form caspase-1. Mature caspase-1 cleaves pro-IL-1β into active IL-1β and promotes the progress of inflammation. Attenuated *S. typhimurium* infection of cancer cells *in vitro* increases cancer cell release of ATP, which can serve as a DAMP signal to activate the NLRP3 inflammasome [15]. Administration of attenuated *S. typhimurium* to tumor-bearing mice results in the upregulation of expression of inflammasome-related genes, including IPAF, NLRP3, and P2X7 [15]. By contrast, treatment of tumor-bearing mice with *E. coli* K-12 strain (MG1655) does not significantly suppress tumor growth and does not activate the inflammasome pathway, despite the detection of similar numbers of bacteria in tumor tissues. These findings suggest that attenuated *S. typhimurium* has great potential for activation of inflammasomes and the induction of anticancer immunity.

6.5.2 Macrophage Polarization

TAMs, which originate from circulating monocytes, are polarized into a classic M1-like or alternative M2-like phenotype in response to different microenvironmental stimuli. M1-like macrophage are induced by interferon (IFN)-γ and LPS and are associated with high expression of nitric oxide synthase (iNOS), whereas M2-like macrophages are induced by Th2 cytokines (IL-4 and IL-13) and are characterized by high expression of anti-inflammatory cytokines, IL-10, mannose receptor (CD206), and arginase [16]. Most TAMs exhibit the characteristics of M2-like macrophages, potentially promoting cancer cell proliferation, stimulating tumor angiogenesis, and enhancing tumor invasion and metastasis [51]. The immunosuppressive activities of TAMs are associated with their secretion of immunosuppressive cytokines, chemokines, and proteases, such as TGF-β, IL-10, CCL17, CCL22, and arginase (Arg-1) [52]. TAMs may also suppress $CD8^+$ T cells by surface expression of inhibitory B7 family molecules such as B7-H1 (programmed death ligand 1, PD-L1) and B7-H4, resulting in T cell exhaustion [53].

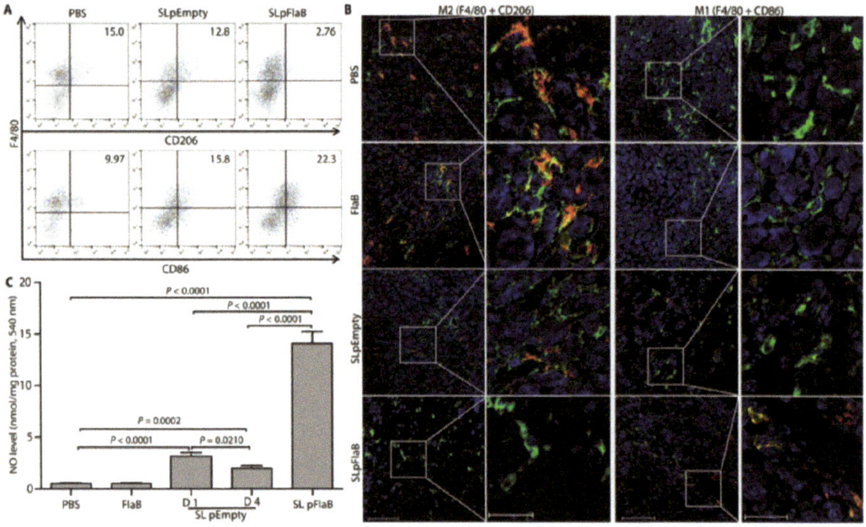

Figure 6.4 M1 and M2 macrophage polarization after treatment with FlaB-secreting bacteria. Samples were prepared from MC38 tumors at 24 h after induction. (A) Samples were triple-stained with antibodies to CD45 (hematopoietic cell marker), F4/80 (macrophage marker), and CD206 (M2-type macrophages) or CD86 (M1-type macrophages) and analyzed by FACS. All the samples were pregated on CD45-positive cells (n = 5; data are representative of three independent experiments). (B) Contiguous sections were doubly stained with F4/80 (green) and CD206 (red) (M2 macrophages) or F4/80 (green) and CD86 (red) (M1 macrophages). Nuclei were stained with DAPI (blue). Merged images are shown at low (scale bar = 50 μm) and high (scale bar = 20 μm) magnification. Data are representative of three individual experiments. (C) Nitric oxide levels were measured in tumor lysates (n = 13) at 1 dpi (D1) and 4 dpi (D4) of SLpEmpty and four days after treatment with PBS, FlaB, or SLpFlaB (24 h after induction). Reprinted from Ref. [6], with permission from AAAS.

Reprogramming of tumor-infiltrating macrophages into M1-like macrophages may enhance anticancer response and improve the efficacy of immunotherapies. TLRs are broadly expressed on macrophages and may be targets for macrophage phenotype conversion. Poly I:C, a dsRNA analog that binds to toll-like receptor 3 (TLR3), was found to convert tumor-promoting to antitumor macrophages [54]. In addition, a toll-like receptor 9 (TLR9) ligand, CpG-oligodeoxynucleotide (ODN), and anti-IL-10R antibody induced infiltrated macrophages to switch from an M2 to an M1 phenotype and triggered an innate response [55]. Colonization of tumor tissues by attenuated *S. typhimurium* decreased the number of M2-like macrophages ($F4/80^+CD206^+$), while increasing the number of M1-like macrophages ($F4/80^+CD86^+$) and the production of nitric oxide (NO) [6]. Treatment with engineered FlaB-expressing *S. typhimurium* further enhanced M1-like macrophage polarization in the tumor microenvironment and significantly increased NO production ($P < 0.0001$) (Fig. 6.4). Moreover, proinflammatory cytokines, including IL-1β, TNF-α, and IL-18, were upregulated in tumor tissues after treatment with engineered *S. typhimurium* [6, 14, 15]. Taken together, these findings showed that FlaB-expressing *S. typhimurium* robustly suppressed tumor growth by modulating the tumor microenvironment to enhance M1-like macrophage polarization.

6.6 Application in Diseases

6.6.1 Cancer Therapy

Cancers are among the most lethal diseases worldwide, causing millions of patient deaths annually. The mainstays of current treatment are surgery, radiation, and chemotherapy. Emerging immunotherapeutic approaches include treatment with antibodies and strategies such as immune checkpoint blockade and adaptive cell transfer. Solid tumors, characterized by hypoxic areas and abnormal angiogenesis, are resistant to these treatments. However, attenuated *S. typhimurium*, a facultative anaerobic bacterial strain, takes advantage of these characteristics and specifically colonizes and proliferates in tumor tissues. These bacteria release high concentrations of PAMPs, which induce anticancer activity by activating host immunity. Bacterial anticancer activity may be enhanced by utilizing attenuated *S. typhimurium* as a delivery and/or expression vector for cancer vaccines, interfering RNA, and anticancer proteins. High numbers of stromal cells in the tumor microenvironment are usually associated with poor patient prognosis and resistance to conventional therapies [56]. However, targeted cancer therapy with engineered *S. typhimurium* secreting oncolytic proteins may overcome this drawback. Cancer immunotherapy using antibody inhibitors to target immune checkpoints has been found to greatly improve patient outcomes [57]. Anticancer efficacy may be further improved by combination therapy. For example, an antigen-specific bacterial vaccine and PD-L1 antibody rescued endogenous T cell dysfunction and resulted in the rejection of established tumors in mice [58]. The features of another facultative anaerobic strain, *E. coli* MG1655, are similar to those of *S. typhimurium*, with the two showing comparable bacterial accumulation in tumor tissues. However, the anticancer activity and the induction of host innate immunity were lower with *E. coli* MG1655 than with genetically engineered *Salmonella* [14, 15].

6.6.2 Myocardial Infarction and Other Diseases

Heart disease is the leading cause of deaths worldwide among both men and women. Many manifestations of heart disease are associated with plaque buildup in the walls of the arteries. Myocardial infarction, also known as heart attack, occurs when blood flow stops within a section of the heart, damaging the cardiac muscles, which become infarcted and hypoxic. Infarcted regions may serve as a harbor that favors the colonization by and proliferation of attenuated ΔppGpp *S. typhimurium*. For example, a rat model of myocardial infarction was generated by ligation of the left anterior descending artery [29]. These rats were subsequently injected with several strains of attenuated *S. typhimurium* and *E. coli* to check the bacterial tropism for myocardial infarction. Although the *E. coli* strains failed to home in on the infarcted areas, some attenuated *S. typhimurium* strains, including attenuated ΔppGpp *S. typhimurium*, exhibited strong targeting and sustained colonization of infarcted areas even nine days after bacterial infection, as monitored by optical

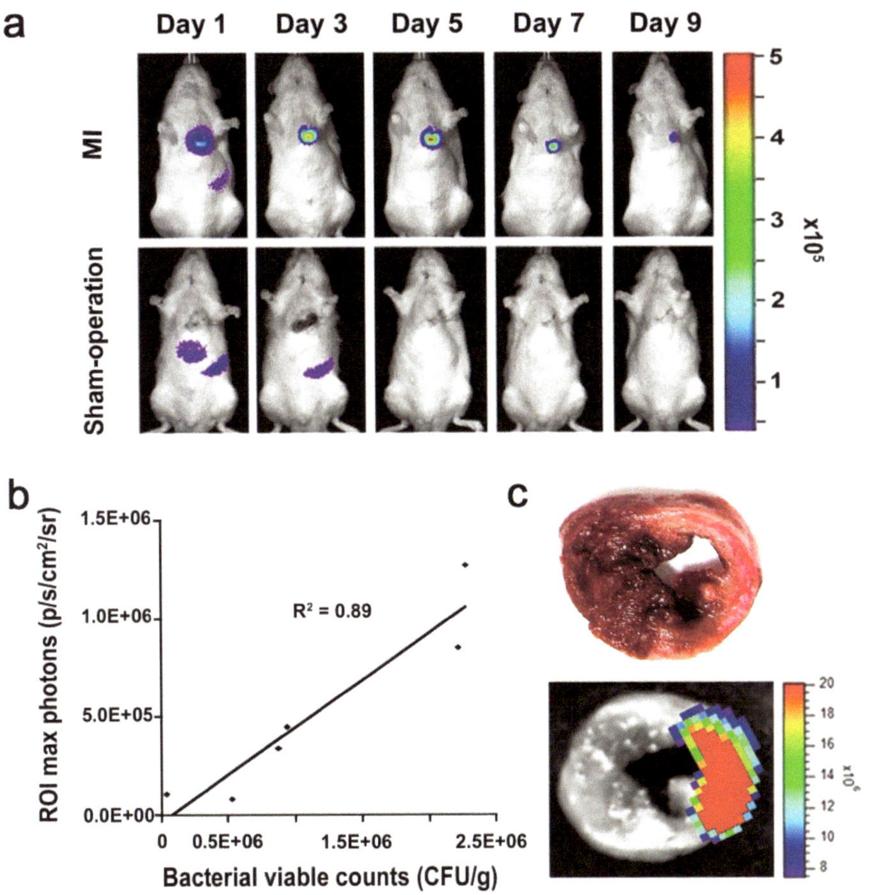

Figure 6.5 Molecular imaging of bacterial tropism for infarcted myocardium (MI). (A) ΔppGpp *S. typhimurium* expressing *lux* (2 × 10^8 CFU) was injected through the tail vein into Sprague–Dawley rats with or without MI (n = 5, each group) 6 h after surgery. (B) Direct comparison between photon flux and bacterial colony counts in MI (n = 21). A robust correlation was observed between the number of bacterial colonies and bacterial bioluminescence signals (R^2 = 0.89). (C) Cross sections of the heart from MI rats five days after inoculation with *Salmonellae*. Thin-slice (1.5 mm) cross sections were prepared and stained with triphenyltetrazolium chloride (top). Bioluminescence imaging using a cooled charge-coupled device camera for 30 sec. (bottom). Note the dull white area of reduced dehydrogenase activity. CFU, colony-forming units; MI, myocardial infarction; ROI, region of interest. Reprinted from Ref. [29], with permission from American Society of Gene & Cell Therapy.

imaging (Fig. 6.5). The numbers of attenuated *S. typhimurium* bacteria remained high in infarcted hearts, even after the clearance of bacteria from normal organs, such as the liver and spleen. Attenuated bacteria engineered to express proangiogenesis and/or growth factors, such as vascular endothelial growth factor (VEGF) and fibroblast growth factor (FGF), may be used for rehabilitation of the infarcted myocardia, whereas bacteria engineered to express a reporter gene may be useful for the diagnosis of myocardial infarction. This approach may also be applied to the diagnosis and treatment of other diseases, such as atherosclerosis.

6.7 Summary

This chapter mainly described an approach to cancer therapy using attenuated ΔppGpp *S. typhimurium*. Bacterial cancer therapy has several advantages over conventional chemotherapy (Table 6.2), including very specific tumor targeting and maintenance of high concentrations of bacteria in tumor tissues for a long period of time. Attenuated *S. typhimurium* can sense the tumor microenvironment and metabolize substrates, enabling better tissue penetration and colonization of areas far from the tumor vasculature. Deep tissue penetration leads to the activation of robust anticancer immunity and effective delivery of anticancer drugs, as well as sequentially destroying quiescent cancer cells that are usually unresponsive to chemotherapy. The ability of attenuated *S. typhimurium* to stimulate host immunity to generate anticancer activity makes this vector ideal for the treatment of pancreatic cancer, which is usually resistant to conventional therapies and shows poor infiltration by immune cells.

The most important advantage of bacterial cancer therapy may be the ability of genetic modification to increase anticancer efficacy. Genetic engineering can result in attenuated strains with good safety profiles and high tumor targeting or targeted delivery of anticancer molecules to enhance tumor-specific killing. Many of our recent studies showed that treatment with genetically engineered *S. typhimurium* carrying cargo molecules resulted in enhanced anticancer activity, without evidence of toxicity. Administration of attenuated ΔppGpp *S. typhimurium* to tumor-bearing mice led to tumor-specific colonization and proliferation and subsequent activation of the inflammasome pathway to secrete proinflammatory cytokines. This, in turn, enhanced M1-like macrophage polarization, resulting in robust anticancer activities. Future development of bacterial cancer therapy should include collaboration with other disciplines, including microbiology, cancer biology, immunology, medical imaging, and clinical oncology. Further studies, including modifications of experimental conditions, are required to accumulate evidence for clinical cancer research.

Acknowledgment

This work was supported by the Pioneer Research Center Program (2015M3C1A3056410) and the Basic Science Research Program (No.2017R1A2B3012157) through the National Research Foundation of Korea (NRF), funded by the Ministry of Science, ICT and Future Planning.

References

1. McCarthy E. F. The toxins of William B. Coley and the treatment of bone and soft-tissue sarcomas. *Iowa Orthopaedic Journal*, 26 (2006) 154–158.
2. Zhu H., Li Z., Mao S., Ma B., Zhou S., Deng L., *et al.* Antitumor effect of sFlt-1 gene therapy system mediated by *Bifidobacterium Infantis* on Lewis lung cancer in mice. *Cancer Gene Therapy*, 18 (2011) 884–896.
3. Roberts N. J., Zhang L., Janku F., Collins A., Bai R. Y., Staedtke V., *et al.* Intratumoral injection of *Clostridium novyi*-NT spores induces antitumor responses. *Science Translational Medicine*, 6 (2014) 249ra111.
4. Toso J. F., Gill V. J., Hwu P., Marincola F. M., Restifo N. P., Schwartzentruber D. J., *et al.* Phase I study of the intravenous administration of attenuated *Salmonella typhimurium* to patients with metastatic melanoma. *Journal of Clinical Oncology*, 20 (2002) 142–152.

5. Zhao M., Yang M., Li X. M., Jiang P., Baranov E., Li S., *et al.* Tumor-targeting bacterial therapy with amino acid auxotrophs of GFP-expressing *Salmonella typhimurium*. *Proceedings of the National Academy of Sciences of the United States of America,* 102 (2005) 755–760.
6. Zheng J. H., Nguyen V. H., Jiang S. N., Park S. H., Tan W., Hong S. H., *et al.* Two-step enhanced cancer immunotherapy with engineered *Salmonella typhimurium* secreting heterologous flagellin. *Science Translational Medicine,* 9 (2017) eaak9537.
7. Jiang S. N., Phan T. X., Nam T. K., Nguyen V. H., Kim H. S., Bom H. S., *et al.* Inhibition of tumor growth and metastasis by a combination of *Escherichia coli*-mediated cytolytic therapy and radiotherapy. *Molecular Therapy,* 18 (2010) 635–642.
8. Min J. J., Nguyen V. H., Kim H. J., Hong Y., Choy H. E. Quantitative bioluminescence imaging of tumor-targeting bacteria in living animals. *Nature Protocols,* 3 (2008) 629–636.
9. Zheng J. H., Min J. J. Targeted cancer therapy using engineered *Salmonella typhimurium*. *Chonnam Medical Journal,* 52 (2016) 173–184.
10. Zhao M., Yang M., Ma H., Li X., Tan X., Li S., *et al.* Targeted therapy with a *Salmonella typhimurium* leucine-arginine auxotroph cures orthotopic human breast tumors in nude mice. *Cancer Research,* 66 (2006) 7647–7652.
11. Jiang S. N., Park S. H., Lee H. J., Zheng J. H., Kim H. S., Bom H. S., *et al.* Engineering of bacteria for the visualization of targeted delivery of a cytolytic anticancer agent. *Molecular Therapy,* 21 (2013) 1985–1995.
12. Park S. H., Zheng J. H., Nguyen V. H., Jiang S. N., Kim D. Y., Szardenings M., *et al.* RGD peptide cell-surface display enhances the targeting and therapeutic efficacy of attenuated *Salmonella*-mediated cancer therapy. *Theranostics,* 6 (2016) 1672–1682.
13. Na H. S., Kim H. J., Lee H. C., Hong Y., Rhee J. H., Choy H. E. Immune response induced by *Salmonella typhimurium* defective in ppGpp synthesis. *Vaccine,* 24 (2006) 2027–2034.
14. Kim J. E., Phan T. X., Nguyen V. H., Dinh-Vu H. V., Zheng J. H., Yun M., *et al. Salmonella typhimurium* suppresses tumor growth via the pro-inflammatory cytokine interleukin-1β. *Theranostics,* 5 (2015) 1328–1342.
15. Phan T. X., Nguyen V. H., Duong M. T., Hong Y., Choy H. E., Min J. J. Activation of inflammasome by attenuated *Salmonella typhimurium*

in bacteria-mediated cancer therapy. *Microbiology and Immunology*, 59 (2015) 664–675.

16. Kaimala S., Mohamed Y. A., Nader N., Issac J., Elkord E., Chouaib S., *et al.* *Salmonella*-mediated tumor regression involves targeting of tumor myeloid suppressor cells causing a shift to M1-like phenotype and reduction in suppressive capacity. *Cancer Immunology, Immunotherapy*, 63 (2014) 587–599.
17. Nguyen V. H., Kim H. S., Ha J. M., Hong Y., Choy H. E., Min J. J. Genetically engineered *Salmonella typhimurium* as an imageable therapeutic probe for cancer. *Cancer Research*, 70 (2010) 18–23.
18. Jeong J. H., Kim K., Lim D., Jeong K., Hong Y., Nguyen V. H., *et al.* Anti-tumoral effect of the mitochondrial target domain of Noxa delivered by an engineered *Salmonella typhimurium*. *PLOS One*, 9 (2014) e80050.
19. Kim K., Jeong J. H., Lim D., Hong Y., Lim H. J., Kim G. J., *et al.* L-asparaginase delivered by *Salmonella typhimurium* suppresses solid tumors. *Molecular Therapy Oncolytics*, 2 (2015) 15007.
20. Lim D., Kim K. S., Kim H., Ko K. C., Song J. J., Choi J. H., *et al.* Anti-tumor activity of an immunotoxin (TGFα-PE38) delivered by attenuated *Salmonella typhimurium*. *Oncotarget*, 8 (2017) 37550–37560.
21. Al-Ramadi B. K., Fernandez-Cabezudo M. J., El-Hasasna H., Al-Salam S., Bashir G., Chouaib S. Potent anti-tumor activity of systemically-administered IL2-expressing *Salmonella* correlates with decreased angiogenesis and enhanced tumor apoptosis. *Clinical Immunology*, 130 (2009) 89–97.
22. Song M., Kim H. J., Kim E. Y., Shin M., Lee H. C., Hong Y., *et al.* ppGpp-dependent stationary phase induction of genes on *Salmonella* pathogenicity island 1. *Journal of Biological Chemistry*, 279 (2004) 34183–34190.
23. Shi L., Yu B., Cai C. H., Huang W., Zheng B. J., Smith D. K., *et al.* Combined prokaryotic-eukaryotic delivery and expression of therapeutic factors through a primed autocatalytic positive-feedback loop. *Journal of Controlled Release*, 222 (2016) 130–140.
24. Tjuvajev J., Blasberg R., Luo X., Zheng L. M., King I., Bermudes D. *Salmonella*-based tumor-targeted cancer therapy: tumor amplified protein expression therapy (TAPET) for diagnostic imaging. *Journal of Controlled Release*, 74 (2001) 313–315.

25. Liu Z., Wang F., Chen X. Integrin $\alpha_v\beta_3$-targeted cancer therapy. *Drug Development Research*, 69 (2008) 329–339.

26. Gilad Y., Noy E., Senderowitz H., Albeck A., Firer M. A., Gellerman G. Dual-drug RGD conjugates provide enhanced cytotoxicity to melanoma and non-small lung cancer cells. *Biopolymers*, (2015) .

27. Xiong X. B., Huang Y., Lu W. L., Zhang X., Zhang H., Nagai T., *et al.* Intracellular delivery of doxorubicin with RGD-modified sterically stabilized liposomes for an improved antitumor efficacy: in vitro and in vivo. *Journal of Pharmaceutical Sciences*, 94 (2005) 1782–1793.

28. Massa P. E., Paniccia A., Monegal A., de Marco A., Rescigno M. *Salmonella* engineered to express CD20-targeting antibodies and a drug-converting enzyme can eradicate human lymphomas. *Blood*, 122 (2013) 705–714.

29. Le U. N., Kim H. S., Kwon J. S., Kim M. Y., Nguyen V. H., Jiang S. N., *et al.* Engineering and visualization of bacteria for targeting infarcted myocardium. *Molecular Therapy*, 19 (2011) 951–959.

30. Ganai S., Arenas R. B., Forbes N. S. Tumour-targeted delivery of TRAIL using *Salmonella typhimurium* enhances breast cancer survival in mice. *British Journal of Cancer*, 101 (2009) 1683–1691.

31. Ryan R. M., Green J., Williams P. J., Tazzyman S., Hunt S., Harmey J. H., *et al.* Bacterial delivery of a novel cytolysin to hypoxic areas of solid tumors. *Gene Therapy*, 16 (2009) 329–339.

32. Swofford C. A., Van Dessel N., Forbes N. S. Quorum-sensing *Salmonella* selectively trigger protein expression within tumors. *Proceedings of the National Academy of Sciences of the United States of America*, 112 (2015) 3457–3462.

33. Hong H., Lim D., Kim G. J., Park S. H., Sik Kim H., Hong Y., *et al.* Targeted deletion of the *ara* operon of *Salmonella typhimurium* enhances L-arabinose accumulation and drives P_{BAD}-promoted expression of anti-cancer toxins and imaging agents. *Cell Cycle*, 13 (2014) 3112–3120.

34.. Galan J. E., Nakayama K., Curtiss R. 3rd. Cloning and characterization of the asd gene of *Salmonella typhimurium*: use in stable maintenance of recombinant plasmids in *Salmonella* vaccine strains. *Gene*, 94 (1990) 29–35.

35. Kim K., Jeong J. H., Lim D., Hong Y., Yun M., Min J. J., *et al.* A novel balanced-lethal host-vector system based on *glmS*. *PLOS One*, 8 (2013) e60511.

36. Wai S. N., Lindmark B., Soderblom T., Takade A., Westermark M., Oscarsson J., *et al.* Vesicle-mediated export and assembly of pore-forming oligomers of the enterobacterial ClyA cytotoxin. *Cell*, 115 (2003) 25–35.

37. Anderson K. G., Stromnes I. M., Greenberg P. D. Obstacles posed by the tumor microenvironment to T cell activity: a case for synergistic therapies. *Cancer Cell*, 31 (2017) 311–325.

38. Cai Z., Sanchez A., Shi Z., Zhang T., Liu M., Zhang D. Activation of Toll-like receptor 5 on breast cancer cells by flagellin suppresses cell proliferation and tumor growth. *Cancer Research*, 71 (2011) 2466–2475.

39. Rhee S. H., Im E., Pothoulakis C. Toll-like receptor 5 engagement modulates tumor development and growth in a mouse xenograft model of human colon cancer. *Gastroenterology*, 135 (2008) 518–528.

40. Lee S. E., Kim S. Y., Jeong B. C., Kim Y. R., Bae S. J., Ahn O. S., *et al.* A bacterial flagellin, *Vibrio vulnificus* FlaB, has a strong mucosal adjuvant activity to induce protective immunity. *Infection and Immunity*, 74 (2006) 694–702.

41. Lee S. E., Hong S. H., Verma V., Lee Y. S., Duong T. N., Jeong K., *et al.* Flagellin is a strong vaginal adjuvant of a therapeutic vaccine for genital cancer. *Oncoimmunology*, 5 (2016) e1081328.

42. Nguyen C. T., Hong S. H., Sin J. I., Vu H. V., Jeong K., Cho K. O., *et al.* Flagellin enhances tumor-specific CD8(+) T cell immune responses through TLR5 stimulation in a therapeutic cancer vaccine model. *Vaccine*, 31 (2013) 3879–3887.

43. De Filippo K., Henderson R. B., Laschinger M., Hogg N. Neutrophil chemokines KC and macrophage-inflammatory protein-2 are newly synthesized by tissue macrophages using distinct TLR signaling pathways. *Journal of Immunology*, 180 (2008) 4308–4315.

44. Wang L., Liu Q., Sun Q., Zhang C., Chen T., Cao X. TLR4 signaling in cancer cells promotes chemoattraction of immature dendritic cells via autocrine CCL20. *Biochemical and Biophysical Research Communications*, 366 (2008) 852–856.

45. Seo Y. W., Woo H. N., Piya S., Moon A. R., Oh J. W., Yun C. W., *et al.* The cell death-inducing activity of the peptide containing Noxa mitochondrial-targeting domain is associated with calcium release. *Cancer Research*, 69 (2009) 8356–8365.

46. Wriston J. C. Jr., Yellin T. O. L-asparaginase: a review. *Advances in Enzymology and Related Areas of Molecular Biology*, 39 (1973) 185–248.

47. Wright S. E., Rewers-Felkins K. A., Quinlin I., Chowdhury N. I., Ahmed J., Eldridge P. W., *et al.* TGFα-PE38 enhances cytotoxic T-lymphocyte killing of breast cancer cells. *Oncology Letters*, 7 (2014) 2113–2117.

48. Ochiai H., Archer G. E., Herndon J. E. 2nd, Kuan C. T., Mitchell D. A., Bigner D. D., *et al.* EGFRvIII-targeted immunotoxin induces antitumor immunity that is inhibited in the absence of CD4+ and CD8+ T cells. *Cancer Immunology, Immunotherapy*, 57 (2008) 115–121.

49. Franchi L., Amer A., Body-Malapel M., Kanneganti T. D., Ozoren N., Jagirdar R., *et al.* Cytosolic flagellin requires Ipaf for activation of caspase-1 and interleukin 1β in salmonella-infected macrophages. *Nature Immunology*, 7 (2006) 576–582.

50. Franchi L., Munoz-Planillo R., Nunez G. Sensing and reacting to microbes through the inflammasomes. *Nature Immunology*, 13 (2012) 325–332.

51. Qian B. Z., Pollard J. W. Macrophage diversity enhances tumor progression and metastasis. *Cell*, 141 (2010) 39–51.

52. Hao N. B., Lu M. H., Fan Y. H., Cao Y. L., Zhang Z. R., Yang S. M. Macrophages in tumor microenvironments and the progression of tumors. *Clinical & Developmental Immunology*, 2012 (2012) 948098.

53. Ruffell B., Affara N. I., Coussens L. M. Differential macrophage programming in the tumor microenvironment. *Trends in Immunology*, 33 (2012) 119–126.

54. Shime H., Matsumoto M., Oshiumi H., Tanaka S., Nakane A., Iwakura Y., *et al.* Toll-like receptor 3 signaling converts tumor-supporting myeloid cells to tumoricidal effectors. *Proceedings of the National Academy of Sciences of the United States of America*, 109 (2012) 2066–2071.

55. Guiducci C., Vicari A. P., Sangaletti S., Trinchieri G., Colombo M. P. Redirecting in vivo elicited tumor infiltrating macrophages and dendritic cells towards tumor rejection. *Cancer Research*, 65 (2005) 3437–3446.

56. Shakya R., Gonda T., Quante M., Salas M., Kim S., Brooks J., *et al.* Hypomethylating therapy in an aggressive stroma-rich model of pancreatic carcinoma. *Cancer Research*, 73 (2013) 885–896.

57. Lussier D. M., Johnson J. L., Hingorani P., Blattman J. N. Combination immunotherapy with α-CTLA-4 and α-PD-L1 antibody blockade

prevents immune escape and leads to complete control of metastatic osteosarcoma. *Journal for Immunotherapy of Cancer*, 3 (2015) 21.

58. Binder D. C., Engels B., Arina A., Yu P., Slauch J. M., Fu Y. X., *et al.* Antigen-specific bacterial vaccine combined with anti-PD-L1 rescues dysfunctional endogenous T cells to reject long-established cancer. *Cancer Immunology Research*, 1 (2013) 123–133.

Chapter 7

Engineering *Escherichia coli* to Combat Cancer

Carlos Piñero-Lambea, David Ruano-Gallego, Gustavo Bodelón, Beatriz Álvarez, and Luis Ángel Fernández

Department of Microbial Biotechnology, Centro Nacional de Biotecnología (CNB-CSIC), Campus Cantoblanco-UAM, Madrid, 28049, Spain

lafdez@cnb.csic.es

This chapter highlights the potential of engineering *E. coli* for the development of powerful therapies against cancer. We review the status of bacterial therapies against cancer and the application of commensal and probiotic *E. coli* strains as vectors for tumor colonization and delivery of therapeutic proteins. We discuss the use of synthetic biology for a complete design of *E. coli* bacteria for tumor therapy, incorporating modular elements and gene circuits responding to tumors. Lastly, we describe the development of modular elements for the specific adhesion of *E. coli* bacteria to tumors and for the injection therapeutic proteins into the tumor cells.

Microbial Infections and Cancer Therapy: Recent Advances
Edited by Ananda M. Chakrabarty and Arsénio M. Fialho

ISBN 978-981-4774-86-4 (Hardcover), 978-1-351-04190-4 (eBook)
www.panstanford.com

7.1 Introduction

7.1.1 Bacterial Therapies against Cancer

At the end of the 19th century, physicians W. Busch and W. Coley reported spontaneous tumor remissions associated with acute infections caused by *Streptococcus pyogenes* [1]. Prompted by these remissions, Coley started to systematically treat sarcoma patients with live *Streptococcus pyogenes* bacteria first and with isolated preparations of bacterial toxins later. Those studies were the foundational stone of bacterial therapies against cancer [2]. The variability in clinical outcomes of Coley's treatment, ranging from complete tumor remission to death, reduced clinical attention to his findings. In 1976 Morales and Eidinger reported successful treatment of human bladder cancer with *Mycobacterium bovis* bacillus Calmette–Guérin (BCG) [3] and its clinical use in the last four decades has demonstrated that intravesical immunotherapy with BCG reduces recurrence and progression in patients with nonmuscle-invasive bladder cancer [4, 5].

The interest in tumor-colonizing microbes gained ground when genetic engineering established the methods to specifically modify bacteria, providing direct control over bacterial virulence and the expression of therapeutic proteins. Preclinical and clinical studies conducted with these bacteria established that different bacterial genera can selectively replicate in tumor tissue and produce different cytoxins and prodrug converting enzymes [6]. Currently, it is well established that the tumor microenvironment provides a safe niche for bacterial replication, as clearance by the immune system is limited and bacterial growth is facilitated by abundant nutrients. In addition, active motility allows microbial cells to reach tumor regions that are currently untreatable with conventional chemotherapies relying on passive diffusion [7, 8]. Thus, taking advantage of their selective replication within solid tumors and preferential colonization of the tumor microenvironment, interested parties have investigated several bacterial genera as anticancer agents. Significantly, preclinical studies with attenuated bacterial strains have resulted in tumor regression and even complete tumor eradication [9].

Natural bacteria can destroy tumor tissue by competing for nutrients, secreting toxins, and/or eliciting host immune responses against malignant cells [6, 10, 11]. The relative importance of each of these processes seems to depend on the bacterial gender, and more precisely on its pathogenic potential. Pathogenic bacteria such as *Salmonella enterica* can kill tumor cells, given their natural armory of cytotoxic molecules. The infection of tumors with microorganisms can elicit strong antitumor immune activation, resulting also in the specific destruction of the malignant cells. The inherent antitumor activity of bacteria is connected to pathogen-associated molecular patterns (PAMPs), like lipopolysaccharide (LPS), flagella, and CpG [9]. It has been proposed that infection of tumors leads to infiltration by lymphocytes and antigen-presenting cells, such as macrophages and dendritic cells. Recognition of PAMPs by specific cellular receptors, (e.g., toll-like receptors) induces production of diverse cytokines, triggering full activation of the immune system and improved antigen presentation [12]. It has been found that invasive *Salmonella typhimurium* has the ability to infect nonphagocytic cells via the expression of a type III secretion system (T3SS). Infected tumor cells present antigenic determinants of bacterial origin, thereby making them targets of anti-*Salmonella*-specific T cells [13]. Tumor-colonizing bacteria have also been shown to recruit inflammatory cells, such as granulocytes and natural killer (NK) cells, both of which are necessary for induction of an antitumor response [14]. Activated CD4+ T cells in the tumor induce interferon (IFN)-γ production, thus enhancing the host antitumor immunity [15]. Processes such as cell apoptosis, tumor necrosis, and autophagy have been implicated in the natural cytotoxic activities of bacteria against tumors [16–20].

Besides the intrinsic antitumor effect, bacteria can be used as shuttle vectors for therapeutic molecules [21]. Engineered bacterial strains can be tailored to specifically target tumor tissue and produce therapeutic agents directly inside the malignant tissue. Thus, combining intrinsic immune-mediated and extrinsic vector-based bacterial therapies represents an attractive alternative strategy for treating cancer patients in the future.

7.1.2 Hypoxic Tumor Microenvironment and Bacterial Colonization

During tumor development, the aggressive growth of neoplastic cells and the associated overexpression of proangiogenic factors lead to the formation of aberrant neovasculature, characterized by immature and hyperpermeable blood vessels failing to deliver sufficient oxygen and nutrients to the rapidly dividing cancer cells [22, 23]. An inadequate oxygen supply produces regions of hypoxia and necrosis at varying degrees. This so-called tumor hypoxia leads to resistance to radiotherapy and anticancer chemotherapy as well as predisposition to increased tumor metastases. Furthermore, the abnormal vasculature in tumors obstructs conventional therapeutic anticancer strategies. This anaerobic nature of hypoxic/necrotic regions found within tumors promotes growth of anaerobic and facultative anaerobic bacteria. This hypoxic tumor microenvironment, along with a localized dysfunction of the immune cells that enhances immunosuppression, is believed to be an important factor involved in the capacity of bacteria to replicate and colonize solid tumors [24, 25]. Several key mechanisms have been proposed that promote bacterial colonization of tumors upon systemic administration. In general, the systemic administration of bacteria induces the production of proinflammatory blood cytokines, such as tumor necrosis factor alpha (TNF-α), which, in turn, induces intratumoral hemorrhage, facilitating the entrapment of bacteria within the tumor [17, 26]. Later, chemotaxis attracts bacteria to quiescent, necrotic, and anaerobic regions. These conditions found in the tumor microenvironment enable bacteria to proliferate protected from clearance by the immune system.

On the basis of their requirements for oxygen, tumor-targeting microbes can be been classified into two groups: obligate anaerobes, such as *Bifidobacterium, Lactobacillus*, and *Clostridium*, and facultative anaerobes, such as *Salmonella*, *Escherichia*, and *Listeria* [1, 27]. Although efficient targeting of solid tumors by anaerobes has been demonstrated, their restriction to anaerobic regions might be disadvantageous when targeting metastases and small tumors without necrotic areas. On the other hand, facultative anaerobes, such as *Escherichia coli* and *Salmonella*, have been shown to colonize oxygenated as well as hypoxic and necrotic tumor regions. The ability of these microbes to grow independently of oxygen enabled their use to target primary tumors and metastases accessible by systemic circulation [28–30]. The active flagellar motility of these bacteria also favors the colonization of solid tumors at distant sites from tumor blood vessels [7, 8, 18].

7.2 *Escherichia coli* as an Anticancer Agent

7.2.1 Tumor Colonization by *E. coli*

Different pathogenic, commensal, probiotic, and laboratory *E. coli* strains have been shown to colonize solid tumors and metastasis in mice, including *E. coli* CFT073, K-12 MG1655, Nissle1917 (EcN), and Symbioflor-2 [30–39]. Stritzker and colleagues compared the efficiency of various pathogenic and nonpathogenic bacterial strains to colonize murine 4T1 tumors upon intravenous (IV) administration, including the pathogenic *Salmonella typhimurium* strains 14028 and SL1344, the enteroinvasive *E. coli* 4608-58 strain, the attenuated *Shigella flexneri* 2a SC602 strain, the uropathogenic *E. coli* CFT073, the nonpathogenic *E. coli* Top10, and the probiotic *E. coli* Nissle 1917 strain [32]. They found that all of these strains were able to efficiently colonize and replicate in tumors, each resulting in more than 1×10^8 colony-forming units (CFU) per gram of tumor tissue. Interestingly, colonization of spleen and liver was significantly lower when *E. coli* strains were used as compared to *Salmonella typhimurium* [32]. Weibel and colleagues analyzed the colonization and biodistribution of *E. coli* K-12 in the murine 4T1 breast carcinoma model upon IV administration of 5×10^6 CFU [30]. The authors showed that *E. coli* cells persisted in 4T1 tumors of immunocompromised as well as immunocompetent mice, from day 3 to 14 after inoculation, with counts ca. 1×10^8 CFU/g of tumor. Bacterial counts in livers and spleens were already low on day 3 after inoculation ($<1 \times 10^2$ CFU/g of tumor). One hour after systemic administration, approximately 1×10^3 CFU reached the tumor tissue, followed by an exponential increase of bacterial CFU. After 72 h, most bacteria were located in the area between the necrotic and the proliferating tumor tissue. The central necrotic tissue was also colonized but with lower bacterial density [30]. These results confirmed a previous report, in which high densities of bacteria were also observed in the border regions between the peripheral proliferative and central necrotic regions of tumors [34]. Weibel also reported that the colonization resulted in a larger avascular necrotic tissue, redistribution of hypoxic areas, and intensified matrix remodeling, as evidenced by collagen IV deposition. Remarkably, bacterial colonization led to site-specific accumulation of tumor-associated macrophages, the generation of an extended fibrotic granuloma-like structure with central necrosis, and the upregulation of TNF-α and matrix metalloproteinase 9 expression. The authors found that, in spite of dramatic inflammatory changes, no tumor regression occurred within two weeks and proposed that the lack of significant tumor growth inhibition was due to a limited or incomplete immune response due to the restricted distribution of bacteria, which thereby trigger only local immune responses [30]. It is also well documented that *E. coli* strains, including K-12 and probiotic EcN and Symbioflor-2, generally show a higher tumor specificity than *Salmonella* strains, with only the transient presence of detectable bacteria in organs such as liver and spleen [30, 32, 38, 39]. Contrary to *Salmonella* strains, reduction in animal body weight and hypertrophy of spleen (splenomegaly) are not observed after inoculation with *E. coli* strains. However, *Salmonella* strains also show a higher intrinsic antitumoral effect than *E. coli* strains against resilient tumors [39]. Interestingly, the antitumoral effect of *E. coli* Symbioflor-2 strain has been enhanced to levels similar to *Salmonella* by depleting neutrophils *in vivo* [39]. Collectively, these observations highlight both the increased biosafety of *E. coli* strains and the need of engineering to increase their antitumoral effects.

7.2.2 Genetic Engineering *E. coli* for Tumor Therapy and Diagnosis

Given the genetic amenability of *E. coli*, this microorganism has been modified to express or deliver anticancer agents for tumor therapy. As reported with other bacteria, many strategies can be followed, such as the expression of enzymes to activate anticancer "prodrugs," secretion of cytotoxic agents, production of cytokines or tumor antigens that promote immune response against cancer cells, delivery of antibodies that interfere with tumor development, and transfer of mammalian expression vectors (i.e., bactofection) encoding for therapeutic molecules or silencing RNAs (for excellent reviews see Refs. [6, 21, 40]). Jiang and collaborators engineered *E. coli* K-12 to produce the cytotoxic protein cytolysin A (ClyA) for killing tumor cells after IV administration of 5 × 10^7 CFU in immunocompetent BALB/c mice bearing CT26 colon carcinoma [36]. Although the engineered *E. coli* induced extensive tumor necrosis through secretion of ClyA, the restriction of bacteria to the hypoxic regions led to insufficient destruction of the rapidly proliferating tumor tissues. Thus, despite the initial growth retardation, the tumors grew thereafter, indicating that the bacterial therapy was insufficient for complete tumor eradication. *E. coli* equipped with genes encoding a different bacterial toxin, the alpha-hemolysin from *Staphylococcus aureus*, boosted the tumor destruction rate [41]. Bacterial-directed enzyme prodrug therapy has been also evaluated to improve the localized release of toxins in tumor areas [42]. For instance, an *E. coli* strain was engineered to produce the enzyme β-glucuronidase, which catalyzed the transformation of a nontoxic compound or prodrug (i.e., 9ACG) into a toxic drug (i.e., 9AC) [43]. In addition to the direct production (or conversion) of toxins, *E. coli* strains have been modified to express proapoptotic factors, cytokines, or deliver DNA molecules encoding tumor antigens (vaccination) and interference RNA (gene silencing) [6, 21, 44–46]. Remarkably, an *E. coli* strain has been validated as an orphan drug by the US Food and Drug Administration (USFDA) for the treatment of familial adenomatous polyposis that transfers to host cells plasmids encoding short-hairpin RNAs (shRNAs) [46]. The final goal of this therapy is to silence the expression of catenin β-1, which is overproduced in several types of cancer.

E. coli strains that have been prescribed to humans as probiotics to treat gastrointestinal disorders are attractive candidates for tumor therapy. A controlled expression of reporter genes in recombinant EcN strains in tumor-bearing mice has been demonstrated [35]. EcN harboring promoter constructs with bacterial *lux* operon was administered either orally to healthy mice or intravenously to tumor-bearing animals. Subsequent to bacterial colonization of tissues, inducer substances were administered via the oral or systemic route. By use of *in vivo* bioluminescence imaging, the time course of reporter gene expression was analyzed. This and other studies lay the foundation for the recombinant *E. coli* strains able to express a therapeutic substance or a diagnostic molecule in the tumor and only after induction of the gene encoding the enzyme by administration of a simple substance. A recent example of this was the generation an EcN biosensor to indicate liver metastasis by producing detectable signals in urine [47]. The motivation was to generate an accessible, highly sensitive, and selective tool for the detection of small metastases that are beyond the reach of existing diagnostic tools. In this study, the orally administered recombinant strains rapidly (within 24 h) translocated across the gastrointestinal tract and specifically replicated within metastatic tumors present in the liver, leading to high levels of *lacZ* expression, which elicit hydrolysis of systemically injected cleavable substrates of β-galactosidase. Cleavage products of the substrates filtered through the renal system into the urine for detection. This microbial diagnostic generated a high-contrast urine signal through selective expansion in liver metastases and high expression of a *lacZ* reporter maintained by engineering a stable plasmid system. EcN robustly colonized tumor tissue in rodent models of liver metastasis after oral delivery but did not colonize healthy organs or fibrotic liver tissue. Remarkably, no deleterious health effects were observed in the mice for more than 12 months after oral delivery [47].

7.3 Synthetic Biology of *E. coli* to Combat Cancer

7.3.1 Synthetic Biology and the Design of Bacteria against Tumors

The field of synthetic biology is now emerging to bring engineering approaches into biomedicine. As researchers build constructs (e.g., synthetic gene networks and programmable organisms) effective synthetic biology therapies are being implemented through rational design to alter mechanisms and processes underlying disease [48–50]. Thus, using tools from synthetic biology, researchers have now the capability to engineer gene circuits that allow bacteria to communicate and express therapeutic or diagnostic molecules inside tumors. In a recent study, bacteria were engineered with artificial genetic circuits for killing cancer cells in three different ways: by expressing genes to produce an antitumor toxin, by expressing genes to activate a host immune response, and by expressing genes to trigger programmed tumor cell death. To prevent potential side effects from these drugs, the researchers added a control circuit based on quorum sensing (QS). Upon reaching a predetermined target level, the bacterial cells released their toxic contents all at once. Following quorum lysis, surviving bacteria reseed the growing population, leading to pulsatile delivery cycles [51].

7.3.2 Synthetic Adhesins to Program the Adhesion of *E. coli*

As discussed in previous sections, it is well established using tumor-bearing mice models that systemic administration of *E. coli* and *Salmonella* strains results in the preferential colonization of solid tumors. However, clinical trials using systemic administration of *Salmonella* for human cancer therapy revealed that the highest bacterial dose that was tolerated was still insufficient for effective colonization [52, 53]. Therefore, it is of high interest to improve the tumor colonization capabilities of bacteria (i.e., requiring lower doses for effective colonization and showing an increased ratio of bacteria in tumors versus healthy organs).

One way to improve bacterial tumor targeting is to engineer bacterial adhesion toward proteins differentially expressed on the surface of cancer cells. Expression of cell surface proteins in cancer cells is dysregulated, leading to the production of tumor-associated cell surface antigens that often correlate with tumor progression and metastasis, being important factors for prognosis and selection of therapy [54, 55]. In this framework, an engineered *E. coli* strain targeting specifically a cell surface-exposed tumor antigen may be an attractive strategy to improve the bacterial colonization efficiency, increasing specificity and biosafety.

A high variety of proteins involved in tissue and surface adhesion (referred to as adhesins) are encoded in the *E. coli* genome, highlighting the importance that host and surface attachment has for this microorganism [56–58]. Adhesins can be subdivided into two major classes: (i) fimbrial adhesins, which constitute a group of filamentous appendages associated to the bacterial surface, and (ii) non-fimbrial adhesins, which are surface-associated proteins, mostly nonmultimeric, that anchor in the bacterial outer membrane (OM). Frequently, fimbrial- and non-fimbrial adhesins of *E. coli* contain immunoglobulin (Ig)-like domains in their structure for recognition of host tissues/cells [59].

Inspired by the modular organization of the natural *E. coli* intimin family of non-fimbrial adhesins (Fig. 7.1A), we developed synthetic adhesins (SAs) capable of mediating specific adhesion of engineered *E. coli* cells to target cells and tumors *in vitro* and *in vivo* [38]. SAs consist in the highly stable β-barrel module derived from an N-terminal fragment of intimin (Int) called Neae (residues 1-654) that tethers the polypeptide in the OM and allows the display on the bacterial surface of a single antibody variable domain (VHH) of high affinity and specificity (Fig. 7.1A). VHHs, also referred to as nanobodies (Nbs), are small antibody fragments comprising a single variable domain from the heavy chain-only antibodies of camelids (e.g., dromedaries and llamas) [60, 61]. Nbs have a number of properties that make them attractive antibody molecules, such as their small size (ca. 14 kDa), simple structure, high affinity and specificity, distinct epitope recognition, high stability, and similarity to human VH sequences.

To engineer synthetic (e.g., non-natural) *E. coli* adhesion, we developed gene expression cassettes consisting in the SA under the control of a constitutive promoter (P_{N25}) for integration as a single copy in the chromosome of *E. coli*. This allows constant expression of the SA in the absence of exogenous inducers and antibiotics for plasmid maintenance. For site-specific integration in the bacterial chromosome we adapted a markerless gene deletion strategy, enabling sequential manipulation of multiple gene loci, leaving no plasmid sequences (i.e., antibiotic resistance genes) in the chromosome [62]. This technology is based on the insertion of a suicide plasmid bearing homology regions (HRs)

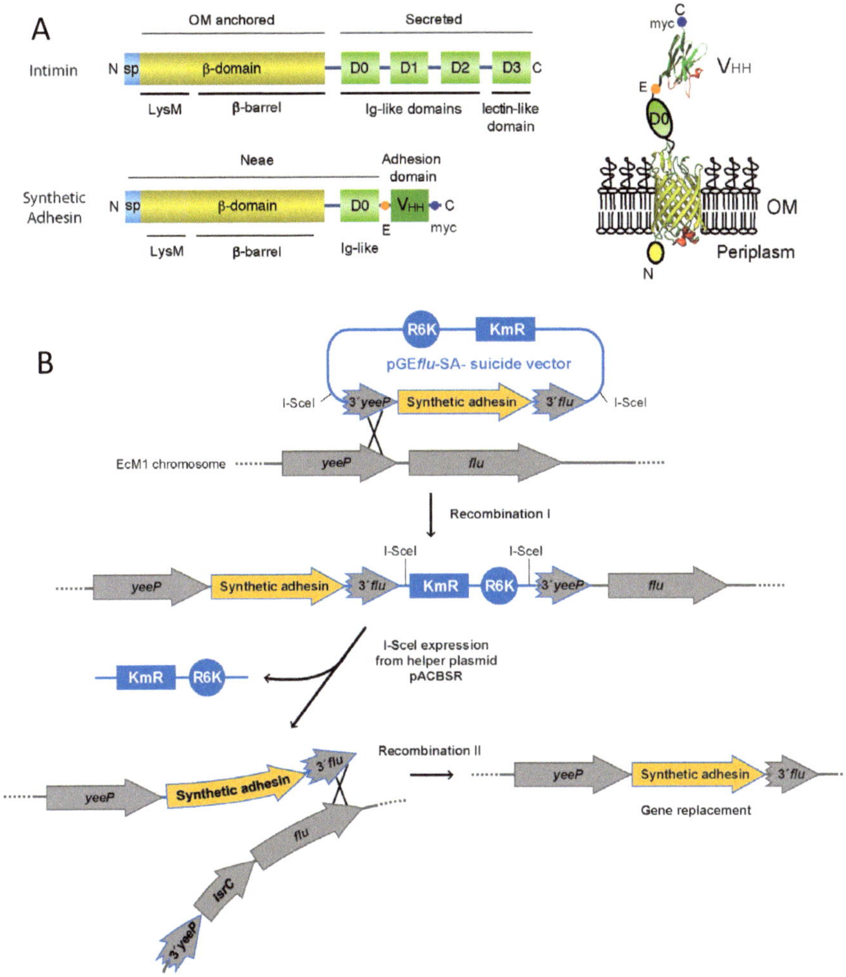

Figure 7.1 Structural organization of the synthetic adhesin and site-specific integration in the chromosome of *E. coli*. (A) Scheme of intimin (polypeptide found in EHEC strains) and synthetic adhesin (SA) fusion. Model of SA polypeptide in the OM (right), with an N-terminal LysM domain in the periplasm, a β-barrel with a linker in the OM, and connecting with C-terminal D0 and VHH domains exposed to the extracellular milieu. (B) Scheme showing the integration of a SA gene in the *flu* locus of the *E. coli* K-12 chromosome. Integration is done using a suicide plasmid containing the pi-dependent R6K origin of replication, a kanamycin resistance gene (Km^R), and a SA gene cassette of the desired specificity under the control of the P_{N25} constitutive promoter. Figure adapted from Ref. [38].

of the targeted gene and the subsequent generation of double-strand breaks by expression of I-SceI restriction endonuclease *in vivo*, which are repaired by homologous recombination, resulting in the specific modification of the targeted gene (Fig. 7.1B). To reduce the natural adhesion capabilities of *E. coli* K-12, the SA cassette was inserted in the chromosome, replacing the *flu* gene, which encodes the antigen 43 adhesin [63]. For the same reason, we used an *E. coli* K-12 strain carrying a deletion of the operon encoding type 1 fimbriae (MG1655Δ*fimA-H*), named EcM1. Type 1 fimbriae are prominent *E. coli* adhesins involved in the recognition of mannosylated glycoproteins found on epithelial cell surfaces [59, 64]. The engineered strains were also tagged with a bioluminescent reporter, the *luxCDABE* operon from *Photorhabdus luminescens* that allows for luminescent visualization without providing exogenous luciferin [65], which was inserted in the *matBCDEF* operon. This operon encodes the meningitis-associated and temperature-regulated Mat fimbriae, also termed *E. coli* common pilus, which is also involved in host cell recognition [66].

The final engineered strains were named EcM1*lux*SAgfp and EcM1*luxS*Atir, having VHHs binding GFP and TirM, respectively, as model antigens. TirM is the extracellular domain (residues 252–360) of the translocated Int receptor enterohemorrhagic *E. coli* O157:H7 (EHEC) [67]. These engineered *E. coli* strains were able to adhere *in vitro* in a highly specific manner to mammalian HeLa-GFP-tm or HeLa-TirM-tm cells, expressing on their surface the target antigen recognized by the SA (Fig. 7.2A and 7.2B). Importantly, the expression of the SAs and the *lux* operon did not affect bacterial growth and was stably maintained without any selection pressure throughout at least 55 bacterial generations (Fig. 7.2C and 7.2D) [38].

7.3.3 Synthetic Adhesins Improve *E. coli* Tumor Targeting

The capability of the engineered *E. coli* strains expressing SAs to colonize experimental tumors was assessed in a tumor xenograft model of athymic nude mice bearing solid tumors of HeLa-GFP-tm cells (200 ≈ 400 mm^3) [38]. In the first term, we tested whether the engineered *E. coli* strains retained their

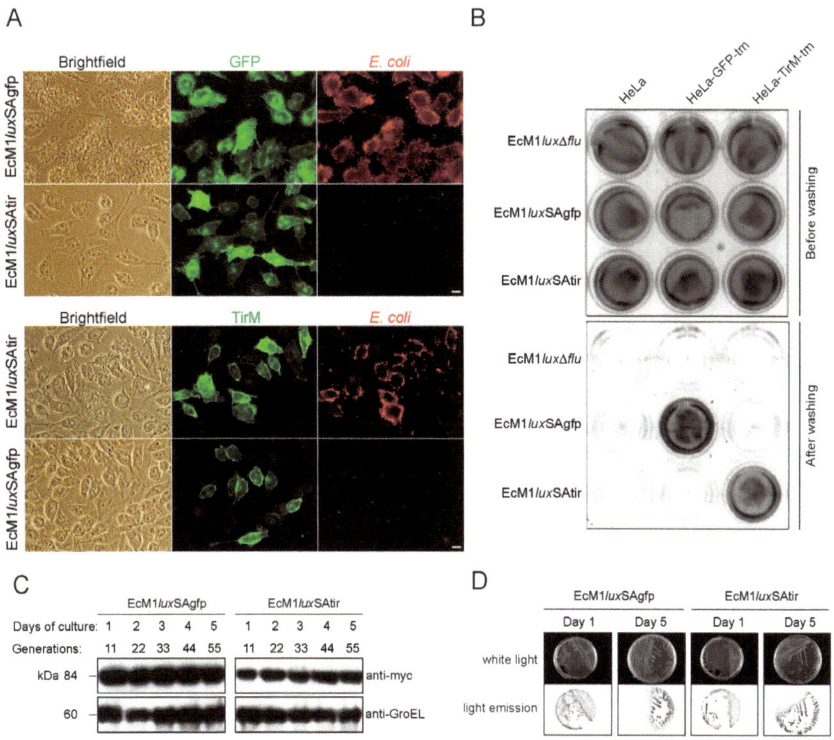

Figure 7.2 Adhesion of *E. coli* expressing synthetic adhesins to target mammalian cells and evaluation of constitutive expression. (A) Light and fluorescence microscopy images of HeLa-GFP-tm cells (upper panels) and HeLa-TirM-tm cells (lower panels) infected with EcM1*lux*SAgfp or EcM1*lux*SAtir bacteria (MOI 300:1), as indicated. Expression of GFP-tm and TirM-tm (containing mWasabi fluorescent protein) on the cell surface is evidenced by their green fluorescence emission. Bacteria were stained with anti–*E. coli* polyclonal serum and anti-IgG-rabbit-Alexa-594 (red). Scale bars represent 10 μm. (B) Bioluminescence assay testing the adhesion of engineered EcM1*lux*Δflu, EcM1*lux*SAgfp, and EcM1*lux*SAtir to target mammalian cells. (C) Western blot analysis of the expression of SAs in EcM1*luxS*Agfp and EcM1*lux*SAtir strains grown in LB cultures for the indicated time. A cytoplasmic GroEL chaperone was used as loading control. (D) Stability of EcM1*lux*SAgfp and EcM1*lux*SAtir bioluminescence. The bacterial strains were grown in liquid LB and diluted with a fresh LB medium (1:2000) for the indicated time. A sample of these cultures was streaked on LB agar plates, and white light and light emission images from the plates were acquired. All individual colonies on the plates show strong bioluminescence. Figure adapted from Ref. [38].

natural ability to colonize tumors. To this end, mice bearing HeLa-GFP-tm tumors were divided into two experimental groups (n = 6), receiving an IV bacterial dose of 1 × 10^7 CFU of either EcM1*lux*SAgfp or EcM1*lux*SAtir strain. Four days after the IV injection, live imaging of the animals showed bioluminescence signals in the tumors from both groups and bacteria were found in high numbers (~10^8 CFU/g) in all tumors from each group (6/6), whereas livers and spleens did not contain detectable bacteria (detection limit ~5 × 10^1 CFU/g) or had low bacterial numbers (<10^3 CFU/g) [38]. This demonstrated that the engineered *E. coli* strains maintained the capacity to colonize solid tumors of HeLa-GFP-tm cells regardless of the specificity of the SA when a high bacterial dose was administered. These results are in agreement with those of Weibel and collaborators, who showed that systemic administration of a single bacterial dose of 5 × 10^6 CFU of wild-type *E. coli* K-12 (strain MG1655) to tumor-bearing mice elicited colonization of >90% of the tumors [30].

Next, we investigated whether the expression of SAs could favor tumor colonization at low bacterial doses. First, we determined that 1 × 10^5 CFU is suboptimal for the colonization of HeLa-GFP-tm tumors by wild-type *E. coli* MG1655, as four days after systemic administration, only one-third of the mice (3/9) showed tumor colonization by bacteria (Fig. 7.3A). This inoculum represents 2% of the dose reported for optimal tumor colonization with wild-type *E. coli* MG1655 [30]. Interestingly, tumors that were colonized had bacterial titers of ~10^8 CFU/g, similar to those found when a high bacterial dose (1 × 10^7 CFU) was employed for inoculation, suggesting that once *E. coli* succeed at an early stage of tumor colonization, the bacteria proliferate, reaching a final titer that is independent of the administered dose.

The ability of EcM1*lux*SAgfp and EcM1*lux*SAtir to colonize HeLa-GFP-tm tumors was compared employing a bacterial dose of 1 × 10^5 CFU, which was suboptimal for wild-type *E. coli* MG1655. As above, EcM1*lux*SAgfp or EcM1*lux*SAtir bacteria were administered intravenously to two groups of mice (n = 9) bearing subcutaneous HeLa-GFP-tm tumors. Four days after inoculation, most of the animals (8/9) inoculated with EcM1*lux*SAgfp had their tumors colonized with high bacterial titers (≥10^8 CFU/g), whereas in the experimental group inoculated with EcM1*lux*SAtir,

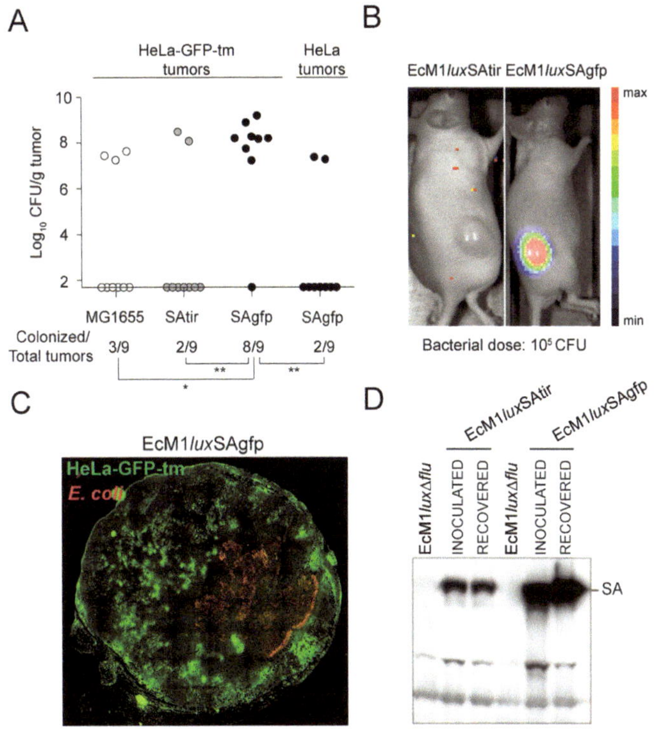

Figure 7.3 *In vivo* colonization of tumors with *E. coli* expressing synthetic adhesins. (A) Bacterial colonization of HeLa-GFP-tm or HeLa tumors by wild-type *E. coli* K-12 (MG1655), EcM1*lux*SAtir (SAtir), and EcM1*lux*SAgfp (SAgfp) strains, as indicated. Each bacterial strain was intravenously administered (1×10^5 CFU/mouse) to tumor-bearing mice (experimental groups n = 9) and four days after administration the number of CFU per gram of tumor (Log10 CFU/g) in each tumor was determined (circles). The ratio of colonized tumors in each group is shown at the bottom, along with the statistical analyses between groups connected with lines. Two-tailed P values of Fisher's exact test are indicated with one asterisk (*) when $P < 0.05$ and two asterisks (**) when $P = 0.015$. (B) Bioluminescence live imaging of HeLa-GFP-tm tumor-bearing mouse infected with 1×10^5 CFU of EcM1*lux*SAtir (left image) and EcM1*lux*SAgfp (right image). The intensities of the bioluminescence signals are represented in pseudocolor according to the scale bar. (C) Histological cross sections of colonized HeLa-GFP-tm solid tumor four days after infection with $\sim 1 \times 10^7$ CFU of EcM1*lux*SAgfp. The bacteria were stained with anti-*E. coli* polyclonal antibodies and anti-rabbit-Alexa-594 antibodies (red). The green color corresponds to the fluorescence of GFP in HeLa-GFP-tm cells. (D) Western blot analysis of SA expression in inoculated and tumor-recovered EcM1*lux*SAtir and EcM1*lux*SAgfp bacteria. Figure adapted from Ref. [38].

less than one-third of the animals (2/9) had colonized tumors (Fig. 7.3A). This differential colonization was also detected by live bioluminescence imaging of the animals (Fig. 7.3B). As a control to evaluate targeting specificity, a dose of 1×10^5 CFU of EcM1*lux*SAgfp was administered systemically to a group (n = 9) of nude mice bearing tumors derived from untransfected HeLa cells. Four days after inoculation, HeLa tumors were colonized with low efficiency (2/9) by EcM1*lux*SAgfp, an identical result to that found with by EcM1*lux*SAtir in HeLa-GFP-tm tumors (Fig. 7.3A). The higher efficiency and specificity in tumor colonization introduced by the SAs allowed a significant reduction (ca. 2 orders of magnitude) of the bacterial dose needed for optimal tumor colonization *in vivo*, an important issue in order to increase the biosafety of bacterial therapies. Histological cross sections of colonized HeLa-GFP-tm tumors revealed that bacteria localized preferentially in the inner regions of the tumors (Fig. 7.3C), mostly at the border with outer regions where tumor cells preferentially proliferate. A similar pattern of bacterial distribution was reported for tumors colonized with wild-type *E. coli* MG1655 [30]. Remarkably, the level of expression of the SAs was identical in the inoculated bacteria and in tumor-recovered bacteria (Fig. 7.3D), showing the stability of the expression of SAs *in vivo.*

7.3.4 Selection of Synthetic Adhesins against Cell Surface Antigens

Libraries of VHHs available in phage display vectors have been used for the selection of high-affinity binders against diverse antigens using biopanning. For SA construction, selected VHHs can be cloned fused to the Neae fragment in the suicide vector for constitutive expression and integration in the chromosome of *E. coli*, as described above. Alternatively, SAs can be directly selected by cloning of VHH libraries fused to the Neae fragment for expression on the surface of *E. coli*. In this process, *E. coli* bacteria displaying the library of VHHs on their surface are incubated with the antigen of interest labeled with the biotin. Bacteria bound to the biotinylated antigen are captured by magnetic cell sorting (MACS) using paramagnetic microbeads coated with streptavidin or antibiotin monoclonal antibody. Growth of antigen-bound bacteria elicits efficient selection of VHHs binding the antigen of interest. Importantly, this *E. coli* display selection enables the direct isolation of SA constructs with the desired antigen specificity, eliminating functional uncertainties of the transfer of VHH sequences from a phage display system to the *E. coli* Neae display system [68, 69]. The *E. coli* display also allows efficient selection of SAs binding tumor cell surface antigens expressed directly on mammalian cells, without purification and biotin labeling. In our laboratory, high-affinity VHHs against the human epidermal growth factor receptor (EGFR), a cell surface receptor overexpressed in many human cancers of epithelial origin, have been selected by screening on a murine cell line transfected with human EGFR [69]. *E. coli* bacteria displaying an immune VHH library raised by immunization of llamas with a human tumor cell line overexpressing EGFR (called A431) were first incubated with the murine mammalian cell line 3T3 to remove nonspecific binders. Next, unbound bacteria were incubated with 3T3 cells transfected with human EGFR. Bacteria bound to the EGFR-expressing cells were grown on LB plates showing selective amplification of bacteria displaying VHHs against human EGFR [69]. An obvious advantage of this methodology is that it enables selection of SAs binding surface antigens expressed on tumor cells. Since this procedure can be done totally on cells, from immunization to selection, it clearly simplifies the isolation of SAs against different cell surface proteins expressed by tumor cells, some of which may be difficult to purify in sufficient amounts and native conformation. In addition, it will open the possibility of using large libraries of VHHs displayed on *E. coli* to screen for SAs binding yet uncharacterized cell surface antigens expressed on human tumors.

7.3.5 Arming Engineered *E. coli* with Protein Injection Nanosyringes

E. coli can be "armed" to act on the tumor cell by inducing its death and/or enhancing the natural cytotoxic activities of immune cells to destroy the tumor [21]. A promising strategy in this regard is the direct delivery of these therapeutic proteins, (e.g., cytotoxins, antibodies, antigens, enzymes, and transcription factors) into the cytoplasm of the tumor and/or immune cells using protein injection systems derived from a bacterial T3SS [70, 71]. The T3SS is found in many gram-negative bacterial pathogens, including *Salmonella, Shigella, Yersinia, Pseudomonas,* and enteropathogenic *E. coli* (EPEC) strains. The T3SS encodes a nanosyringe-like supramolecular protein complex, known as injectisome, which is assembled by over 20 different polypeptides and spans the bacterial envelope to make contact with the host cell [70, 72]. Injectisomes translocate to the cytoplasm of the infected cell a number of bacterial proteins that participate in the infection process, known as effectors. Effectors exert multiple functions, such as reorganization of the cytoskeleton, modulation of the immune response, and apoptosis [73–76]. Delivery to a mammalian cell of a heterologous protein fused to an N-terminal sequence of a natural effector was first demonstrated by the translocation of adenylate cyclase using *Yersinia pseudotuberculosis* [77]. Later, attenuated strains of *Salmonella, Pseudomonas, Yersinia,* and EPEC, among others, have been used to translocate heterologous proteins, such as antigens for vaccination [78–80], antibody fragments [81, 82], transcription factors [83, 84], enzymes for genome edition [85, 86], and proapoptotic peptides [87].

The use of attenuated pathogenic bacteria for protein translocation poses serious biosafety concerns in therapeutic applications since these strains may still have some degree of pathogenicity. Furthermore, the attenuated strains used in the reported studies also translocate their own natural effectors in addition to the protein(s) of interest. These limitations can be overcome by expressing the T3SS in a nonpathogenic bacterial strain devoid of an endogenous T3SS, like commensal, probiotic, and laboratory strains of *E. coli* (e.g., K-12). Studies in which genomic regions encoding T3SS from different pathogens were cloned in *E. coli* K-12 reported weak expression of injectisomes, poor translocation, and bacterial toxicity [88, 89]. More recently, two independent studies have achieved the efficient and functional expression in *E. coli* K-12 of T3SS injectisomes from *Shigella flexneri* [90] and EPEC [91]. The work by Reeves and colleagues [90] used an inducible plasmid system for the expression of *S. flexneri* T3SS in *E. coli* K-12. Our own work obtained the inducible expression of EPEC injectisomes in *E. coli* K-12 using a markerless strategy to integrate in the chromosome the genes needed for the assembly of a function T3SS [91]. Engineered inducible operons for chromosomal integration were constructed avoiding endogenous regulators, promoters, and effectors of EPEC (see below). There are also some differences between both systems that can be relevant for specific applications. *E. coli* K-12 bacteria expressing *Shigella* T3SS injectisomes and a small set of *Shigella* effectors become internalized into the mammalian cell and escape from vacuoles to the cytosol, similarly to wild type *Shigella flexneri* [92]. Importantly, the ability to escape from the vacuoles is provided by the T3SS injectisomes of *Shigella*, even in the absence of effectors [92]. In contrast, *E. coli* K-12 bacteria expressing the T3SS injectisomes of EPEC, an extracellular pathogen, remain extracellular during protein translocation [91]. In addition, EPEC injectisomes contain a long extracellular filament, of up to 700 nm, allowing protein translocation to occur at a distance even when target cells are shielded by extracellular mucins (e.g., enterocytes) [93, 94].

7.3.6 Constructing SIEC Bacteria

We chose the filamentous injectisomes of EPEC for expression in *E. coli* K-12 because of their distinctive properties (i.e., extracellular injection and long filament) and demonstrated the capacity to translocate antibody fragments [81]. The assembly of EPEC injectisomes and their encoding genes are well characterized [94]. Other EPEC-related pathogens, such as EHEC and *Citrobacter rodentium*, also encode similar filamentous injectisomes. These bacteria form part of the attaching and effacing (A/E) family of enteric pathogens causing diarrheal diseases [75, 95, 96]. These bacteria infect the small and large intestines of humans and animals, causing A/E lesions characterized by the intimate attachment of the bacteria to the enterocytes and the disruption (effacement) of the absorptive microvilli surface [97, 98]. All genes required for the assembly of the T3SS injectisome of EPEC and other A/E pathogens are present in the locus for enterocyte effacement (LEE) island [88], a genomic locus organized in five main operons and other smaller transcriptional units. Twenty-seven proteins encoded in the LEE participate in the assembly of the filamentous injectisomes of EPEC, including chaperones and proteins regulating injection [94]. This complexity has hindered the transfer of all genes required for assembly of EPEC injectisomes in *E. coli* K-12. In a previous study, the whole LEE of EPEC was cloned in *E. coli* K-12 in a cosmid but resulted in poor assembly of the T3SS [88]. Hence, we assessed the possibility of engineering an *E. coli* K-12 strain expressing functional injectisomes from EPEC using a synthetic approach.

The projected synthetic injector *E. coli* (SIEC) strain would have integrated in the bacterial chromosome all genes required for the assembly of EPEC injectisomes under the control of an inducible promoter, such as the Ptac, which can be induced with isopropyl-β-D-1-thiogalactopyranoside (IPTG) [99] (Fig. 7.4A). In our approach, gene integration was conducted by a markerless strategy [62] used previously for integration of SAs and *lux* operon [38]. This strategy renders the resulting engineered bacteria free of antibiotic resistance genes and mobile elements (i.e., plasmids) and allows a stable, controlled expression of the injectisomes.

In the design of the engineered LEE operons (eLEEs), we discarded genes encoding effectors and transcriptional regulators and also the natural promoters of the LEE operons, selecting only the genes encoding injectisome structural proteins (*escK*, *escL*, *escR*, *escS*, *escT*, *escU*, *escC*, *escJ*, *escI*, *escV*, *escN*, *escO*, *escP*, *escQ*, *escC*, and *escF*), assembly checkpoint regulators (*sepD*, *sepL*, and *cesL*), chaperones (*escE*, *cesAB*, *cesD*, *cesD2*, and *escG*), and the translocators of the T3SS substrates (*espA*, *espB*, and *espD*) [94] (Fig. 7.4B). We maintained the original gene order found in the native LEE operons, excluding effector genes, amplifying from the start codon of the first selected gene of the operon to the stop codon of the last one. This implied the deletion of native promoters, transcriptional terminators, and ribosome binding sites (RBS) found in these operons, which were replaced by a strong RBS (RBS264). The design resulted in five transcriptional units attending to the genome organization of the LEE: eLEE1, eLEE2, eLEE3, eLEE4, and eEscD (Fig. 7.4C).

Similarly to SAs, we selected the strain *E. coli* K-12 MG1655 lacking type 1 fimbriae (EcM1) as the parental strain of SIEC. We integrated the eLEEs in loci encoding natural and cryptic adhesins of K-12 [56–58] as potential integration sites. Before integrating the eLEE operons, we determined the expression of a GFP reporter in different adhesin loci. Upon determination by

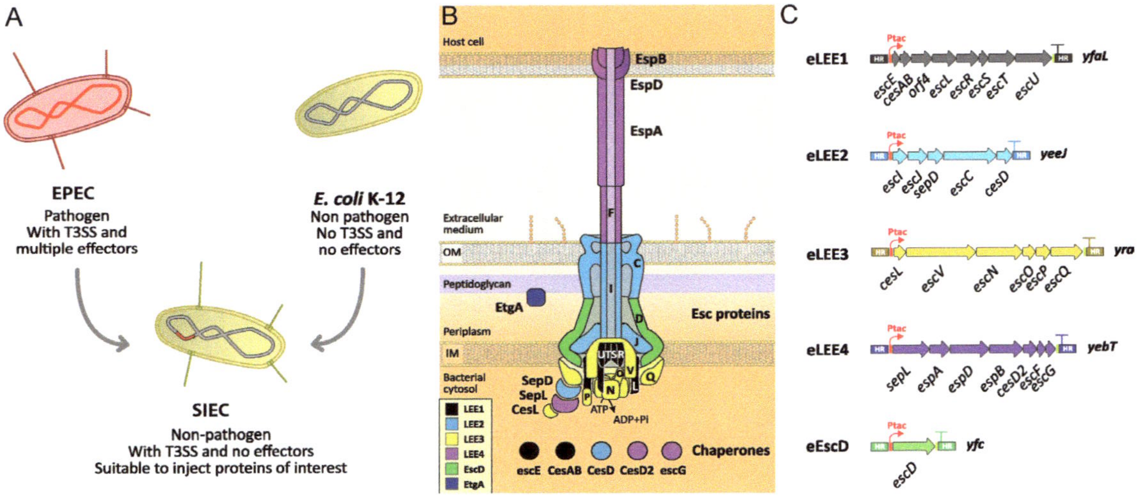

Figure 7.4 Strategy for the generation of SIEC. (A) Scheme showing the properties of interest of EPEC and *E. coli* K-12 MG1655 strains that make them appealing for the generation of SIEC strain. (B) Model showing the structure of EPEC injectisomes comprising a basal body anchored to the bacterial envelope and an extracellular needle terminated with a long extracellular filament. The scheme indicates the proposed location of proteins that assemble the injectisome basal body (Esc proteins) in the bacterial inner and outer membranes (IM and OM), the cytoplasmic ATPase (EscN), the components of the cytoplasmic switch complex (SepD, SepL, and CesL), the proteins building the extracellular needle (EscF) and filament (EspA), and those forming the translocation pore in the host plasma membrane (EspB and EspD). Cytoplasmic chaperones and the peptidoglycan (PG)-associated transglycosylase (EtgA) are also indicated. Each protein is colored according to its encoding operon (color code as in A). (C) Scheme showing the structure of the engineered operons integrated in the chromosome of *E. coli* K-12. The Ptac promoter, transcriptional terminator and flanking HRs of the *loci* used for integration (*yfaL*, *yeeJ*, *yra*, *yebT*, and *yfc*) are indicated. Figure adapted from Ref. [91].

flow cytometry of the fluorescence intensities, *yeeJ*, *yebT*, *yra*, *yfaL*, and *yfc* loci were selected for the integration of the five eLEE operons. In addition, to maintain the relative expression hierarchy of the natural LEE operons, we chose an integration site for each eLEE operon according to the relative expression of LEE operons in EPEC [100, 101]. Taking all the information together, *yeeJ* was assigned to eLEE2, *yebT* to eLEE4, *yra* to eLEE3, *yfaL* to eLEE1, and *yfc* to eEscD. As a control strain, we also constructed a promoterless version of eLEE1, named eLEE1*, that lacks the Ptac promoter. Integration of the operons was done sequentially, starting with the eLEE2 operon, followed by eLEE3, eEscD, the promoterless eLEE1*, and lastly eLEE4. Upon integration of these operons we obtained strain SIECΔp1, which contains all eLEEs under the Ptac except eLEE1*. Finally, we integrated the Ptac upstream of the eLEE1* to obtain the final SIEC strain, containing all eLEEs under the control of Ptac [91].

7.3.7 SIEC Bacteria Assembles Functional Injectisomes

We confirmed that SIEC was able to express EPEC injectisomes from the different operons integrated in its chromosome. This was initially carried out by Western blot analysis of the bacterial protein lysates from induced cultures of SIEC (Fig. 7.5A). In parallel, we analyzed bacterial proteins from wild-type EPEC, EPECΔ*escN* (a mutant lacking the essential ATPase EscN of the T3SS), uninduced SIEC, SIECΔp1, and parental EcM1 strains. This analysis confirmed the expression of the OM secretin EscC and the inner-ring-forming protein EscJ (from eLEE2 operon), the protein EscD (from a single transcriptional unit), the ATPase EscN that energizes the system (from eLEE3), and the translocators EspB and EspA (from eLEE4). Interestingly, the expression levels of these proteins in the induced SIEC strain were similar to or even higher (for EscD, EspB, and EspA) than those produced by the wild-type EPEC strain (Fig. 7.5A). Importantly, we also determined that the expression of the eLEE operons did not affect the growth and viability of SIEC strain when compared with the parental strain EcM1. Maintaining bacterial viability and growth after engineering is a crucial element for future applications *in vivo*.

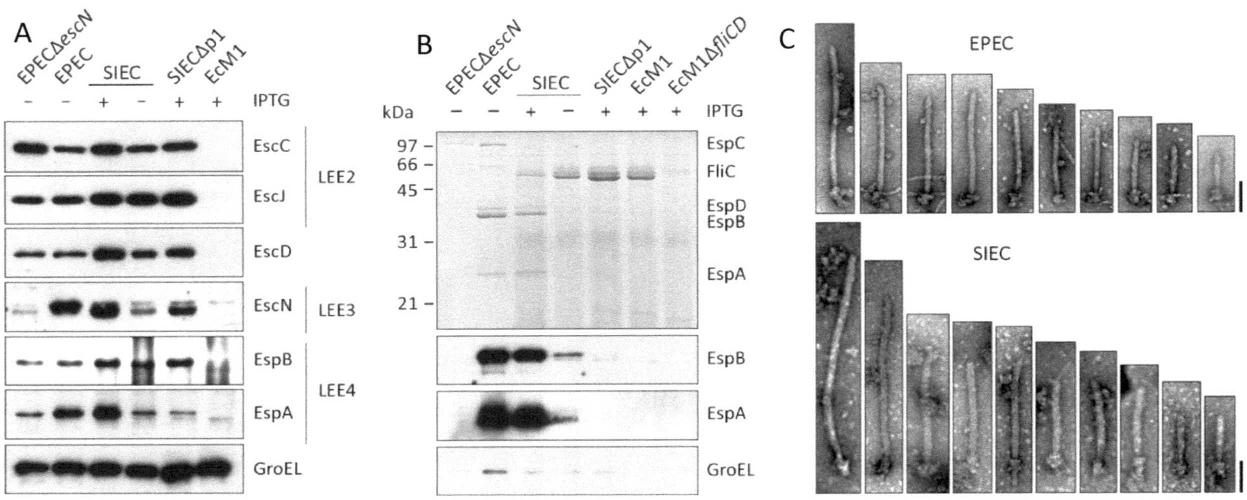

Figure 7.5 SIEC bacteria express filamentous injectisomes upon induction. (A) Western blot of the bacterial whole-cell protein extracts from the indicated bacterial strains (EPECΔ*escN*, EPEC, SIEC, SIECΔp1, and EcM1), induced (+) or not (–) with IPTG, detecting proteins of the T3SS (EscC, EscJ, EscD, EscN, EspB, and EspA), and GroEL as a loading control. The identity of each protein band is indicated on the right, along with the encoding operon. (B) Coomassie staining and Western blot of proteins in culture media of the indicated strains (EPEC, EPECΔ*escN*, SIEC, SIECΔp1, EcM1, and EcM1Δ*fliCD*) induced (+) or not (–) with IPTG. Anti-EspA, -EspB, and -GroEL antibodies were used in Western blot. Detection of cytoplasmic GroEL was used to control for the absence of bacterial lysis. The protein bands of T3SS translocators EspA, EspB, and EspD; of autotransporter EspC; and flagellin (FliC) are labeled on the right. Molecular weight markers are indicated on the left (in kDa). (C) TEM micrographs showing representative injectisome-like particles visualized in negatively stained protein samples after injectisome purification from induced EPEC and SIEC bacteria, as indicated. Injectisome particles are aligned at their basal bodies to show the different lengths of their filaments. Scale bars represent 50 nm. Figure adapted from Ref. [91].

When the basal needle complex of EPEC injectisomes is assembled, it mediates the secretion of the translocator proteins EspB, EspD, and EspA. EspA forms the extracellular filaments that extend up to 700 nm from the basal complex of the injectisome. EspB and EspD get located on the tip of EspA filaments and later form the translocon pore in the plasma membrane of the mammalian cell for injection of proteins (reviewed in Ref. [94]). Bacteria expressing a functional needle complex are able to secrete EspA, EspB, and EspD proteins. Analysis of the proteins found in the culture media of IPTG-induced SIEC strain allowed the detection of EspA, EspB, and EspD (Fig. 7.5B). Importantly, in the absence of an inducer, the proteins EspB, EspD, and EspA were not efficiently secreted by SIEC. Likewise, the strain SIECΔp1 was defective for the secretion of EspA, EspB, and EspD proteins. In addition, assembly of EPEC injectisomes in the SIEC strain was also supported by visualization of EspA filaments on the surface of induced SIEC bacteria using electron microscopy. Injectisomes could be purified and visualized by electron microscopy from the induced SIEC strain as well as the wild-type EPEC (Fig. 7.5C).

We also demonstrated that the levels of injectisomes produced by SIEC were much higher than those produced by the parental EcM1 transformed with a cosmid carrying the entire LEE of EPEC (named pCVD462) [91]. In addition to the higher expression, SIEC has benefits such as a controlled inducible expression, the absence of LEE effectors, the lack of antibiotic-resistant genes, and a high genetic stability due to the chromosomal integration of the eLEEs.

7.3.8 SIEC Bacteria Translocate Proteins to Tumor Cells

We also demonstrated that SIEC was capable of protein translocation into mammalian cells. As a first approach, we measured the formation of the EspB/D translocation pore in the plasma membrane by quantifying the lysis of red blood cells by bacteria [91]. This assay had been previously used to quantitate the assembly of functional injectisomes by EPEC strains [102]. The hemolytic activity determined for the induced SIEC strain reached ca. 70% of that detected with wild-type EPEC, indicating that EspB and EspD translocators secreted by SIEC were capable of forming pores on mammalian plasma membranes.

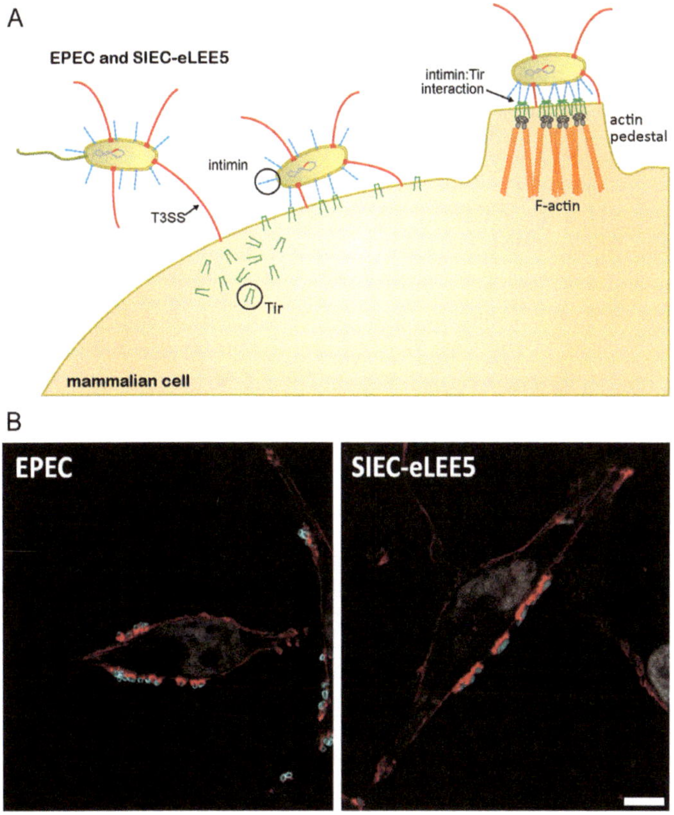

Figure 7.6 Translocation of Tir protein into HeLa cells by the injectisomes of SIEC. (A) Scheme showing intimate adhesion of EPEC and SIEC-eLEE5 bacteria to mammalian cells. The bacterium injects Tir into the cytoplasm through the T3SS. Tir exposes on the membrane of the eukaryotic cell its central domain and is recognized by the C-terminal lectin-like domain of intimin. The Int:Tir interaction induces the clustering of Tir, leading to an intimate attachment of the bacteria and the polymerization of filamentous actin at the site of bacterial attachment, referred to as actin pedestals. (B) Confocal fluorescence microscopy images of HeLa cells infected with the bacterial strains EPEC and SIEC-eLEE5 and stained with TRITC-conjugated phalloidin (red) to visualize F-actin and DAPI (gray) to visualize DNA and nuclei. EPEC bacteria are labeled with anti-intimin 280 and Alexa 488–conjugated anti-rabbit antibodies (cyan). Fluorescence signals of SIEC bacteria expressing GFP are also colored in cyan. Strong red fluorescence signals are clearly visible beneath adhered EPEC and SIEC-eLEE5 bacteria, indicating F-actin pedestal formation triggered by translocated Tir protein. Figure adapted from Ref. [91].

Next, we demonstrated that SIEC was able to inject a biologically active effector protein into tumor HeLa cells. During infection EPEC bacteria translocate their own specific receptor Tir (*t*ranslocated *i*ntimin *r*eceptor) to the infected cells. The translocated Tir gets inserted in the host plasma membrane, and its extracellular domain is recognized by the OM protein Int exposed on the bacterial surface [98, 103]. The Int-Tir interaction leads to the intimate attachment of the bacteria to the infected host cell and triggers a localized F-actin polymerization underneath the attached bacteria that produces actin-rich pedestal-like protrusions of the host plasma membrane at the sites of bacterial intimate adhesion (Fig. 7.6A). These actin-rich accumulations are visible by fluorescence microscopy after staining of infected cells with a fluorophore phalloidin conjugate [97]. To test whether SIEC could inject Tir effector, we integrated an additional eLEE operon (called eLEE5) encoding Tir, Int, and the Tir-specific chaperone CesT in the *flu* locus (Antigen 43) of SIEC and SIECΔp1. Following integration, we obtained strains SIEC-eLEE5 and SIECΔp1-eLEE5, in which we confirmed the expression of Int and Tir.

HeLa cells were infected with SIEC-eLEE5 bacteria, which adhered intimately to the cells and induced intense actin accumulation beneath the bound bacteria, similar to the actin pedestals triggered by EPEC (Fig. 7.6A). As expected, infection with control strains SIECΔp1-eLEE5 and EPECΔ*escN* bacteria did not trigger actin pedestal formation. SIECΔp1-eLEE5 were unable to bind to HeLa cells and were efficiently washed out from the preparations before fluorescence staining. Hence, SIEC-eLEE5, similarly to EPEC, is able to inject functional Tir into HeLa cells, leading to strong intimate bacterial adhesion and formation of actin pedestals.

7.4 Conclusions and Future Perspectives

SAs and a controlled expression of T3SS protein delivery systems in *E. coli* K-12 represent two desirable milestones to improve bacterial therapies against cancer. These two technologies, in combination with the development of logic genetic circuits for controlled expression, integration of environmental signals and memory, metabolic engineering, and other developments of synthetic biology, might allow the ultimate development of "smart" *E. coli* bacteria that distinguish between healthy and tumor cells and deliver different therapeutic molecules for specific tumors, following the concept of personalized medicine [49, 50, 104–107]. Additional interesting elements of engineering in *E. coli* to improve tumor targeting include bacterial chemotaxis and metabolism, to generate a strong cancer-cell metabolic dependence for bacterial growth [6, 8, 108]. The incorporation of QS genetic circuits activated by bacterial density could also assist in the controlled release of cytotoxins at the tumor site [109]. These QS systems can be coupled to a controlled death of the bacterium *in vivo*, increasing its biosafety [51]. Biosafety is of major importance for the actual application of bacterial therapies in the clinic [110, 111]. Fortunately, different approaches already exist to increase biosafety of the engineered bacteria, from the simple incorporation of auxotrophies to complex engineering to generate bacterial dependence of unnatural amino acids or nucleotides [112, 113]. Altogether, these developments are paving the way for the future clinical use of bacteria as an additional part of the global medical weaponry against human cancer.

Acknowledgment

Work in the laboratory of LAF is supported by research grants from the Spanish *Ministerio de Ciencia, Innovación y Universidad* BIO2017-89081R, and the European Research Council ERC-2012-ADG_20120314.

References

1. Pawelek J. M., Low K. B., Bermudes D. Bacteria as tumour-targeting vectors. *The Lancet Oncology*, 4 (2003) 548–556.
2. Piñero-Lambea C., Ruano-Gallego D., Fernández L. Á. Engineered bacteria as therapeutic agents. *Current Opinion in Biotechnology*, 35 (2015) 94–102.
3. Morales A., Eidinger D. Bacillus Calmette–Guerin in the treatment of adenocarcinoma of the kidney. *Journal of Urology*, 115 (1976) 377–380.

4. Gandhi N. M., Morales A., Lamm D. L. Bacillus Calmette–Guerin immunotherapy for genitourinary cancer. *British Journal of Urology International*, 112 (2013) 288–289 doi:10.1111/j.1464-410X.2012.11754.x.

5. Kamat A. M., Flaig T. W., Grossman H. B., Konety B., Lamm D., O'Donnell M. A., *et al.* Expert consensus document: consensus statement on best practice management regarding the use of intravesical immunotherapy with BCG for bladder cancer. *Nature Reviews Urology*, 12 (2015) 225–235.

6. Forbes N. S. Engineering the perfect (bacterial) cancer therapy. *Nature Reviews Cancer*, 10 (2010) 785–794.

7. Toley B. J., Forbes N. S. Motility is critical for effective distribution and accumulation of bacteria in tumor tissue. *Integrative Biology (Camb)*, 4 (2012) 165–176.

8. Thornlow D. N., Brackett E. L., Gigas J. M., Van Dessel N., Forbes N. S. Persistent enhancement of bacterial motility increases tumor penetration. *Biotechnology and Bioengineering*, (2015) doi:10.1002/bit.25645.

9. Felgner S., Kocijancic D., Frahm M., Weiss S. Bacteria in cancer therapy: renaissance of an old concept. *International Journal of Microbiology*, 2016 (2016) 8451728.

10. Sznol M., Lin S. L., Bermudes D., Zheng L. M., King I. Use of preferentially replicating bacteria for the treatment of cancer. *Journal of Clinical Investigation*, 105 (2000) 1027–1030.

11. St Jean A. T., Zhang M., Forbes N. S. Bacterial therapies: completing the cancer treatment toolbox. *Current Opinion in Biotechnology*, 19 (2008) 511–517.

12. Vance R. E., Isberg R. R., Portnoy D. A. Patterns of pathogenesis: discrimination of pathogenic and nonpathogenic microbes by the innate immune system. *Cell Host & Microbe*, 6 (2009) 10–21.

13. Avogadri F., Martinoli C., Petrovska L., Chiodoni C., Transidico P., Bronte V., *et al.* Cancer immunotherapy based on killing of *Salmonella*-infected tumor cells. *Cancer Research*, 65 (2005) 3920–3927.

14. Westphal K., Leschner S., Jablonska J., Loessner H., Weiss S. Containment of tumor-colonizing bacteria by host neutrophils. *Cancer Research*, 68 (2008) 2952–2960.

15. Shahabi V., Maciag P. C., Rivera S., Wallecha A. Live, attenuated strains of *Listeria* and *Salmonella* as vaccine vectors in cancer treatment. *Bioengineered Bugs*, 1 (2010) 235–243.

16. Liu B., Jiang Y., Dong T., Zhao M., Wu J., Li L., *et al.* Blockage of autophagy pathway enhances *Salmonella* tumor-targeting. *Oncotarget*, 7 (2016) 22873–22882 doi:10.18632/oncotarget.8251.

17. Zhang M., Swofford C. A., Forbes N. S. Lipid A controls the robustness of intratumoral accumulation of attenuated *Salmonella* in mice. *International Journal of Cancer*, 135 (2014) 647–657.

18. Ganai S., Arenas R. B., Sauer J. P., Bentley B., Forbes N. S. In tumors *Salmonella* migrate away from vasculature toward the transition zone and induce apoptosis. *Cancer Gene Therapy*, 18 (2011) 457–466.

19. Kasinskas R. W., Forbes N. S. *Salmonella typhimurium* lacking ribose chemoreceptors localize in tumor quiescence and induce apoptosis. *Cancer Research*, 67 (2007) 3201–3209.

20. Jia L. J., Wei D. P., Sun Q. M., Huang Y., Wu Q., Hua Z. C. Oral delivery of tumor-targeting *Salmonella* for cancer therapy in murine tumor models. *Cancer Science*, 98 (2007) 1107–1112.

21. Van Dessel N., Swofford C. A., Forbes N. S. Potent and tumor specific: arming bacteria with therapeutic proteins. *Therapeutic Delivery*, 6 (2015) 385–399.

22. Wilson W. R., Hay M. P. Targeting hypoxia in cancer therapy. *Nature Reviews Cancer*, 11 (2011) 393–410.

23. Brown J. M., Wilson W. R. Exploiting tumour hypoxia in cancer treatment. *Nature Reviews Cancer*, 4 (2004) 437–447.

24. Yu Y. A., Zhang Q., Szalay A. A. Establishment and characterization of conditions required for tumor colonization by intravenously delivered bacteria. *Biotechnology and Bioengineering*, 100 (2008) 567–578.

25. Maeda H. The link between infection and cancer: tumor vasculature, free radicals, and drug delivery to tumors via the EPR effect. *Cancer Science*, 104 (2013) 779–789.

26. Leschner S., Westphal K., Dietrich N., Viegas N., Jablonska J., Lyszkiewicz M., *et al.* Tumor invasion of *Salmonella enterica serovar Typhimurium* is accompanied by strong hemorrhage promoted by TNF-α. *Plos ONE*, 4 (2009) e6692.

27. Zu C., Wang J. Tumor-colonizing bacteria: A potential tumor targeting therapy. *Critical Reviews in Microbiology*, 40 (2013) 225–235 doi:10.3109/1040841x.2013.776511.

28. Pawelek J. M., Low K. B., Bermudes D. Tumor-targeted *Salmonella* as a novel anticancer vector. *Cancer Research*, 57 (1997) 4537–4544.

29. Forbes N. S., Munn L. L., Fukumura D., Jain R. K. Sparse initial entrapment of systemically injected *Salmonella typhimurium* leads

to heterogeneous accumulation within tumors. *Cancer Research*, 63 (2003) 5188–5193.

30. Weibel S., Stritzker J., Eck M., Goebel W., Szalay A. A. Colonization of experimental murine breast tumours by *Escherichia coli* K-12 significantly alters the tumour microenvironment. *Cellular Microbiology*, 10 (2008) 1235–1248.
31. Yu Y. A., Shabahang S., Timiryasova T. M., Zhang Q., Beltz R., Gentschev I., *et al.* Visualization of tumors and metastases in live animals with bacteria and vaccinia virus encoding light-emitting proteins. *Nature Biotechnology*, 22 (2004) 313–320.
32. Stritzker J., Weibel S., Hill P. J., Oelschlaeger T. A., Goebel W., Szalay A. A. Tumor-specific colonization, tissue distribution, and gene induction by probiotic *Escherichia coli* Nissle 1917 in live mice. *International Journal of Medical Microbiology*, 297 (2007) 151–162.
33. Brader P., Stritzker J., Riedl C. C., Zanzonico P., Cai S., Burnazi E. M., Ghani E. R., *et al. Escherichia coli* Nissle 1917 facilitates tumor detection by positron emission tomography and optical imaging. *Clinical Cancer Research*, 14 (2008) 2295–2302.
34. Min J. J., Kim H. J., Park J. H., Moon S., Jeong J. H., Hong Y. J., *et al.* Noninvasive real-time imaging of tumors and metastases using tumor-targeting light-emitting *Escherichia coli*. *Molecular Imaging and Biology*, 10 (2008) 54–61.
35. Loessner H., Leschner S., Endmann A., Westphal K., Wolf K., Kochruebe K., *et al.* Drug-inducible remote control of gene expression by probiotic *Escherichia coli* Nissle 1917 in intestine, tumor and gall bladder of mice. *Microbes and Infection*, 11 (2009) 1097–1105.
36. Jiang S. N., Phan T. X., Nam T. K., Nguyen V. H., Kim H. S., Bom H. S., *et al.* Inhibition of tumor growth and metastasis by a combination of *Escherichia coli*-mediated cytolytic therapy and radiotherapy. *Molecular Therapy*, 18 (2010) 635–642.
37. Zhang Y., Zhang Y., Xia L., Zhang X., Ding X., Yan F., *et al. Escherichia coli* Nissle 1917 targets and restrains mouse B16 melanoma and 4T1 breast tumor through the expression of azurin protein. *Applied and Environmental Microbiology*, 78 (2012) 7603–7610 doi:10.1128/AEM.01390-12.
38. Piñero-Lambea C., Bodelón G., Fernández-Periáñez R., Cuesta A. M., Álvarez-Vallina L., Fernández L. A. Programming controlled adhesion

of *E. coli* to target surfaces, cells, and tumors with synthetic adhesins. *ACS Synthetic Biology*, 4 (2015) 463–473.

39. Kocijancic D., Felgner S., Frahm M., Komoll R. M., Iljazovic A., Pawar V., *et al.* Therapy of solid tumors using probiotic Symbioflor-2: restraints and potential. *Oncotarget*, 7 (2016) 22605–22622.
40. Hosseinidoust Z., Mostaghaci B., Yasa O., Park B.-W., Singh A. V., Sitti M. Bioengineered and biohybrid bacteria-based systems for drug delivery. *Advanced Drug Delivery Reviews*, (2016) doi: 10.1016/j.addr.2016.09.007.
41. St Jean A. T., Swofford C. A., Panteli J. T., Brentzel Z. J., Forbes N. S. Bacterial delivery of *Staphylococcus aureus* α-hemolysin causes regression and necrosis in murine tumors. *Molecular Therapy*, 22 (2014) 1266–1274.
42. Lehouritis P., Springer C., Tangney M. Bacterial-directed enzyme prodrug therapy. *Journal of Controlled Release*, 170 (2013) 120–131.
43. Lehouritis P., Stanton M., McCarthy F. O., Jeavons M., Tangney M. Activation of multiple chemotherapeutic prodrugs by the natural enzymolome of tumour-localised probiotic bacteria. *Journal of Controlled Release*, 222 (2015) 9–17.
44. Radford K. J., Higgins D. E., Pasquini S., Cheadle E. J., Carta L., Jackson A. M., *et al.* A recombinant *E. coli* vaccine to promote MHC class I-dependent antigen presentation: application to cancer immunotherapy. *Gene Therapy*, 9 (2002) 1455–1463.
45. Critchley R. J., Jezzard S., Radford K. J., Goussard S., Lemoine N. R., Grillot-Courvalin C., *et al.* Potential therapeutic applications of recombinant, invasive *E. coli*. *Gene Therapy*, 11 (2004) 1224–1233.
46. Xiang S., Fruehauf J., Li C. J. Short hairpin RNA-expressing bacteria elicit RNA interference in mammals. *Nature Biotechnology*, 24 (2006) 697–702.
47. Danino T., Prindle A., Kwong G. A., Skalak M., Li H., Allen K., *et al.* Programmable probiotics for detection of cancer in urine. *Science Translational Medicine*, 7 (2015) 289ra284.
48. Hasty J. Engineered microbes for therapeutic applications. *ACS Synthetic Biology*, 1 (2012) 438–439.
49. Church G. M., Elowitz M. B., Smolke C. D., Voigt C. A., Weiss R. Realizing the potential of synthetic biology. *Nature Reviews Molecular Cell Biology*, 15 (2014) 289–294.

50. Cameron D. E., Bashor C. J., Collins J. J. A brief history of synthetic biology. *Nature Reviews Microbiology*, 12 (2014) 381–390 doi:10.1038/nrmicro3239.
51. Din M. O., Danino T., Prindle A., Skalak M., Selimkhanov J., Allen K., *et al.* Synchronized cycles of bacterial lysis for in vivo delivery. *Nature*, 536 (2016) 81–85.
52. Toso J. F., Gill V. J., Hwu P., Marincola F. M., Restifo N. P., Schwartzentruber D. J., *et al.* Phase I study of the intravenous administration of attenuated *Salmonella typhimurium* to patients with metastatic melanoma. *Journal of Clinical Oncology*, 20 (2002) 142–152.
53. Heimann D. M., Rosenberg S. A. Continuous intravenous administration of live genetically modified *Salmonella typhimurium* in patients with metastatic melanoma. *Journal of Immunotherapy*, 26 (2003) 179–180.
54. Ludwig J. A., Weinstein J. N. Biomarkers in cancer staging, prognosis and treatment selection. *Nature Reviews Cancer*, 5 (2005) 845–856.
55. Scott A. M., Wolchok J. D., Old L. J. Antibody therapy of cancer. *Nature Reviews Cancer*, 12 (2012) 278–287.
56. Korea C. G., Ghigo J. M., Beloin C. The sweet connection: Solving the riddle of multiple sugar-binding fimbrial adhesins in *Escherichia coli*. Multiple *E. coli* fimbriae form a versatile arsenal of sugar-binding lectins potentially involved in surface-colonisation and tissue tropism. *BioEssays*, 33 (2011) 300–311.
57. Korea C. G., Badouraly R., Prevost M. C., Ghigo J. M., Beloin C. *Escherichia coli* K-12 possesses multiple cryptic but functional chaperone-usher fimbriae with distinct surface specificities. *Environmental Microbiology*, 12 (2010) 1957–1977.
58. Roux A., Beloin C., Ghigo J. M. Combined inactivation and expression strategy to study gene function under physiological conditions: application to identification of new *Escherichia coli* adhesins. *Journal of Bacteriology*, 187 (2005) 1001–1013.
59. Bodelón G., Palomino C., Fernández L. A. Immunoglobulin domains in *Escherichia coli* and other enterobacteria: from pathogenesis to applications in antibody technologies. *FEMS Microbiol Reviews*, 37 (2013) 204–250.
60. Muyldermans S., Cambillau C., Wyns L. Recognition of antigens by single-domain antibody fragments: the superfluous luxury of paired domains. *Trends in Biochemical Sciences*, 26 (2001) 230–235.

61. Muyldermans S. Nanobodies: natural single-domain antibodies. *Annual Review of Biochemistry*, 82 (2013) 775–797.

62. Posfai G., Kolisnychenko V., Bereczki Z., Blattner F. R. Markerless gene replacement in *Escherichia coli* stimulated by a double-strand break in the chromosome. *Nucleic Acids Research*, 27 (1999) 4409–4415.

63. van der Woude M. W., Henderson I. R. Regulation and function of Ag43 (flu). *Annual Review of Microbiology*, 62 (2008) 153–169.

64. Lillington J., Geibel S., Waksman G. Biogenesis and adhesion of type 1 and P pili. *Biochimica Et Biophysica Acta*, 1840 (2014) 2783–2793 doi:10.1016/j.bbagen.2014.04.021.

65. Winson M. K., Swift S., Hill P. J., Sims C. M., Griesmayr G., Bycroft B. W., *et al.* Engineering the *luxCDABE* genes from *Photorhabdus luminescens* to provide a bioluminescent reporter for constitutive and promoter probe plasmids and mini-Tn5 constructs. *FEMS Microbiology Letters*, 163 (1998) 193–202.

66. Rendon M. A., Saldana Z., Erdem A. L., Monteiro-Neto V., Vazquez A., Kaper J. B., *et al.* Commensal and pathogenic *Escherichia coli* use a common pilus adherence factor for epithelial cell colonization. *Proceedings of the National Academy of Sciences of the United States of America*, 104 (2007) 10637–10642.

67. Frankel G., Phillips A. D., Trabulsi L. R., Knutton S., Dougan G., Matthews S. Intimin and the host cell—is it bound to end in Tir(s)? *Trends in Microbiology*, 9 (2001) 214–218.

68. Salema V., Marín E., Martínez-Arteaga R., Ruano-Gallego D., Fraile S., Margolles Y., *et al.* Selection of single domain antibodies from immune libraries displayed on the surface of *E. coli* cells with two β-domains of opposite topologies. *PLOS One*, 8 (2013) e75126.

69. Salema V., Mañas C., Cerdán L., Piñero-Lambea C., Marín E., Roovers R. C., *et al.* High affinity nanobodies against human epidermal growth factor receptor selected on cells by *E. coli* display. *mAbs* 8 (2016) 1286–1301.

70. Portaliou A. G., Tsolis K. C., Loos M. S., Zorzini V., Economou A. Type III secretion: building and operating a remarkable nanomachine. *Trends in Biochemical Sciences*, 41 (2016) 175–189.

71. Galán J. E., Lara-Tejero M., Marlovits T. C., Wagner S. Bacterial type III secretion systems: specialized nanomachines for protein delivery into target cells. *Annual Review of Microbiology*, 68 (2014) 415–438.

72. Cornelis G. R. The type III secretion injectisome. *Nature Reviews Microbiology*, 4 (2006) 811–825.

73. Raymond B., Young J. C., Pallett M., Endres R. G., Clements A., Frankel G. Subversion of trafficking, apoptosis, and innate immunity by type III secretion system effectors. *Trends in Microbiology*, 21 (2013) 430–441.

74. Wall D. M., McCormick B. A. Bacterial secreted effectors and caspase-3 interactions. *Cellular Microbiology*, (2014) doi:10.1111/cmi.12368.

75. Santos A. S., Finlay B. B. Bringing down the host: enteropathogenic and enterohaemorrhagic *Escherichia coli* effector-mediated subversion of host innate immune pathways. *Cellular Microbiology*, 17 (2015) 318–332.

76. Ratner D., Orning M. P., Lien E. Bacterial secretion systems and regulation of inflammasome activation. *Journal of Leukocyte Biology*, 101 (2016) 165–181 doi:10.1189/jlb.4MR0716-330R.

77. Sory M. P., Cornelis G. R. Translocation of a hybrid Yop E-adenylate cyclase from *Yersinia enterocolitica* into HeLa cells. *Molecular Microbiology*, 14 (1994) 583–594.

78. Rüssmann H., Shams H., Poblete F., Fu Y., Galan J. E., Donis R. O. Delivery of epitopes by the *Salmonella* type III secretion system for vaccine development. *Science*, 281 (1998) 565–568.

79. Igwe E. I., Geginat G., Russmann H. Concomitant cytosolic delivery of two immunodominant listerial antigens by *Salmonella enterica serovar typhimurium* confers superior protection against murine listeriosis. *Infection and Immunity*, 70 (2002) 7114–7119.

80. Panthel K., Meinel K. M., Sevil Domenech V. E., Trulzsch K., Russmann H. *Salmonella* type III-mediated heterologous antigen delivery: a versatile oral vaccination strategy to induce cellular immunity against infectious agents and tumors. *International Journal of Medical Microbiology*, 298 (2008) 99–103.

81. Blanco-Toribio A., Muyldermans S., Frankel G., Fernández L. A. Direct injection of functional single-domain antibodies from *E. coli* into human cells. *PLOS One*, 5 (2010) e15227.

82. Van Impe K., Bethuyne J., Cool S., Impens F., Ruano-Gallego D., De Wever O., *et al.* A nanobody targeting the F-actin capping protein CapG restrains breast cancer metastasis. *Breast Cancer Research*, 15 (2013) R116.

83. Bichsel C., Neeld D., Hamazaki T., Chang L. J., Yang L. J., Terada N., *et al.* Direct reprogramming of fibroblasts to myocytes via bacterial injection of MyoD protein. *Cell Reprogram*, 15 (2013) 117–125.

84. Berthoin L., Toussaint B., Garban F., Le Gouellec A., Caulier B., Polack B., *et al.* Targeted release of transcription factors for cell reprogramming by a natural micro-syringe. *International Journal of Pharmaceutics*, 513 (2016) 678–687.

85. Bichsel C., Neeld D. K., Hamazaki T., Wu D., Chang L.-J., Yang L., *et al.* Bacterial delivery of nuclear proteins into pluripotent and differentiated cells. *PLOS One*, 6 (2011) e16465.

86. Jia J., Jin Y., Bian T., Wu D., Yang L., Terada N., *et al.* Bacterial delivery of TALEN proteins for human genome editing. *PLOS One*, 9 (2014) e91547.

87. Ittig S. J., Schmutz C., Kasper C. A., Amstutz M., Schmidt A., Sauteur L., *et al.* A bacterial type III secretion-based protein delivery tool for broad applications in cell biology. *Journal of Cell Biology*, 211 (2015) 913–931.

88. McDaniel T. K., Kaper J. B. A cloned pathogenicity island from enteropathogenic *Escherichia coli* confers the attaching and effacing phenotype on *E. coli* K-12. *Molecular Microbiology*, 23 (1997) 399–407.

89. Akeda Y., Kimura T., Yamasaki A., Kodama T., Iida T., Honda T., *et al.* Functional cloning of *Vibrio parahaemolyticus* type III secretion system 1 in *Escherichia coli* K-12 strain as a molecular syringe. *Biochemical and Biophysical Research Communications*, 427 (2012) 242–247 doi:10.1016/j.bbrc.2012.09.018.

90. Reeves A. Z., Spears W. E., Du J., Tan K. Y., Wagers A. J., Lesser C. F. Engineering *Escherichia coli* into a protein delivery system for mammalian cells. *ACS Synthetic Biology*, 4 (2015) 644–654.

91. Ruano-Gallego D., Álvarez B., Fernández L. Á. Engineering the controlled assembly of filamentous injectisomes in *E. coli* K-12 for protein translocation into mammalian cells. *ACS Synthetic Biology*, 4 (2015) 1030–1041.

92. Du J., Reeves A. Z., Klein J. A., Twedt D. J., Knodler L. A., Lesser C. F. The type III secretion system apparatus determines the intracellular niche of bacterial pathogens. *Proceedings of the National Academy of Sciences of the United States of America*, 113 (2016) 4794–4799 doi:10.1073/pnas.1520699113.

93. Sekiya K., Ohishi M., Ogino T., Tamano K., Sasakawa C., Abe A. Supermolecular structure of the enteropathogenic *Escherichia coli* type III secretion system and its direct interaction with the EspA-sheath-like structure. *Proceedings of the National Academy of Sciences of the United States of America*, 98 (2001) 11638–11643.

94. Gaytán M. O., Martínez-Santos V. I., Soto E., González-Pedrajo B. Type three secretion system in attaching and effacing pathogens. *Frontiers in Cellular and Infection Microbiology*, 6 (2016) 129.

95. Frankel G., Phillips A. D., Rosenshine I., Dougan G., Kaper J. B., Knutton S. Enteropathogenic and enterohaemorrhagic *Escherichia coli*: more subversive elements. *Molecular Microbiology*, 30 (1998) 911–921.

96. Kaper J. B., Nataro J. P., Mobley H. L. Pathogenic *Escherichia coli*. *Nature Reviews Microbiology*, 2 (2004) 123–139.

97. Lai Y., Rosenshine I., Leong J. M., Frankel G. Intimate host attachment: enteropathogenic and enterohaemorrhagic *Escherichia coli*. *Cellular Microbiology*, 15 (2013) 1796–1808.

98. Frankel G., Phillips A. D. Attaching effacing *Escherichia coli* and paradigms of Tir-triggered actin polymerization: getting off the pedestal. *Cellular Microbiology*, 10 (2008) 549–556.

99. de Boer H. A., Comstock L. J., Vasser M. The *tac* promoter: A functional hybrid derived from the *trp* and *lac* promoters. *Proceedings of the National Academy of Sciences of the United States of America*, 80 (1983) 21–25.

100. Bustamante V. H., Santana F. J., Calva E., Puente J. L. Transcriptional regulation of type III secretion genes in enteropathogenic *Escherichia coli*: Ler antagonizes H-NS-dependent repression. *Molecular Microbiology*, 39 (2001) 664–678.

101. Leverton L. Q., Kaper J. B. Temporal expression of enteropathogenic *Escherichia coli* virulence genes in an in vitro model of infection. *Infection and Immunity*, 73 (2005) 1034–1043.

102. García-Gómez E., Espinosa N., de la Mora J., Dreyfus G., González-Pedrajo B. The muramidase EtgA from enteropathogenic *Escherichia coli* is required for efficient type III secretion. *Microbiology*, 157 (2011) 1145–1160.

103. Kenny B., DeVinney R., Stein M., Reinscheid D. J., Frey E. A., Finlay B. B. Enteropathogenic *E. coli* (EPEC) transfers its receptor for intimate adherence into mammalian cells. *Cell*, 91 (1997) 511–520.

104. Farzadfard F., Lu T. K. Genomically encoded analog memory with precise in vivo DNA writing in living cell populations. *Science*, 346 (2014) 1256272.

105. Siuti P., Yazbek J., Lu T. K. Synthetic circuits integrating logic and memory in living cells. *Nature Biotechnology*, 31 (2013) 448–452.

106. Courbet A., Endy D., Renard E., Molina F., Bonnet J. Detection of pathological biomarkers in human clinical samples via amplifying genetic switches and logic gates. *Science Translational Medicine*, 7 (2015) 289ra283.

107. Nielsen A. A. K., Der B. S., Shin J., Vaidyanathan P., Paralanov V., Strychalski E. A., *et al.* Genetic circuit design automation. *Science*, 352 (2016) aac7341.

108. Zhang M., Forbes N. S. Trg-deficient *Salmonella* colonize quiescent tumor regions by exclusively penetrating or proliferating. *Journal of Controlled Release*, 199 (2015) 180–189.

109. Swofford C. A., Van Dessel N., Forbes N. S. Quorum-sensing *Salmonella* selectively trigger protein expression within tumors. *Proceedings of the National Academy of Sciences of the United States of America*, 112 (2015) 3457–3462 doi:10.1073/pnas.1414558112.

110. Braat H., Rottiers P., Hommes D. W., Huyghebaert N., Remaut E., Remon J. P., *et al.* A phase I trial with transgenic bacteria expressing interleukin-10 in Crohn's disease. *Science Translational Medicine*, 4 (2006) 754–759.

111. Limaye S. A., Haddad R. I., Cilli F., Sonis S. T., Colevas A. D., Brennan M. T., *et al.* Phase 1b, multicenter, single blinded, placebo-controlled, sequential dose escalation study to assess the safety and tolerability of topically applied AG013 in subjects with locally advanced head and neck cancer receiving induction chemotherapy. *Cancer*, 119 (2013) 4268–4276.

112. Mandell D. J., Lajoie M. J., Mee M. T., Takeuchi R., Kuznetsov G., Norville J. E., *et al.* Biocontainment of genetically modified organisms by synthetic protein design. *Nature*, 518 (2015) 55–60.

113. Marlière P., Patrouix J., Döring V., Herdewijn P., Tricot S., Cruveiller S., *et al.* Chemical evolution of a bacterium's genome. *Angewandte Chemie International Edition*, 50 (2011) 7109–7114.

Chapter 8

Live *P. aeruginosa* as a Cancer Vaccine Vector

Y. Wang,[a] B. Polack,[b] and B. Toussaint[b]

[a]*Université Grenoble Alpes, CNRS, Grenoble INP, TIMC-IMAG, F38000 Grenoble, France*
[b]*Université Grenoble Alpes, CNRS, Grenoble INP, CHU Grenoble Alpes, TIMC-IMAG, F38000 Grenoble, France*

btoussaint@chu-grenoble.fr

8.1 Introduction

The study of the lifestyle of pathogenic bacteria allows scientists to discover the strategies developed by these to resist numerous defense mechanisms of the infected hosts. Some of these microbial strategies can be diverted from their natural function by "biomimicry" approaches and thus become potential new therapeutic tools.

Among the different molecular systems used by bacteria to exert their virulence, there is a complex family of protein secretion systems. These secretion systems allow the bacteria to secrete into the surrounding environment or to inject into the host cells proteins whose activity will be beneficial for the survival

Microbial Infections and Cancer Therapy: Recent Advances
Edited by Ananda M. Chakrabarty and Arsénio M. Fialho

ISBN 978-981-4774-86-4 (Hardcover), 978-1-351-04190-4 (eBook)
www.panstanford.com

or spreading of the bacteria. Many different types of secretion or injection systems exist that differ not only in function but also in the secretion mechanisms used [1]. Some secretion systems, such as the type 3 secretion system (T3SS), allow the injection of proteins into target cells of the host. The T3SS is widespread in gram-negative bacteria and is commonly considered as one major virulence factor of these bacteria. The opportunistic pathogen *P. aeruginosa* is responsible for severe acute infections in immunocompromised patients or in intensive care, as well as chronic pulmonary infections in patients with cystic fibrosis. It has several secretion systems, including a T3SS. To establish infections, *P. aeruginosa* employs a large arsenal of determinants of virulence, including its T3SS, which has been widely studied [2]. Thirty-six genes encoded in five operons clustered in the chromosome of *P. aeruginosa* are involved in the biogenesis and regulation of the type 3 delivery machine. At least six other genes scattered around the chromosome encode the effector proteins and their chaperones. It is possible to establish six classes of different proteins involved in the T3SS: the proteins regulating the expression of the genes of the regulon, the proteins that constitute the needle complex that transports exotoxins from the bacterial cytosol to the outside, the proteins that transfer secreted proteins into host cells (translocon), the proteins regulating the secretion process, the chaperone proteins that facilitate the secretion of exotoxins, and finally the proteins injected into the host cells called effector proteins or exotoxins (Fig. 8.1). *P. aeruginosa* has four types of effector proteins: ExoS, ExoT, ExoU, and ExoY. These proteins exert their activities in the target cells of the host. Targeted cells could be immune cells or epithelial cells. This is not the place to detail the different activities of the *P. aeruginosa* exotoxins but, for example, the ExoS toxin has two types of activities: amino-terminal Rho-GAP and C-terminal ADP-ribosyltransferase activities [3]. We were the first to demonstrate that, thanks to its T3SS, *P. aeruginosa* can escape the bactericidal action of polynuclear neutrophils by inducing the rapid death of these by an oncotic process [4–6].

It was from that moment that we began work to demonstrate that we can use the ability of *P. aeruginosa* to inject proteins into immune cells in therapeutic applications.

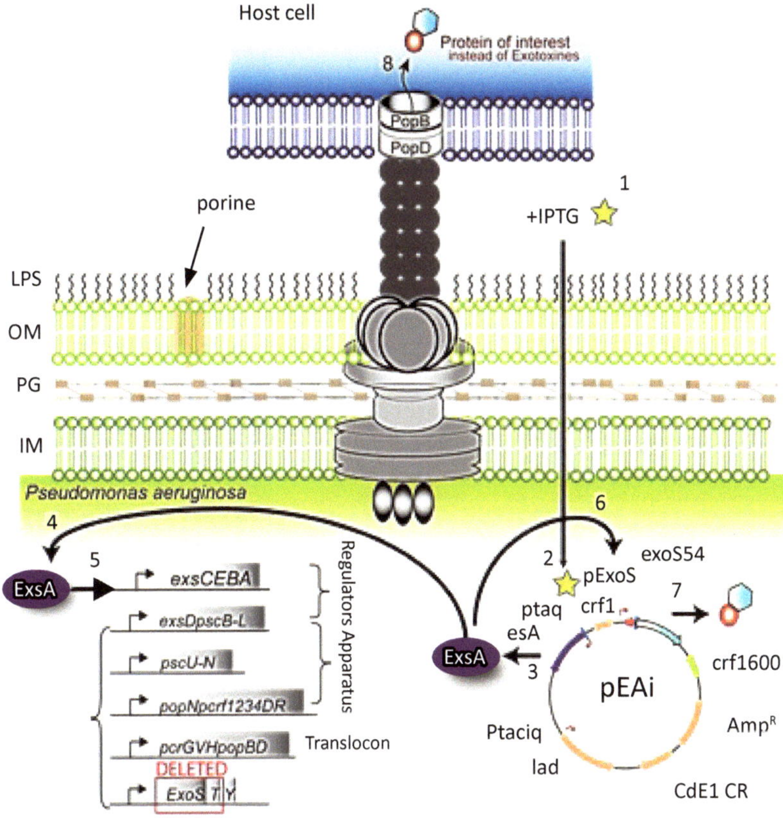

Figure 8.1 The type 3 secretion system of *P. aeruginosa* and its subversion for protein delivery inside cells. The regulatory circuit is as follows: (1–3) Addition of isopropyl β-D-1-thiogalactopyranoside (IPTG) activates ExsA production via Ptaq on pEAi plasmid. ExsA, the major activator of the type 3 secretion system, induces formation of injectisome and production of the protein of interest fused to secretion tag (S54) (Patent WO2005/049644). (8) The proteins of interest are translocated directly into the cytoplasm of eukaryotic cells upon contact between bacteria and cells. The major exotoxins (ExoS and T) of *P. aeruginosa* have been deleted.

8.2 How to Make a *P. aeruginosa* Strain a Powerful Tool for Protein Delivery

Since CHA, our *P. aeruginosa* strains, were able to inject into the cytosol of PMN cells the ExoS and ExoT toxins of, respectively, 49 and 53 kDa (453 and 457 amino acids) [7], we decided to evaluate *P. aeruginosa*'s ability to inject proteins into target cells. Indeed, direct protein transfer into the cytosol of a target cell in order to restore or modulate a cellular function is a limiting step in cell therapy. Furthermore, the T3SS seemed the optimal system for this purpose, as eukaryote cell contact is needed for the full activation of the secretory pathway. Rüssmann *et al.*, using the T3SS of *Salmonella*, previously employed this approach. However, they injected chimeric proteins made of the whole SptP toxin containing nine amino acids inserted in its middle [8]. Therefore, we tried to inject quite a big protein of 67 kDa, the cytosolic $p67^{phox}$ protein of the nicotinamide-adenine-dinucleotide-phosphate (NADPH) oxidase complex generating superoxide radicals during the respiratory burst of phagocytes [9]. This choice was driven by the presence in the laboratory of a group studying chronic granulomatous disease (CGD), where oxidase activity is abolished and which is characterized by severe and recurrent infections. Indeed, activation of the respiratory burst involves assembly of four cytosolic components ($p47^{phox}$, $p67^{phox}$, $p40^{phox}$, and a small monomeric G-protein Rac1 or Rac2) with a transmembrane heterodimeric glycoprotein, flavocytochrome b_{558}, which is constituted of two subunits, $p22^{phox}$ and $gp91^{phox}$. Molecular lesions in the genes encoding $p47^{phox}$, $p67^{phox}$, $p22^{phox}$, or $gp91^{phox}$ result in CGD. Since NADPH oxidase is also expressed, though at a lower level, in B lymphocytes, we had an Epstein–Barr virus (EBV)-immortalized cell line obtained from a patient with CGD due to $p67^{phox}$ deficiency. Therefore, we decided to fuse the $p67^{phox}$ protein to a part of the ExoS toxin as it was secreted in a greater quantity by our CHA strain than by fused to ExoT. To that aim, we constructed a plasmid containing the 129 first amino acids of ExoS fused to $p67^{phox}$ and we constructed *Orf*1, the putative chaperone for ExoS.

8.2.1 *P. aeruginosa*'s T3SS Is Able to Secrete an Active Bacterial-Human Hybrid Protein Using T3SS

The first step was to prove that our hybrid $ExoS_{129}$-$p67^{phox}$ protein was produced by our *P. aeruginosa* strain, and the second one was to confirm that *P. aeruginosa* was able to secrete that big protein through its T3SS. Using antibody to $p67^{phox}$ and Western blot we detected $ExoS_{129}$-$p67^{phox}$ both in the sonicated bacterial pellet and in the culture supernatant when the T3SS was artificially activated upon calcium chelation. Furthermore, we observed a nice time increase of $ExoS_{129}$-$p67^{phox}$ in both media.

The second step was to prove that the purified $ExoS_{129}$-$p67^{phox}$ hybrid protein was still active. We then used it to complement a medium composed of purified cytochrome b_{558} and the cytosolic factors isolated from a $p67^{phox}$-deficient patient. $ExoS_{129}$-$p67^{phox}$ hybrid protein was as efficient as recombinant $p67^{phox}$ to get a functional NADPH oxidase enzyme complex.

8.2.2 The Secreted Hybrid Protein Is Active in a Human Cell Line

The third step was to evaluate the ability of our *P. aeruginosa* strain to translocate the $ExoS_{129}$-$p67^{phox}$ hybrid protein into a target cell. Upon coincubation of *P. aeruginosa* and EBV-B lymphocytes, the $ExoS_{129}$-$p67^{phox}$ hybrid protein was found in the cytosol by Western blot.

The last step was to evaluate the ability of *P. aeruginosa* to reconstitute NADPH oxidase activity into EBV-B lymphocytes from the $p67^{phox}$-deficient CGD patient. Indeed, *P. aeruginosa* was able, upon translocation of our $ExoS_{129}$-$p67^{phox}$ hybrid protein, to reconstitute the NADPH oxidase activity to approximately 40% of normal at multiplicity of infection (MOI) of 5 or 10. It was not possible to increase this effect as our strain still contained the ExoS and ExoT toxin [10].

However, we had determined that (i) it was possible to use the T3SS of *P. aeruginosa* to inject rather big proteins, (ii) it was compulsory to reduce the toxicity of the bacterial strain and therefore to be able to realize iterative gene knockout, (iii) it was necessary to optimize efficiency by determining the best translocation sequence, and (iv) since we observed variation in the activity of the T3SS it was necessary to be able to maintain it at an optimal activation level.

8.2.3 Detoxification of *P. aeruginosa*: An Iterative Gene Knockout Method

To perform multiple knockouts to remove toxic genes from *P. aeruginosa*, it was compulsory to recycle selection markers in order to be able to use iteratively the most efficient selection system and generate a strain without resistance to antibiotics. To that aim, we combined the sacB-based negative selection system with a *cre-lox* antibiotic marker recycling method. This methodology allowed allelic exchange between a target gene and a gentamicin cassette flanked by the two lox sequences. A tetracycline plasmid expressing the crerecombinase was then introduced in the mutant strain to catalyze the excision of the lox-flanked resistance marker. In addition, we demonstrated the efficiency of the combination of these two methods in *P. aeruginosa* by successively deleting ExoS and ExoT, the two genetically independent toxins of the T3SS that were present in our *P. aeruginosa* strain. Therefore, we succeeded in creating a less toxic strain with multiple mutations without modifying the antibiotic resistance profile of the new strain compared to that of the parental strain [11].

8.2.4 A Remote Control for *P. aeruginosa*

We then tackled the problem of T3SS activity variation from experiment to experiment. Indeed, the T3SS is activated during the exponential phase of growth but can attain a noninducible phenotype. This bistability, as suggested by the presence of a positive feedback circuit in the regulatory network controlling T3SS expression, may be due to an epigenetic switch allowing heritable phenotypic modifications. Using the generalized logical method, we designed a minimal model of the T3SS regulatory network that could support the epigenetic hypothesis and studied its dynamics, which helped to define a discriminating experimental scenario sufficient to validate the epigenetic hypothesis. A mathematical framework based on formal methods from computer science allowed a rigorous validation and certification of parameters of this model leading to epigenetic behavior. Experiments suggested by the formal method require pulsing ExsA by application of an external stimulus and observing the change in phenotype and its stability when the stimulus is removed. To pulse ExsA, we added an additional *exsA* gene, under the control of an inducible promoter, to a noninducible *P. aeruginosa* strain. In the construction, transcription of *exsA* is under the control of the p*tac* promoter repressed by the LacI protein produced in large amounts because of the presence of the *lac*^{iq} gene. Under inducing conditions, transcriptional repression by LacI is inhibited, permitting overexpression of the *exsA* gene from the p*tac* promoter. This induction is immediately released when the medium of the inducer is depleted. Using this approach, we demonstrated that a noninducible strain of *P. aeruginosa* can stably acquire the capacity to be induced by calcium depletion for the T3SS after a short pulse of the regulatory protein. Finally, the increased cytotoxicity of a strain after this epigenetic switch was demonstrated *in vivo* in an acute pulmonary infection model. Therefore, with the constructed plasmid we designed a sort of remote control of the T3SS in *P. aeruginosa* [12, 13].

8.2.5 Determination of the Optimal T3SS Secretion Sequence for Hybrid Proteins

To increase the secretion of hybrid proteins, we determined the minimal length of the leading sequence of ExoS for optimal secretion. Starting from our leading sequence of 129 amino acids, we constructed fusion proteins with the 96, 54, 42, 30, and 17 first amino acids of ExoS. The optimal length-to-concentration ratio was observed with the $ExoS_{54}$ fusion protein (Fig. 8.2A). There was no secretion when trying to reduce the length of the leading amino acid sequence of ExoS as no secretion was observed with the $ExoS_{42}$, $ExoS_{30}$, and $ExoS_{17}$ fusion protein constructs. We evaluated also the ability of ExoT fusion proteins to be secreted. $ExoT_{54}$ was efficiently secreted at a level that was higher than the 129 or 96 fusion constructs. However, levels of secretion were higher using $ExoS_{54}$ fusion proteins [14]. Finally, to formally identify the chaperone of ExoS, we analyzed the role of the postulated chaperone termed *Orf*1 that shares a promoter with ExoS, though expressed in the reverse direction. Using a pull-down assay, we showed that *Orf*1 binds to ExoS and ExoT. Then, by allelic exchange, we constructed the mutant with the deletion of gene *Orf*1. A secretion profile analysis showed that *Orf*1 was necessary for the optimal secretion of ExoS and ExoT, probably by maintaining ExoS or ExoT in a secretion-prone conformation. We proposed to name *Orf*1 as SpcS for "specific *Pseudomonas* chaperone for ExoS" [15].

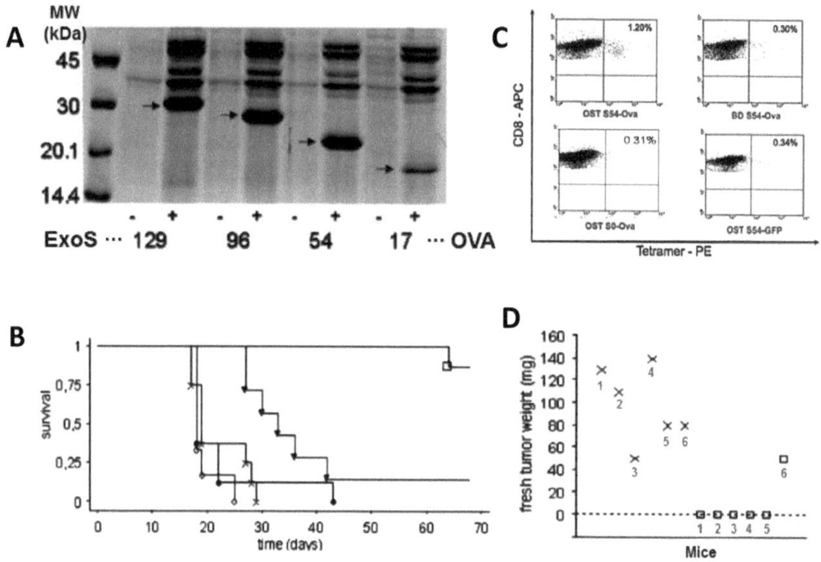

Figure 8.2 Proof of concept of active and specific immunotherapy by the T3SS of *P. aeruginosa.* (A) Secretion of ExoS-OVA through T3SS: CHA-OST strains transformed with pEAi-ExoS (129, 96, 54, or 17)-OVA were grown in the absence (–) or presence (+) of EGTA to induce T3SS activation; then culture supernatants were analyzed by SDS-PAGE (proteins of interest are marked with arrows). (B) Quantification of antiovalbumin peptide SIINFEKL–specific CD8+ lymphocytes: C57BL/6 mice were injected with different bacterial strains 14 and 5 days before analysis and splenocytes were freshly harvested and quantified by flow cytometry using anti-CD8-FITC and H-2Kb ovalbumin$_{257-264}$ (SIINFEKL) in conjunction with the HLA type I tetramer-PE. Dead cells were excluded from analysis after viability assessment using propidium iodide staining. The dot plots are representative of repeated experiments in separate animals. (C) Prophylactic tumor challenge: C57BL/6 mice were injected two times with different bacterial vectors, 14 days and 7 days before the challenge, with a B16-OVA tumor (day 0), when the survival curve started to be registered: (□) CHA-OST S54-OVA, *n* = 8; (○) CHA-OST S0-OVA, *n* = 6; (▼) CHA-BD S54-OVA, *n* = 7; (×) CHA-OST S54-GFP, *n* = 8; (•) PBS, *n* = 8. Animals were sacrificed when the tumor diameter exceeded 1 cm. (D) Curative tumor challenge: C57BL/6 mice received an intravenous tumor challenge with B16-OVA on day 0 and then were injected with either CHA-OST S54-OVA or CHA-OST S54-GFP on days 5 and 12. Animals were sacrificed on day 16, and metastatic intrathoracic tumors (if any) were weighed. (•) CHA-OST S54-PVA; (○) CHA-OST S54-GFP.

Therefore, we made the proof of concept that the T3SS of *P. aeruginosa* could be subverted to obtain a live strain able to inject proteins inside target cells (Fig. 8.1). We will see hereafter how to use this tool for cancer immunotherapy.

8.3 Proof of Concept of Active and Specific Immunotherapy by *P. aeruginosa* T3SS

The triggering of a cellular immune reaction (cytotoxic T lymphocyte) against an antigen of interest (tumor associated antigen) requires that the specific lymphocytes be stimulated by the presentation of peptides derived from this antigen by the dendritic cells (DCs) and that this presentation be accompanied by delivery by DCs to these lymphocytes of costimulation signals. Obtaining such antigen presentation is the goal of the vast majority of the active and specific immunotherapy approaches. Many techniques for administering antigens to an organism have been developed: injection of whole proteins, injection of antigenic peptides, injection of DNA sequences coding for antigenic proteins, and use of genetically modified virus. Many studies have shown that these injections should be accompanied by molecules that activate the immune system: these adjuvants are indispensable for the expression by DCs of molecules involved in costimulation, in the absence of which there is no response or even an undesirable toleration response. DC activation has been revealed to be particularly stimulable by the ligands of certain toll-like receptors (TLRs), in particular molecules of bacterial origin (LPS, flagellin, bacterial DNA, etc.). Thus, because of their intrinsically adjuvant character, the study of antigen delivery by entire bacterial vectors began about 20 years ago [16].

Numerous modes of antigen delivery by different bacterial tools have been considered, including the T3SS. In this strategy, the bacterial vectors are used to both inject antigenic proteins into the cytoplasm of immune cells and deliver a bacterial activation signal. Encouraging results, particularly with *Salmonella typhimurium* [8], have opened the door to the exploration of other vectors.

Because of the knowledge of the *P. aeruginosa* T3SS acquired by our laboratory, thanks to several works described above, we tried to vectorize antigens of interest by ensuring that the bacterium delivers antigenic proteins to the DCs through its T3SS. We first decided to make the proof of concept of this approach using the well-characterized murine melanoma B16 transformed by an exogenous antigen ovalbumine. The strain CHA studied in the laboratory was attenuated by deletion of the exotoxins encoding genes to yield the CHA-OST strain. Different variants of pEAI plasmid allowing the production of a chimeric protein that contains the first 129, 96, 54, or 17 amino acids of ExoS fused to an ovalbumin fragment that contains the murine CD8 epitope SIINFEKL were introduced into the CHA-OST strain.

We first revealed that the 54 ExoS N-terminal sequence is the minimal sequence that allowed a strong secretion of OVA fragment through the T3SS (Fig. 8.2A). We decided to keep on following work [17] using the S54-OVA construct.

8.3.1 *Ex Vivo* Experiments

We evaluated whether exposure of DCs to *P. aeruginosa* delivering the fusion protein allows DC maturation and activation. We induced the expression of S54-OVA in the CHA-OST strain by addition of IPTG and then incubated bacteria for 1 h with DCs from C57BL/6 (MHC-I H-2Kb) mice. Within 24 h more than 90% of DCs were activated as they expressed MHC-II at their surface.

We then evaluated whether exposure of DCs to the CHA-OST (S54-OVA) vector induces antigen presentation by DCs to specific CD8+ T lymphocytes *ex vivo*. To do that, we constructed control *P. aeruginosa* strains. The first control strain, CHA-OST S0-OVA, possesses a pEAI plasmid that allows expression of the OVA fragment not fused to ExoS54 amino-terminal part. In that strain, the T3SS is fully functional but the OVA fragment could not be secreted/injected through it. The second control strain, CHA-BDS54-OVA, has been obtained by deletion of popB and popD genes that encode essential proteins of the translocon of the T3SS. This strain contains pEAI, which allows expression of the ExoS54-tagged OVA fragment that should not be injected in DCs as the translocon is not functional. We incubated DCs from C57BL/6 mice for 3 h, with each of the three strains after IPTG preinduction of the T3SS. We then harvested the DCs and incubated them with B3Z hybridoma cells having a T cell receptor (TCR) specific to the ovalbumin 257–264 peptide (SIINFEKL) presented by MHC-I H-2Kb. TCR-mediated B3Z activation was obtained after incubation with DCs that had been exposed to CHA-OST S54-OVA. In contrast, we observed no activation after exposure of DCs to phosphate-buffered saline (PBS), CHA-OST S0-OVA, and CHA-BDS54-OVA. These *ex vivo* experiments demonstrated that specific antigen delivery via the fully functional *P. aeruginosa* T3SS was well suitable for MHC-I presentation and activation of DCs.

8.3.2 Vaccinal and Therapeutic Efficiency of BacVac in a Mouse Model of Melanoma

We have evaluated the *in vivo* prophylactic and therapeutic vaccinal effects of the bacterial vector using a murine melanoma model. We used the CHA-OSTS54-OVA as the vaccine candidate and CHA-OSTS0-OVA and CHA-BDS54-OVA as control strains, as well as another control, CHA-OST S54GFP, that produces green fluorescent protein fused with an ExoS54 amino terminal part.

We first used a prophylactic setting for experiments that comprises a first immunization with 5×10^6 living bacteria on day 14, a boost with the same amount on day 7, and subcutaneous implantation of B16 (OVA) melanoma cells on day 0. In a first series of experiments, the mice were immunized as described above and 5 days after the boost they were sacrificed and splenocytes recovered to measure by a specific tetramer the population of CD8 cells specific of OVA epitopes SIINFEKL. An activation of CD8 specific of OVA epitopes was seen only when mice where immunized with CHA-OSTS54-OVA (Fig. 8.2B). In a second series of experiments, after immunization and implantation of melanoma cells mice were followed for tumor growth and euthanized when the melanoma tumor reached 1 cm diameter. We demonstrated that prophylactic inoculation with CHA-OSTS54-OVA protected the mice against the growth of tumors consisting of B16-OVA melanoma cells (Fig. 8.2C). In contrast, mice injected with the control strains developed tumors within 3 weeks.

Complete regression of an established tumor is difficult to achieve. We verified the antitumor effect of the strain in a therapeutic setting assay of an established metastatic tumor model. B16-OVA melanoma cells (10 cells) were injected intravenously at day 1, and vaccine strains were injected subcutaneously on days 5 and 12. The mice were sacrificed on day 16. The results indicated the absence of intrathoracic metastatic tumors in five of six mice vaccinated with the strain CHA-OST S54-OVA, whereas all of the mice vaccinated with a strain translocating the control antigen GFP had numerous metastatic tumors (Fig. 8.2D).

In summary we have demonstrated that the T3SS of *P. aeruginosa* delivers *in vivo* an antigenic peptide into antigen presenting cells and triggers an efficient cytotoxic immune response toward cells expressing this antigen.

8.4 Optimization of T3SS-Based Bacterial Vector for Clinical Use

The proof of the concept of using *P. aeruginosa* as an *in vivo* antigen delivery tool having been made, it appeared to us necessary to continue the development of this bacterial vector with the aim of future clinical use. For this we have modified the plasmid pEAi. To be able to combine several different protein antigens, we optimized the vaccination scheme, determined a chemically defined culture medium, and finally improved the safety of the strain by different attenuation methods.

8.4.1 Bi-antigen Delivery Pattern Design

During recent years, several studies reported that multiantigen immunization is more efficient than immunization by a vaccine with a single antigen because the latter pattern can prime diverse T lymphocyte responses and stimulate immunity to a broad array of antigens. Actually, this pattern has been applied in the design of cancer vaccines and its efficiencies have been validated not only in animal experiments but also in human trials [1, 18–21]. Thus, multiantigen delivery could be also a great strategy for optimizing the performance of our bacterial vector.

We started the new pattern design with a bi-antigen delivering model [22]. Generally, a bi-antigen cloning vector was constructed on the basis of a single-antigen expression plasmid; each fusion protein expression cassette contained a ribosome binding site and a STOP codon, and thus two fusion proteins could be cotranscribed and individually translated (Fig. 8.3A). First, we investigated *in vitro* fusion protein expression and the secretion ability of a bi-antigen vector. The results obtained from several bi-antigen delivering strains were identical: both fusion proteins were well expressed and secreted by bi-antigen vectors, whereas fusion proteins were slightly less secreted when they were cloned at the second position, probably because of a lower level of translation. So we wondered whether the position-dependent protein secretion would later affect antigen-specific immune response activation; we used OVA as a model antigen and cloned it at either the first or the second position in the bi-antigen vector to determine the influence of the antigen cloning position on antigen delivery and presentation. The results of the B3Z activation assay didn't show any evident difference related to the OVA cloning position, which indicated that DCs' activation and antigen presentation were not directly antigen quantity dependent. Thereby, we further assessed the bi-antigen vector through an *in vivo* tumor challenge; here, we tested the bi-antigen vector directly in a natural tumor model (glioblastoma, GL261) subcutaneously implanted with the self-antigens TRP2 and GP100. The results were encouraging. Both in the prophylactic and in the therapeutic assay, bi-antigen strains provided more efficient protection. Tumor onset was more effectively delayed and tumor growth progression was more evidently reduced in the bi-antigen strain-vaccinated group than in the single-antigen strain-vaccinated groups. Moreover, the bi-antigen strain demonstrated a performance similar to that of combined single-antigen strains.

All these results reveal the advantages of the new bi-antigen delivering vector. The first advantage is better efficiency: vaccinations with a bi-antigen vector delivering double antigens provided better tumor protection than either single-antigen immunization. The second advantage is the simplicity: in contrast to the individual preparations for two vaccines, the bi-antigen vector is processed at one time. The third advantage is the security: the therapeutic dose would be half reduced compared to the admission of two single-antigen delivering vaccines. All these benefits confer more potential to the bi-antigen delivering bacterial vector in antitumor immunotherapy.

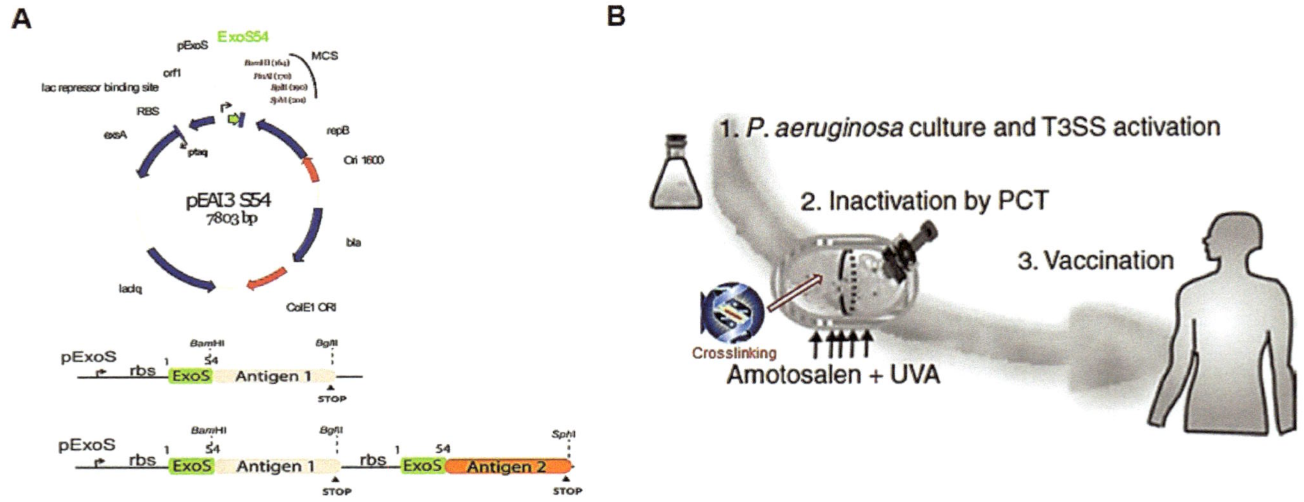

Figure 8.3 Development of *P. aeruginosa* T3SS–based vaccine vector: (A) T3SS-based bi-antigen delivering bacterial vector: the bi-antigen coexpression vector was constructed with a single-antigen expression vector (pEAI-S54) in which the first antigen was cloned at BamHI/BglII sites and the second S54-PADRE-antigen fusion protein expression cassette containing an ribosome-binding site, fusion protein, and STOP codon was added to the single-antigen expression plasmid at BglII/SphI sites located downstream from the first antigen. (B) T3SS-based KBMA bacterial vector: The KMBA vector was constructed on the basis of deletion of two *uvr* genes (A and B). The Δ*uvrAB* mutant strain is first cultivated under T3SS-inducing conditions. The protein used for vaccination is overexpressed by bacteria before bacterial inactivation with PCT in the presence of amotosalen. Then, *P. aeruginosa* is injected subcutaneously (s.c.), and its active T3SS allows protein injection into the host cells.

8.4.2 Virulence Attenuation

Although the potential use of the CHA-OST strain as a vaccine carrier has been proven, its instinct toxicity might limit its clinical applications. So virulence attenuation of bacterial vector should be further optimized.

For this purpose, we explored the effects of the deletion of the *aroA* gene, which encodes a key enzyme in aromatic amino acid synthesis, and two genes (*lasI* and *rhlI*) that participate in the quorum sensing (QS) system [23]. In fact, *aroA* deletion could lead to the auxotrophy of aromatic amino acids and has been successfully used to elaborate attenuated *P. aeruginosa* strains for the purpose of anti-*Pseudomonas* vaccination [24]; *P. aeruginosa* QS inactivation has been shown to be associated with virulence attenuation in various animal models for injury or illness, including those for pneumonia [25, 26], burns [27], and pyelonephritis [28]. For genes knockout, we used the *cre-lox* system that we previously mentioned. By successive mutations, we generated three attenuated mutants from CHA-OST: CHA-OA (ΔexoS ΔexoT ΔaroA), CHA-OAL (ΔexoS ΔexoT ΔaroA ΔlasI), and CHA-ORL (ΔexoS ΔexoT ΔrhlI ΔlasI). All mutants were genetically verified and confirmed by polymerase chain reaction (PCR).

To evaluate these mutants, we first detected their phenotype characters. We observed that because of the deletion of *aroA*, CHA-OA and CHA-OAL grew slower than CHA-OST and CHA-ORL both in Lysogeny Broth (LB)-rich medium and Vogel Bonner (VB)-minimum medium, while QS inactivation didn't impact the bacterial growth rate. Then, fusion protein secretion by different mutants has also been verified *in vitro* under a calcium deprivation condition. We found that QS activation did not influence the T3SS function of the CHA-ORL strain. On the other hand, it is encouraging to find that even the growth of *aroA*-deleted strains is impacted; they can always secret fusion protein at a higher level, which confirmed the T3SS functionality of *aroA*-deleted mutants. After that, to confirm the vaccine potential of these mutants, we continued to test *in vivo* their toxicities and also their antitumor protection performance. On being compared with CHA-OST, CHA-ORL showed a little but not significantly lower toxicity; but the *aroA*-deleted mutant demonstrated greatly reduced toxicities; the lethal doses of CHA-OA and CHA-OAL are 100 times higher than that of CHA-OST. This reduced *in vivo* toxicity of *aroA* mutants is along with their slower growth rates conferred by the deletion of *aroA* gene, which might also influence the synthesis of some important signal molecules for *P. aeruginosa* virulence.

Thereby, we demonstrated that *aroA* deletion of *P. aeruginosa* could confer greatly reduced toxicity and a higher T3SS functional level so that *aroA*-deleted mutants are good potential vaccine vectors. The CHA-OAL strain that combined deletions of *aroA* and *lasI* genes gains a more enhanced performance so it should be an ideal candidate for further development. Moreover, we were attracted by some preliminary results that showed that the immunization schedule (dose and frequency) might influence the efficiency of antitumor vaccination, which guided us for later optimization of the performance of our bacterial vector.

8.4.3 Chemically Defined Growth Medium

Even the results gained from the CHA-OAL strain were encouraging. All these results were obtained in a complex not chemically defined LB. For clinical applications, beside the safety and the efficacy, the production process of the bacterial vector complying with the current good manufacturing practices grade is also indispensable. Also, CHA-OAL demonstrated uncontrollable growth defects in the LB medium. All these defects made us look for a new chemically defined medium for bacterial vector preparation. A chemically defined medium, M9, is one of the standard minimal mediums for bacterial culture. One other chemically defined medium compounded by DeBell *et al.* has been proved to be ideal for exotoxin *A* production by *P. aeruginosa* [29]. On the bases of these two kinds of medium, we still applied chemically defined synthetic yeast extracts and enhanced Mg^{2+} and Ca^{2+} portions to yield a new chemically defined medium, M9-TheREx [22]. Adaptation by progressive medium replacement led to a greatly increased CHA-OAL growth rate in the M9-TheREx medium compared with that in the LB medium (mean doubling time during exponential growth: 43 min. in M9-TheREx and 88 min. in LB). To make sure that the adaption and the new growth conditions modified the phenotypical characters and/or the vaccine potential of the CHA-OAL strain, we verified its T3SS characteristics *in vitro* and also evaluated its toxicity *in vivo*. We confirmed that the change of growth condition didn't impact this attenuated strain; it still has low toxicity and still maintains a good T3SS functionality.

Evidently, instinct T3SS efficacy, high safety, and good manufacturing practices in the chemically defined medium provide this attenuated strain more potential for future development. We renamed this strain CHA-CLIN1.

8.4.4 Optimization of Vaccination Scheme and Vaccination Mode

Many recent studies have indicated that the CD8+ T cell response is a dynamic process that can be divided into four phases: (i) cytotoxic T lymphocytes' (CTLs') expansion phase, which generally lasts 7 to 8 days after the infection, (ii) CTLs' contract phase, which lasts about 2 to 3 weeks, (iii) memory T cell maintenance phase, during which memory T cells can be maintained at stable levels throughout the life of the mouse and for many years in humans, and (iv) the rapid recalling CTL response after re-exposure to the pathogen [30–32]. Meanwhile, the progressive-differentiation model has been proposed for sustained expansion during the primary response to the antigen. According to this model, accumulated stimulation of CD8+ T cells by the antigen may induce successive rounds of division/differentiation [33].

In a previous work, we remarked that the efficiency of antitumor vaccination was related to the vaccine dose but could also be modulated by changing the frequency of vaccinations [23]; we would like to further optimize the performance of our bacterial vector in this way. We began our trials with the CHA-OST strain, always using OVA as the model antigen [22]. With an increase in the vaccination frequency and a reduction in the vaccination interval, we found that the expansion phase of CD8+ T cell–mediated response was obviously prolonged, the level of the specific CTL CD8+ response was enhanced, and this response persisted for a longer time. On the basis of these findings, we evaluated *in vivo* the performance of the new vaccination scheme and assessed the therapeutic efficacy of our bacterial vector. We gained consistent results: increasing the frequency of the vaccinations and reducing their intervals were conducive to better antitumor protection; particularly due to the modulated vaccination scheme, we demonstrated for the first time the therapeutic vaccination potential of our bacterial vector. Hence, our assumption was confirmed. Appropriate immunization frequency and interval are both important for programming a primary immune response to an antigen. On the other hand, in the fight of the immune system against cancer, a long-lasting and effective CD8+ T cell memory is also crucial. Therefore, we inoculated mice with OVA-presenting B16 tumor cells 3 months after vaccination to assess the remaining T cells' response *ex vivo* by ELISpot and estimate the long-term contribution of vaccination *in vivo* by a tumor challenge. By this way, the important memory T response induced by our bacterial vector was confirmed. Moreover, the modulation of the vaccination scheme could regulate not only the acute CD8+ T cells response but also CD8+ T cell memory.

Previously, in spite of the low toxicity demonstrated by the CHA-CLIN1 strain, it still presented weaker antitumor protection efficacy *in vivo*. Nevertheless, we tried to improve its vaccine performance by modulating the vaccination scheme; no interesting results were obtained. Therefore, we needed to find the solution in another way. Because the *aroA* gene encodes an enzyme essential for the synthesis of aromatic amino acids that are generally not available in host tissues, the deletion of *aroA* both restrains the bacterial growth and inhibits the pathogenic dissemination in mammalians. Indeed, we previously verified the absence of dissemination of the CHA-OAL strain after a subcutaneous injection; no bacteria were found in organs such as blood, liver, spleen, and kidney [23]. This absence of dissemination could restrain the immunogenicity and efficiency of the vaccine. Thus, we wondered whether vaccinations of mice at multiple loci might facilitate the dissemination and enhance the immunogenicity of our vaccine [19]. Both *ex vivo* immune-monitoring and *in vivo* tumor protection experiments demonstrated that a simple increase in vaccination frequency did not significantly optimize vaccination performance, whereas vaccinations at multiple loci could promote the artificial dissemination of bacteria, which led to a reinforced immune response and provided nearly the same prophylactic and therapeutic efficiencies as the CHA-OST strain. In this way, the efficiency of the CHA-CLIN1 strain–mediated vaccination has been really improved. Its efficiency might even be enhanced by modulating the vaccination scheme.

So high efficacy, satisfactory safety, and good manufacturing practices ensure that this attenuated strain is more suitable for future clinical applications.

8.4.5 Design of the Killed but Metabolically Active Procedure

Although the auxotrophic strain CHA-CLIN1 has been well elaborated and its potential as a vaccine vector has been confirmed, the residual virulence might still concern physicians and patients. Actually, the potential risks of reversion to a virulent state, viability/propagation in environments other than the intestines, and unintentional transfer to other individuals are unacceptable. One novel concept, killed but metabolically active (KBMA) bacterial mutant, developed by Brockstedt *et al.* [34] has helped us to apply this strategy in the development of our *P. aeruginosa* 's T3SS-based vaccine.

A KBMA vector is based on bacterial nucleotide excision repair (NER) mutants. In fact, several mechanisms, such as NER, base excision repair (BER), and DNA mismatch repair (MMR), could be applied when DNA damage occurs constantly. Among these mechanisms, NER is a particularly important excision mechanism that removes DNA damage induced by ultraviolet light (UV). When UV-induced DNA damage is recognized, UvrABC endonuclease, a multienzyme complex, will permit the removal of a short single-stranded DNA segment that contains the lesion. The undamaged single-stranded DNA remains, and DNA polymerase uses it as a template to synthesize a short complementary sequence to complete NER and form a double-stranded DNA. The subunits for UvrABC endonuclease are encoded by *uvrA, uvrB,* and *uvrC* genes. Brockstedt *et al.*'s work showed that the deletion of two *uvr* genes (A and B) rendered bacteria sensitive to psoralen-induced crosslinking [34]. That means the Δ*uvrAB* mutant cannot replicate after photochemical treatment (PCT) with psoralen and long-wavelength ultraviolet light (UVA) because of the presence of infrequent, randomly distributed, psoralen-induced crosslinks. However, they are still metabolically active and can still express its genes, secrete proteins, and induce an innate and adaptive immune response.

We wondered whether this PCT could be applied to *P. aeruginosa* bacteria and whether it will preserve T3SS function. To confirm this assumption, we made an *uvrAB* deletion mutant in *P. aeruginosa* (CHA-OSTAB) using the *cre-lox* system [35]. For vaccination experiments, in general, this antigen-delivering Δ*uvrAB* mutant is first cultivated under T3SS-inducing conditions to ensure the overexpression of fusion protein by bacteria. Before injection *in vivo*, bacterial cells will be inactivated by the PCT in the presence of amotosalen. Then, bacterial vector is injected subcutaneously (Fig. 8.3). To investigate this novel *P. aeruginosa* T3SS–based vector, first, we have verified the toxicity and safety of this vector. In theory, KBMA bacterial cells are killed and should not be replicable and cannot form a colony on *Pseudomonas* isolation agar (PIA) plates. We injected mice with either savage or KBMA bacterial cells. When live *P. aeruginosa* was injected, bacteria were recovered on PIA plates from various organs, such as the lymph nodes, spleen, liver, skin, lungs, and kidneys. In contrast, no replicating bacteria were detected in the animals when they were injected with KBMA *P. aeruginosa.* These results indicate that the attenuation process of bacteria is irreversible *in vivo*. As an attenuated strain, it is safe even at a high dose of the injection (5×10^7). Besides, it also demonstrated a less reactogenic profile *in vivo*.

After that, we verified the T3SS efficacy of this Δ*uvrAB* mutant. It was always capable of expressing and secreting S54-fusion protein, which indicates the maintenance of a functional T3SS microsyringe. So we continued to assess *ex vivo* the immune response activated by the KBMA vector. Our results revealed that this kind of vector is capable of activating and maturating DCs and delivering antigen to the latter, which can induce an efficient CD8+ CTL–mediated immune response. This finding is coherent to the results obtained in tumor challenge experiments. An antigen-specific immune response induced by the KBMA vector was sufficient to inhibit the formation of tumor in the prophylactic mode and also prolong well the survival period in the therapeutic tumor challenge.

So, by this work, we developed a new *P. aeruginosa* T3SS-based KBMA vaccine vector that is always capable of delivering greater amounts of antigen to DCs *in vivo* but induces a decreased systemic response. The distinct quality of this kind of vector for clinical use is that no live bacteria will be released into the environment and the patient has no risk of developing an infection. This character should be attractive for clinical applications.

8.4.5.1 Comparison of the immune response induced by live attenuated bacteria and KBMA bacteria

At this stage of vector development, we have two different strategies for *in vivo* antigen delivery by *P. aeruginosa*: either virulence attenuation of live strain, such as OST and OAL, or the KBMA inactivation mode. To be able to compare the two strategies, we have carried out the analysis of the immune response in the B16 (OVA) melanoma model and we have particularly studied the long-term response [36]. We used the optimized vaccination scheme defined previously with multiple injections. We compared OSTAB S54-OVA and KBMA S54-OVA vaccine strains using two controlled strains. The first control strain was the live OST strain transformed with plasmid pEAI (OST S54-EI) without the OVA antigen. The second control strain was OST transformed with pEAI-OVA but heat-killed before injection (HK S54-OVA).

We first examined the kinetics of OVA-specific CD8+ T cells in blood after vaccination with an OVA tetramer (Fig. 8.4A). The number of cells increases steadily after each injection of S54-OVA or KBMA S54-OVA, reaches a peak at about 8 days after the last injection, and then gradually decreases, reaching a stable value that is practically identical for both strains.

To evaluate the functionality of the generated tumor-specific CD8+ T cells, cytokines secretion and expression of the degranulation marker (CD107a) were investigated after splenocytes stimulation with the immune-dominant MHC-I restricted OVA peptide (SIINFEKL epitope). A tumor-specific CD8+ T cell response induced by OSTAB S54-OVA and KBMA S54-OVA vaccines displays a high degree of polyfunctionality (Fig. 8.4B).

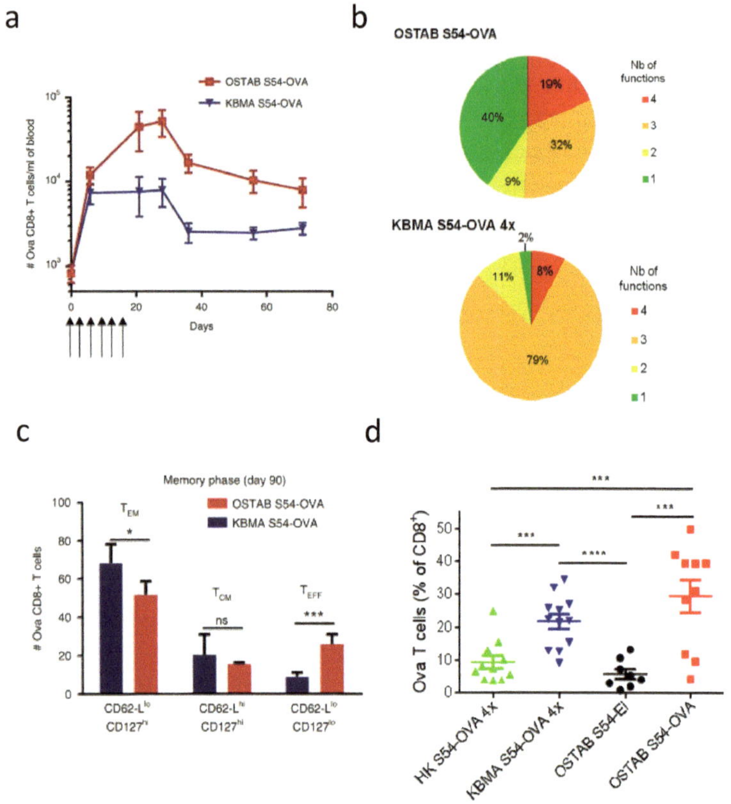

Figure 8.4 Multiple immunizations with OSTAB S54-OVA or KBMA S54-OVA initiate a strong and long-lasting OVA-specific immune response. (A) Kinetic profile of OVA-specific CD8+ T cells (absolute number) in the blood (down). *n* = 5 or 6 mice per group per time point. Mean ± SEM. (B) Pie charts represent the spectrum of functions (cytokines and/or degranulation marker) among responding CD8+ T cells to OVA peptide stimulation, in KBMA and OSTAB groups. Each slice of pie represents the percentage of cells expressing between 1 and 4 effector functions. (C) Mean percentage of memory (CD62-L^{low} $CD127^{hi}$ or CD62-L^{hi} $CD127^{hi}$) and effector (CD62-L^{low} $CD127^{low}$) OVA-specific CD8+ T cell subpopulations at 90 days in splenocytes upon immunization with Pa-OVA vaccines. T_{EM}: effector memory OVA–specific CD8+ T cells; T_{CM}: central memory OVA–specific CD8+ T cells; T_{EFF}: OVA-specific effector CD8+ T cells. Mean ± SEM. *$P < 0.05$, ***$P < 0.001$ determined by the unpaired student's *t*-test. (D) immunizations with OSTAB S54-OVA or KBMA S54-OVA yielded a strong intratumoral OVA $CD8^+$ T cell infiltration in comparison with control groups HK S54-OVA and OST S54-Ei ($P < 0.001$ or $P < 0.0001$). ** $P < 0.01$, *** $P < 0.001$ determined by the student's *t*-test.

We also investigated the tumor-specific CD8+ T cell response in splenocytes both at the effector phase (day 29) and during the memory phase far after the last vaccination (day 90). Just after the immunization period, a majority of tumor-specific CD8+ T cells seemed to take on the $CD127^{hi}$ memory phenotype (data not shown). During the memory phase, these tumor-specific CD8+ T cells evolved into predominant $CD62\text{-}L^{low}$ $CD127^{hi}$ in groups treated with OSTAB S54-OVA or KBMA S54-OVA. This is strongly in favor of the development of a major effector-memory response T_{EM} (day 90, Fig. 8.4C). This means that even 70 days after the last immunization, a T cell memory response is present with both groups. It has to be noticed that we observed the presence of a similar central-memory T_{CM} pool in each group.

In a second series of experiments B16 (OVA) cells were injected subcutaneously into mice before immunization. At first the tumors were recovered when they reached an identical size of 5 mm diameter and analysis of intratumoral OVA-specific CD8+ T cells was performed. There was a significant tumor infiltrate of OVA-specific cells similar between OST strains S54-OVA and KBMA S54-OVA and significantly higher than that obtained with HK S54-OVA or OST S54-Ei strains (Fig. 8.4D). Finally, when the tumor was implanted at day 90 after immunization, similar good protection against tumor growth was observed in both OVA-vaccinated groups (70% of the mice did not develop any tumor) whereas 100% of the mice immunized with the control strains developed a tumor.

All of these last results indicate that the efficacy of the live attenuated strain or the KBMA strain is similar in terms of causing a specific long-term cytotoxic response. However, the use of the KBMA strain provides a level of safety that can satisfy safety requirements for clinical use.

8.5 Conclusion

We have clearly demonstrated here that it is possible to combine knowledge in microbiology and genetic engineering techniques to make a live bacterium a tool for injecting proteins into human cells. This tool can have different applications even though we have focused in this work on the delivery of antigens in the presenting cells. Another application developed in the laboratory was the use of this natural syringe for the delivery into differentiated cells of the various transcription factors known to initiate cell reprogramming in order to obtain induced pluripotent stem cells without foreign genetic material [37].

The development of active and cancer-specific immunotherapy is based on the existence of the antigenic signature of tumors. Nevertheless, the development of effective treatment requires an important search for vectorization approaches capable of provoking a specific, strong, and long-lasting immune response. Bacteria constitute an opportunity for this research because they possess molecular danger signals and can allow the synthesis of the antigenic proteins and their delivery into the good compartment of the presenting cells. We have given here an example of the development over more than 10 years of an approach of vectorization of antigens based on the use of the T3SS of *Pseudomonas aeruginosa* that has been engineered. Other bacterial species have been used, such as *Listeria monocytogenes* live attenuated antigen delivery tool, which is already the subject of clinical trials in different cancers. Studies are still needed to improve the effectiveness and limit the virulence of these live bacterial vectors. The use of active and specific immunotherapy (ASI) combined with other approaches, such as immune checkpoint inhibitors, will probably in the coming years achieve major results in the fight against cancer.

References

1. Steele J. C., Rao A., Marsden J. R., Armstrong C. J., Berhane S., Billingham L. J., *et al.* Phase I/II trial of a dendritic cell vaccine transfected with DNA encoding melan A and gp100 for patients with metastatic melanoma. *Gene Therapy,* 18(6) (2011) 584–593.
2. Hauser A. R. The type III secretion system of *Pseudomonas aeruginosa*: infection by injection. *Nature Reviews Microbiology,* 7(9) (2009) 654–665.
3. Barbieri J. T., Sun J. *Pseudomonas aeruginosa* ExoS and ExoT. *Reviews of Physiology, Biochemistry and Pharmacology,* 152 (2004) 79–92.
4. Dacheux D., Attree I., Schneider C., Toussaint B. Cell death of human polymorphonuclear neutrophils induced by a *Pseudomonas*

aeruginosa cystic fibrosis isolate requires a functional type III secretion system. *Infection and Immunity,* 67(11) (1999) 6164–6167.

5. Dacheux D., Toussaint B., Richard M., Brochier G., Croize J., Attree I. *Pseudomonas aeruginosa* cystic fibrosis isolates induce rapid, type III secretion-dependent, but ExoU-independent, oncosis of macrophages and polymorphonuclear neutrophils. *Infection and Immunity,* 68(5) (2000) 2916–2924.
6. Dacheux D., Attree I., Toussaint B. Expression of ExsA in trans confers type III secretion system-dependent cytotoxicity on noncytotoxic *Pseudomonas aeruginosa* cystic fibrosis isolates. *Infection and Immunity,* 69(1) (2001) 538–542.
7. Frank D. W. The exoenzyme S regulon of *Pseudomonas aeruginosa. Molecular Microbiology,* 26(4) (1997) 621–629.
8. Rüssmann H., Shams H., Poblete F., Fu Y., Galán J. E., Donis R. O. Delivery of epitopes by the *Salmonella* type III secretion system for vaccine development. *Science,* 281(5376) (1998) 565–568.
9. Morel F., Doussière J., Vignais P. V. The superoxide-generating oxidase of phagocytic cells: Physiological, molecular and pathological aspects. *European Journal of Biochemistry,* 201 (1991) 523–546.
10. Polack B., Vergnaud S., Paclet M. H., Lamotte D., Toussaint B., Morel F. Protein delivery by *Pseudomonas* type III secretion system: Ex vivo complementation of $p67^{phox}$-deficient chronic granulomatous disease. *Biochemical and Biophysical Research Communications,* 275(3) (2000) 854–858.
11. Quénée L., Lamotte D., Polack B. Combined sacB-based negative selection and *cre-lox* antibiotic marker recycling for efficient gene deletion in *Pseudomonas aeruginosa. BioTechniques,* 38(1) (2005) 63–67.
12. Filopon D., Mérieau A., Bernot G., Comet J. P., Leberre R., Guery B., Polack B., Guespin-Michel J. Epigenetic acquisition of inducibility of type III cytotoxicity in *P. aeruginosa. BMC Bioinformatics,* 7 (2006) 272.
13. Guespin-Michel J. F., Bernot G., Comet J. P., Mérieau A., Richard A., Hulen C., Polack B. Epigenesis and dynamic similarity in two regulatory networks in *Pseudomonas aeruginosa. Acta Biotheoretica,* 52(4) (2004) 379–390.
14. Derouazi M., Toussaint B., Quenee L., Epaulard O., Guillaume M., Marlu R., Polack B. High yield production of secreted active proteins by the *Pseudomonas aeruginosa* type III secretion system. *Applied and Environmental Microbiology,* 74(11) (2008) 3601–3604.

15. Shen D. K., Quénée L., Bonnet M., Kuhn L., Derouazi M., Lamotte D., Toussaint B., Polack B. Orf1/SpcS chaperones ExoS for the type three secretion by *Pseudomonas aeruginosa. Biomedical and Environmental Sciences,* 21(2) (2008) 103–109.
16. Chabalgoity J. A., Dougan G., Mastroeni P., Aspinall R. J. Live bacteria as the basis for immunotherapies against cancer. *Expert Review of Vaccines,* 1(4) (2002) 495–505.
17. Epaulard O., Toussaint B., Quenee L., Derouazi M., Bosco N., Villiers C., *et al.* Anti-tumor immunotherapy via antigen delivery from a live attenuated genetically engineered *Pseudomonas aeruginosa* type III secretion system-based vector. *Molecular Therapy,* 14(5) (2006) 656–661.
18. Berinstein N. L. Strategies to enhance the therapeutic activity of cancer vaccines: using melanoma as a model. *Annals of the New York Academy of Sciences,* 1174 (2009) 107–117.
19. Chianese-Bullock K. A., Lewis S. T., Sherman N. E., Shannon J. D., Slingluff CL Jr. Multi-peptide vaccines vialed as peptide mixtures can be stable reagents for use in peptide-based immune therapies. *Vaccine,* 27(11) (2009) 1764–1770.
20. Signori E., Iurescia S., Massi E., Fioretti D., Chiarella P., De Robertis M., *et al.* DNA vaccination strategies for anti-tumour effective gene therapy protocols. *Cancer Immunology, Immunotherapy,* 59(10) (2010) 1583–1591.
21. Wagner S., Jasinska J., Breiteneder H., Kundi M., Pehamberger H., Scheiner O., Zielinski C. C., Wiedermann U. Delayed tumor onset and reduced tumor growth progression after immunization with a Her-2/neu multi-peptide vaccine and IL-12 in c-*neu* transgenic mice. *Breast Cancer Research and Treatment,* 106(1) (2007) 29–38.
22. Wang Y., Gouëllec A. L., Chaker H., Asrih H., Polack B., Toussaint B. Optimization of antitumor immunotherapy mediated by type III secretion system-based live attenuated bacterial vectors. *Journal of Immunotherapy,* 35(3) (2012) 223–234.
23. Epaulard O., Derouazi M., Margerit C., Marlu R., Filopon D., Polack B., *et al.* Optimization of a type III secretion system-based *Pseudomonas aeruginosa* live vector for antigen delivery. *Clinical and Vaccine Immunology,* 15(2) (2008) 308–313.
24. Priebe G. P., Meluleni G. J., Coleman F. T., Goldberg J. B., Pier G. B. Protection against fatal *Pseudomonas aeruginosa* pneumonia in mice after nasal immunization with a live, attenuated aroA deletion mutant. *Infection and Immunity,* 71 (2003) 1453–1461.

25. Lesprit P., Faurisson F., Join-Lambert O., Roudot-Thoraval F., Foglino C., Vissuzaine M., Carbon C. Role of the quorum-sensing system in experimental pneumonia due to *Pseudomonas aeruginosa* in rats. *American Journal of Respiratory and Critical Care Medicine,* 167 (2003) 1478–1482.

26. Pearson J. P., Feldman M., Iglewski B. H., Prince A. *Pseudomonas aeruginosa* cell-to-cell signalling is required for virulence in a model of acute pulmonary infection. *Infection and Immunity,* 68 (2000) 4331–4334.

27. Rumbaugh K. P., Griswold J. A., Iglewski B. H., Hamood A. N. Contribution of QS to the virulence of *Pseudomonas aeruginosa* in burn wound infections. *Infection and Immunity,* 67 (1999) 5854–5862.

28. Mittal R., Sharma S., Shhibber S., Harjai K. Contribution of quorum-sensing systems to virulence of *Pseudomonas aeruginosa* in an experimental pyelonephritis model. *Journal of Microbiology, Immunology and Infection,* 39 (2006) 302–309.

29. DeBell R. M. Production of exotoxin A by *Pseudomonas aeruginosa* in a chemically defined medium. *Infection and Immunity,* 24 (1979) 132–138.

30. Butz E. A., Bevan M. J. Massive expansion of antigen-specific CD8+ T cells during an acute virus infection. *Immunity,* 8 (1998) 167–175.

31. Kaech S. M., Wherry E. J., Ahmed R. Effector and memory T-cell differentiation: implications for vaccine development. *Nature Reviews Immunology,* 2 (2002) 251–262.

32. Williams M. A., Bevan M. J. Effector and memory CTL differentiation. *Annual Review of Immunology,* 25 (2007) 171–192.

33. Lanzavecchia A., Sallusto F. Progressive differentiation and selection of the fittest in the immune response. *Nature Reviews Immunology,* 2 (2002) 982–987.

34. Brockstedt D. G., Bahjat K. S., Giedlin M. A., Liu W., Leong M., Luckett W., *et al.* Killed but metabolically active microbes: a new vaccine paradigm for eliciting effector T-cell responses and protective immunity. *Nature Medicine,* 11(8) (2005) 853–860.

35. Le Gouëllec A., Chauchet X., Laurin D., Aspord C., Verove J., Wang Y., *et al.* A safe bacterial microsyringe for in vivo antigen delivery and immunotherapy. *Molecular Therapy,* 21(5) (2013) 1076–1086.

36. Chauchet X., Hannani D., Djebali S., Laurin D., Polack B., Marvel J., *et al.* Poly-functional and long-lasting anticancer immune response elicited by a safe attenuated *Pseudomonas aeruginosa* vector for antigens delivery. *Molecular Therapy Oncolytics,* 3 (2016) 16033.

37. Berthoin L., Toussaint B., Garban F., Le Gouellec A., Caulier B., Polack B., *et al.* Targeted release of transcription factors for cell reprogramming by a natural micro-syringe. *International Journal of Pharmaceutics,* 513(1–2) (2016) 678–687.

Chapter 9

The Anticancer Potential of the Bacterial Protein Azurin and Its Derived Peptide p28

Ana Rita Garizo,[a] Nuno Bernardes,[a] Ananda M. Chakrabarty,[b] and Arsénio M. Fialho[a,c]

[a]*iBB-Institute for Bioengineering and Biosciences, Biological Sciences Research Group, Av. Rovisco Pais 1, 1049-001 Lisbon, Portugal*
[b]*Department of Microbiology & Immunology, University of Illinois College of Medicine, Chicago, IL 60612, USA*
[c]*Department of Bioengineering, Instituto Superior Técnico, University of Lisbon, Lisbon, Portugal*

afialho@tecnico.ulisboa.pt

During the last decade, the use of microbes or their purified products as cancer therapeutic agents is gaining much attention. Several recent reports highlight the use of live or attenuated bacteria as delivery systems of heterologous products for cancer targeting and treatment. Such biological systems explore the natural propensity of certain bacteria to colonize cancer tissues. In parallel, efforts have been made to identify bioactive molecules from microbial sources able to act as anticancer agents. This is

Microbial Infections and Cancer Therapy: Recent Advances
Edited by Ananda M. Chakrabarty and Arsénio M. Fialho

ISBN 978-981-4774-86-4 (Hardcover), 978-1-351-04190-4 (eBook)
www.panstanford.com

the case of the bacterial protein azurin from *Pseudomonas aeruginosa*. Here we provide an overview of current knowledge regarding the use of this protein and its derived peptide p28 as anticancer agents.

9.1 Introduction

On the basis of World Health Organization projections, in 2030, the number of people expected to die of cancer will be around 11.4 million. This expectation is supported by the rapid increase of the population age and urges rapid responses from oncologists, public health professionals, policy makers, and researchers. Conventional cancer treatments, based on chemotherapy plus radiotherapy, often fail to achieve full cancer remission. To circumvent this problem, the implementation of alternative cancer treatments is urgently needed. Among those, the use of life microbes as anticancer agents has been studied in various modalities (solo or in combination with conventional treatments), showing promising results [1].

The regression of cancer in humans and animals exposed to microbial pathogens agents has been verified more than 100 years ago [2]. In 1909, William Coley used bacterial culture supernatants of *Streptococcus pyogenes* and *Serratia marcescens* to treat patients with malignant cancer. This preparation was administrated in approximately 1200 patients, leading to tumor regression in some cases, of which 30 healed completely [3]. Nowadays, it is assumed that the central factor responsible for this therapeutic effect was increased tumor necrosis factor-α secretion in the body of the patient [4].

Several reports have shown that microorganisms can replicate at the tumor locations, under hypoxic conditions (low concentration of oxygen), and also that microorganisms can stimulate the host's immune system during the infections, blocking cancer progression [5].

Another example of a microbial pathogen strain that causes such effects is *Mycobacterium bovis*, which in 1976 was widely used in the treatment of superficial bladder cancer [6]. Besides this, bacterial pathogens agents such as *Listeria monocytogenes* were tested as vaccine vectors for cancer prevention, since they induced the exposition of antigens on the cellular surface, leading to an immune response against cancer cells [7]. With this, it was believed that infection with bacterial pathogen agents causes the activation of macrophages and lymphocytes, resulting in the production of cytotoxic agents with anticancer properties [5]. However, the introduction of live bacteria on the human organism to treat cancer can produce significant side reactions, which may cause serious and eventually fatal infections that are presumed to be the result of the liberation of toxic bacterial products and limiting, that way, their use [7, 8].

9.2 Bacterial Protein Azurin

Currently, the investigation has been directed to segregated soluble factors by bacteria, such as enzymes, secondary metabolites, proteins, or derived peptides and toxins, which may act specifically on cancer cells, being potential anticancer agents [1, 5]. An example of this factor is a small water-soluble protein secreted by *P. aeruginosa*, called azurin (14 kDa; 128 amino acids), which is composed of one α-helix and eight β-sheets, forming a β-barrel motif. On its surface it contains three distinct binding regions: one face with two charged clusters (one large negative nearby one small positive) and a prominent neutral aromatic-rich hydrophobic patch. This arrangement, centered on Phe114, occupies a region around the copper center. Azurin is part of a group of type I redox proteins, which have an ion copper in their constitution, named cupredoxins (Fig. 9.1; [4, 9–15]). It is known that this protein is involved in the transport of electrons during the denitrification of these organisms [16].

Beyond this, azurin has structural similarity with variable domains of immunoglobulins and the ability to mediate high-affinity interactions with unrelated proteins of mammalian origin. Functionally, the structural features revealed by the protein azurin give to it the property of a natural scaffold protein [17]. This property can be exploited through a phage display technology by randomized substitution of selected residues within the pre-existing binding sites of azurin, the overall structural integrity of the β-sandwich scaffold being conserved, aiming to generate azurin variants displaying multiple picomolar affinities to predefined targets relevant in cancers. The implementation of this strategy would lead to directed studies of azurin-engineered variants in cancer therapy, either alone or in conjunction with chemotherapeutics [18].

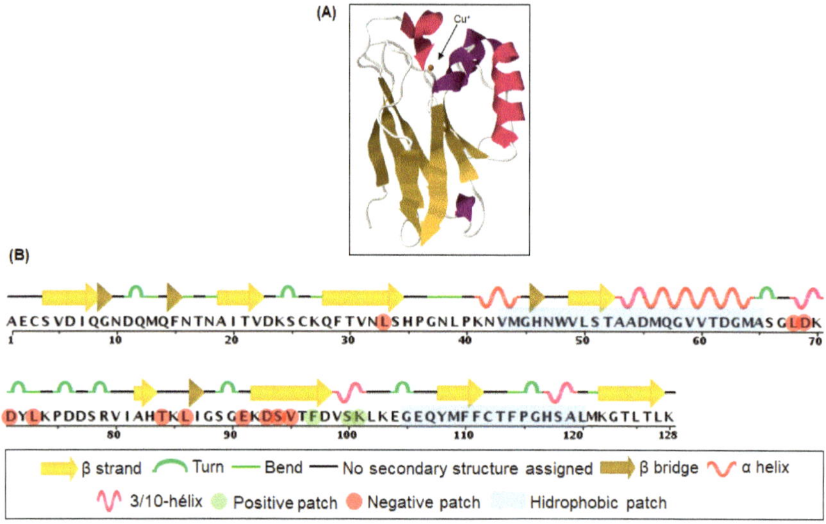

Figure 9.1 (A) Molecular structure of azurin from *Pseudomonas aeruginosa* (PDB_1JZG). This protein is composed of one α-helix (pink) and eight β-sheets (yellow). It is also possible to observe the copper center, a typical component of the cupredoxin protein group. (B) Azurin protein sequence (128 amino acids) and representation of its secondary structure elements (helices: pink; β-sheets: yellow). The green, red, and blue areas correspond to positive, negative, and hydrophobic patches on its surface (based on UniProtKB P00282).

In addition, azurin appears to have selective capacities to be internalized in cancer cells. This event seems dependent on discrete heterogeneous microdomains, denominated lipid rafts (10–200 nm). These regions are less fluid than the surrounding bulk plasma membrane and enriched in cholesterol, sphingolipids, and certain types of proteins, acting as platforms for cellular signaling. Lipid rafts are divided into two types: planar lipid rafts lack specific morphological features, as opposed to *caveolae*, which are nonplanar lipid rafts. In the case of planar lipid rafts, these are constituted of flotillin proteins. On the other hand, *caveolae* are characterized by an abundance of caveolin and cavin proteins. Levels of these microdomains are increased in melanomas, prostate, and breast cancers, which suggests that these structures may play a functional role during tumorigenesis [18–22].

9.3 Entry Mechanism of Azurin/p28 into Human Cells and Subsequent Effects

The mechanism of entry for azurin into cancer cells is still not fully understood. The first hints suggested that azurin enters into mammal cells through the penetration of the plasma membrane via *caveolae*-mediated endocytic pathways, colocalized with caveolin-1, and reaches late endosomes, lysosomes, and the Golgi associated with *caveolae* [23, 24].

Currently, it is known that a peptide derived from azurin called p28 (50–77 amino acids) or protein entry domain (PED) is *per se*, at least in part, responsible for mediating the entrance of the entire protein into cells. This peptide has an overall net negative charge and forms an extended amphipathic α-helix with both hydrophobic amino acids (50–66) and hydrophilic amino acids (67–77). PED was further refined, by reducing the N-terminal to amino acids 50–67 (p18), and it was found that this minimal fragment can be translocated to the inside of human cancer cells [11, 23].

Upon entering cancer cells, azurin is directed to the nucleus and connects with high affinity through the region of p28 to a hydrophobic region inside of the DNA-binding domain of tumor-suppressor protein p53 (21 kDa; 393 amino acids). This binding forms a complex without altering the conformation of p53, blocking its binding with the E3 ubiquitin ligase Cop1, thereby inhibiting the proteasomal degradation of p53 [16, 25, 26]. p53 is involved in numerous cellular processes, including transcription, DNA repair, genomic stability, and cell cycle control, being able to induce cellular death by apoptosis. In human cancers, this protein can suffer from inactivation by oncogenes [27, 28] and it is known that the E3 ubiquitin ligase Cop1 is overexpressed in breast, ovarian, and hepatocellular carcinomas [29], which contributes to the accelerated degradation of the p53 protein and attenuation of the tumor-suppressor function of p53 [30]. In addition, mutations within the DNA-binding domain of this protein are found in >50% of human cancers and may significantly modify the p53 secondary structure, impairing its function [31].

Experiments with isothermal calorimetry demonstrated that azurin binds to the NH_2-terminal domain of p53 with nanomolar affinity in a 4:1 stoichiometry, as well to the DNA-binding domain of this protein [28]. A few studies, supported by site-directed mutagenesis, suggest that a specific region of azurin has been implicated in this complex formation. This region (Met-44 to Met-64) forms a hydrophobic patch and is located within the p28 peptide [32]. Thus, with the inhibition of proteasomal degradation of p53 occurs a raise of the cytoplasmic and nuclear levels of this protein, and consequently, increased DNA binding activity. The levels of the cyclin-dependent kinase inhibitors p21 and p27 also increase, which in turn reduces the intracellular levels of cyclin-dependent kinase 2 (CDK2) and cyclin A1, essential proteins in the mitotic process, as well as Forkhead box M1 (FOXM1), a transcription factor for G_2/M progression. Since these components are involved in controlling the cell cycle, the reduction in their levels interrupts this process at the G_2/M phase, thus leading to apoptosis (Fig. 9.2; [16]). With this, it was possible to understand that the use of azurin/p28 can be a good therapeutic option for the regression of tumors.

Additionally, it is documented that the p28 penetration rate into cancer cells decreases after the elimination of cholesterol on the plasma membranes using methyl-β-cyclodextrin (~60%) and after treatments with nocodazole or with monensin, which disrupt membrane caveolar by disruption of the microtubules and inhibit the activity of endosomes and lysosomes, respectively. This suggests that this peptide and possibly the entire protein penetrate the plasma membrane via *caveolae*-mediated endocytic pathways. It is also known that this process is not dependent on membrane-bound glycosaminoglycans or on clathrins [16, 23].

In addition to all this, it is possible that *N*-glycosylated proteins may have a role at least in the initial steps of recognition [23].

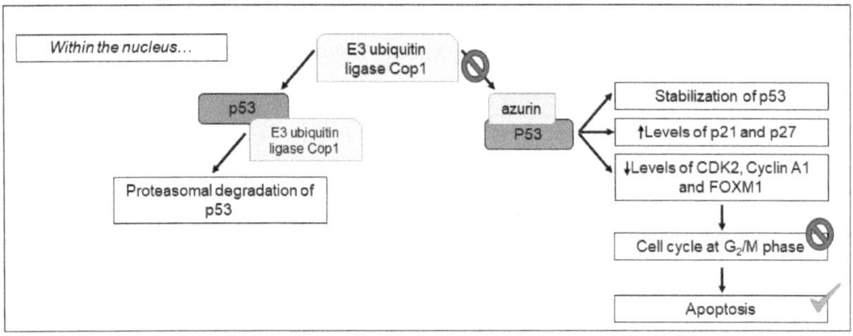

Figure 9.2 Azurin mode of action. After the entrance of azurin into cancer cells, it is processed in the nucleus and binds to the DNA-binding domain of p53, where it blocks the binding of the E3 ubiquitin ligase Cop1. This event inhibits the proteasomal degradation of p53 and induces its stabilization, thereby upregulating the cyclin-dependent kinase inhibitors p21 and p27, which in turn reduces the intracellular levels of CDK2, cyclin A1, and FOXM1. The decrease in these levels interrupts cell cycle at the G2/M phase, leading to apoptosis of cancer cells.

It is still important to note that azurin shows a preferred internalization to the cancer cells rather than the normal ones. Once inside in these cells, the apo and holo forms of this protein are similar in their effects, supporting a copper-independent mechanism of action [11, 33]. It is also known that the position of D-amino acid substitutions within the α-helical backbone and the strength of the substitutions that alter chirality may be critical to the overall entry of p28 but not the preferential nature of its penetration. That way, the application of this bacterial protein and its derived peptide p28 on cancer therapy will identify a new way to fight this disease [34].

9.4 Azurin Mode of Action in the Levels of Cadherin Proteins

Cell invasion is a crucial step in cancer progression. The ability of cancer cells to adhere to other cells, as well as to the surrounding extracellular matrix components, is different from the normal cells [35, 36].

Currently, it is recognized that the P-cadherin overexpression, a cell–cell adhesion molecule expressed in breast tissues that belongs to the type I cadherin family, occurs in 30% of invasive breast carcinomas [37, 38]. Studies have shown that increase in the expression of P-cadherin promotes invasive effects in breast cancer cells, which can be, at least in part, attributed to the release of a soluble form of P-cadherin (sP-cad) to the extracellular media. This occurs because the P-cadherin expression interferes with the normal invasive suppressive function of E-cadherin. However, it was found that P-cadherin overexpression is correlated to increased cell motility, cell migration, and cell invasion [39], which is only observed in cell systems that are also positive for E-cadherin expression. In highly invasive melanoma, which lacks the expression of E-cadherin, P-cadherin expression can induce cell-to-cell contacts and decrease invasion [40].

Studies showed that the administration of azurin in MCF-7/AZ breast cancer cells that overexpress P-cadherin decreases cellular invasion. In cell lines of p53 wild type and mutant, this effect is associated with the decrease in the levels of P-cadherin protein, without affecting the E-cadherin expression. Furthermore, it causes a down-regulation of genes coding for cell surface receptors, which translates into a deficient regulation from the intracellular signaling cascades (Figs. 9.3 and 9.4; [15, 41]).

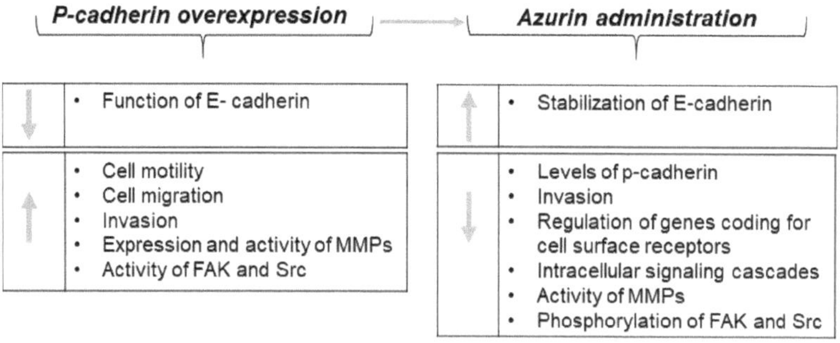

Figure 9.3 Consequences of P-cadherin overexpression and effects of azurin administration on cancer cells.

It was also verified that P-cadherin overexpression is associated with increased expression and activity of matrix metalloproteases (MMPs), namely MMP-1 and MMP-2 [39], as well as the activation of the intracellular nonreceptor tyrosine kinases FAK and Src, which regulate a wide number of signaling pathways involved in cell spreading, adhesion, migration, invasion, survival, proliferation, differentiation, and angiogenesis (Fig. 9.3; [41]). In fact, several tumorigenic processes are mediated by MMPs, namely the breakdown of extracellular components, which accounts greatly for the ability of tumor cells to invade the surrounding tissues through extensive matrix remodeling [42].

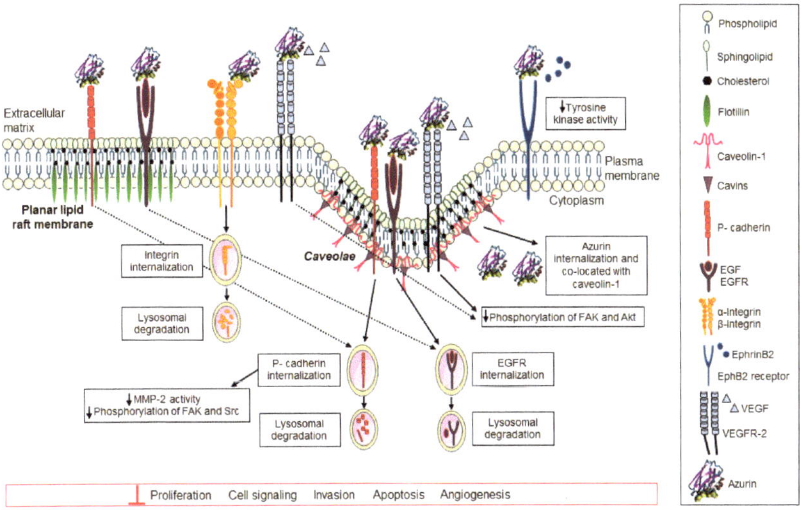

Figure 9.4 Proposed mechanisms of action of azurin against cancer cells. Azurin penetrates into plasma membrane via *caveolae*-mediated endocytic pathways, and/or it can bind to cell-surface receptors. These events interfere in proliferation, cell signaling, invasion, and apoptosis of cancer cells, as well as inhibit angiogenesis.

In 2013, a study assessed the activity of MMP-2 by gelatin zymography in the conditioned media of these breast cancer cells treated with azurin and observed a decrease in its activity. In the same study, it was observed that the decrease in P-cadherin caused by azurin was parallel to a decrease in the phosphorylated levels of FAK and Src nonreceptor proteins, without any alteration in total FAK and Src protein levels (Figs 9.3 and 9.4). It is known that FAK is necessary to the regulation of invadopodia in ovarian carcinoma cells and to promote breast cancer cell invasion [15].

Additionally, in v-Src-transformed fibroblast cells, FAK promotes the formation of a v-Src-Cas-Crk-Dock180 complex, which leads to an elevated expression of MMP-2 and MMP-9 [43]. Also Src, when activated, can facilitate motility and invasion through reorganization of the actin cytoskeleton and disruption of normal cell–cell and cell–matrix adhesion [44].

9.5 Interaction between Azurin/p28 and Surface Receptors in Cancer Cells and Other Activities

In 2014, Bernardes *et al.* revealed through microarray analyses that in MCF-7 breast cancer cells treated with azurin occurred an up-regulation of genes associated with cellular processes, such as vesicle transport and pathways associated with lysosomes, as well as an increased expression of genes associated with endocytosis, membrane organization, and endosome transport. Also, azurin caused a reduction in the expression of an important number of genes coding for cell surface receptors, as it was previously said, resulting in a down-regulation of their downstream signaling, which usually sustains cell proliferation and aberrant constitutive signaling [41]. It is known that cancer cells have the capability to grow, even in the absence of external growth stimulatory signals, frequently by overexpressing growth factor receptor tyrosine kinases [45]. Some of these receptors, for example, epidermal growth factor receptor (EGFR), when activated, stimulate signaling pathways involved in cell growth, survival, and migration. EGFR is located normally on the plasma membrane in lipid rafts [46]. The tyrosine kinase receptors can become extremely active by genomic amplification or overexpression or by mechanisms that inhibit their degradation upon their endocytosis. That way, this deregulation can lead to excessive accumulation of these receptors on the surface of cancer cells [47].

Still in this study, upon treatment with azurin of MCF-7/AZ breast cancer cells with overexpression of P-cadherin, reduction in the expression of the *EGRF* gene was observed. *EGRF* is frequently overexpressed in triple-negative basal-like (TNBL) breast cancers. That way, this study suggests that the most aggressive cellular phenotype that appears on breast cancer cells with a high expression of P-cadherin is tightly connected with the regulation of several receptors on the cellular surface, which may in part be controlled by the azurin treatment (Fig. 9.4; [41]).

More recent, Bernardes *et al.* showed that azurin modulates the levels and localization of β1-integrin, affecting the downstream signaling cascade and the invasiveness of NSCLC A549 cells (Fig. 9.4; [48]).

Azurin is also able to bind to several Eph receptor tyrosine kinases, a family of extracellular receptor proteins known to be upregulated in many tumors. This protein binds to the EphB2 receptor, interfering with its phosphorylation at the tyrosine residue, which in turn interferes with the binding to the ligand ephrinB2, resulting in the inhibition of cell signaling and cancer growth. It was suggested that such events occurred due to structural similarities between azurin and the ligand ephrinB2 (Fig. 9.4; [49]).

In cancer cells, the removal of functional receptors from cell surface and their targeting to lysosome was suggested to be an important mechanism by which their permanent activation and consequent tumorigenesis are prevented [47].

It has also been reported that p28 can inhibit cancer-induced angiogenesis by reducing vascular endothelial growth factor receptor 2 (VEGFR-2) tyrosine kinase activity. Consequently, this inhibition reduces the phosphorylation of the VEGFR-2 downstream targets FAK and Akt (Fig. 9.4; [24]).

Azurin/p28 can also interfere in oncogenic transformation to prevent precancerous lesion formation in mouse alveolar and ductal mammary glands exposed to a 7,12-dimethylbenz(a)anthracene carcinogen (DMBA) [50].

9.6 Azurin/p28 Application in the Treatment of Cancer

There are many reasons that support the theory that azurin has the potential to act as an anticancer agent. Besides its preferential entry into cancer cells, no adverse side effects were observed in in vivo studies [11, 51, 52]. As mentioned above, this protein also can mediate specific high-affinity interactions with various unrelated mammalian proteins relevant in cancer, conferring on it the property of a natural scaffold protein, which is probably the most important characteristic of this protein [17]. This ability to act on multiple targets is important since it might be harder to trigger resistance by the cells. Another advantage of this bacterial protein is that azurin is a water-soluble molecule with a hydrophobic patch and this might help in its tissue penetration and clearance from the bloodstream [9]. In addition to all this, azurin can be easily hyperexpressed in *Escherichia coli*, which makes the process of production very cheap [15]. All these reasons make azurin an attractive molecule to be used in cancer therapy.

Although it has been previously reported that the introduction of live bacteria on the human organism to treat cancer can have side effects, a study was recently done with *Salmonella typhimurium* to deliver a tumoricidal combination therapy of p53 and azurin that induces apoptosis in an intracranial rat model of an aggressive glioblastoma tumor. This strain has active motility in extracellular space and within brain tumors, the capability of expressing apoptotic proteins within the tumor and also a mutation in the *msbB* gene that impedes systemic toxicity. In this study, 19% of treated rats showed that the tumor growth was retarded. Beyond this, proteomic analysis clearly showed a restored neural environment in treated rats relative to control untreated animals. With this, *S. typhimurium* in conjunction with its expression of azurin within the tumor opens a versatile avenue to overcome diffusion barriers in glioblastoma [53].

Preclinical pharmacological studies using p28, which is easier to be chemically synthesized with a higher degree of purity, provided significant evidence that there is no apparent toxicity or immune response in the patients with solid tumors p53+/+, on which no observed adverse effect level (NOAEL) and maximum tolerated dose (MTD) were established [52]. With these results, it can be concluded that azurin has low immunogenicity, being a nonantibody recognized protein and for that, it is not susceptible to immune attack, even though it is a bacterial protein.

As a lead compound supported by CDG therapeutics, p28 has finished phase I clinical trial, which defined it as an anticancer agent under an investigational new drug application

(IND 77.754) approved by the Food and Drug Administration (FDA) [52]. Recent studies have also shown that intravenous administration of p28 was safe and well tolerated and led to some tumor regressing effect in children (age 3 to 21) with progressive central nervous system malignancies [54]. Moreover, it is important to reveal that the azurin-p28 peptide has been approved as an orphan drug by the FDA agency. Subsequent studies will focus on the establishment of an adequate dose for phase II clinical trial, in obtaining a pharmacokinetic profile, determining potential immunogenicity, and if possible assessing preliminary antitumor activity [52].

However, there are other domains in azurin with anticancer property [49] that should provide better efficacy and will likely make azurin less susceptible to resistance development, provided lack of toxicity of azurin in animals and cancer patients can be demonstrated, as has been done for p28 [55].

Given azurin's propensity for both therapeutic and cancer preventive activity, a weekly or biweekly injection of azurin in vulnerable people, for example, women with a family history of breast or ovarian cancers and with diagnosed *BRCA1/BRCA2* mutations, may be one way to prevent, or greatly reduce, the onset of cancer in such people. Other pathways of administration azurin for cancer treatment, such as oral, are currently being investigated [56].

In addition to all this, azurin or its derived peptide 28 can be fluorescently labeled, providing good diagnostic markers to locate tumors inside the body since it preferentially moves toward cancer cells [56].

9.7 Effects of Azurin/p28 Treatment in Combination with Drugs on Cancer Cells

Nowadays, chemotherapy includes DNA-damaging and antimitotic agents. DNA-damaging agents intercalate with DNA, inducing double strand breaks that induce ataxia-telangiectasia mutated (ATM)-dependent nuclear accumulation of p53 [57]. In addition, the apoptotic pathway via Bcl-2/Bax and the caspase cascade, as well as the necrotic pathway through toll-like receptors are targets for DNA-damaging agents [58]. On the other hand, antimitotic agents bind to the β-tubulin subunits of microtubules. This interaction leads to prolonged activation of the mitotic spindle checkpoint and mitotic arrest, followed by mitotic slippage and induction of apoptosis. These agents, also called taxanes, still induce post-transcriptional acetylation and phosphorylation of p53, which leads to its intracellular increase, upregulation of p21 protein, and inhibition of the cell cycle and also leads to apoptosis [59].

Unfortunately, with the consecutive application of these agents, cancer cells acquire resistance. Beyond this, these drugs can also lead to significant toxicity that may force treatment to become dose limiting [58]. With this, new therapeutic strategies, more effective in killing cancer cells but also more selective, are needed to increase the efficiency and decrease the toxic side effects associated with administration of drugs [48].

One of these strategies is based on the combinatorial use of the peptide p28 or the full protein azurin with chemotherapeutic drugs. Yamada *et al.* [58] have shown that the dual administration of p28 with sublethal concentrations of DNA-damaging drugs, like doxorubicin, dacarbazine, and temozolamide, and antimitotic agents, such as paclitaxel and docetaxel, has the potential to improve their singular therapeutic effectiveness. This study suggests that the combinatorial formulations act by stabilizing the tumor-suppressor protein p53 and thereby inducing a sequence of cellular events (induction of p21, reduction of CDK2, and inhibition of cell cycle at G2/M phase), leading to apoptosis. Altogether, these results reinforce the success of using alternative therapies to enhance the efficacy of chemotherapeutic agents while reducing dose-related toxicity [58].

In addition, a recent study also assessed the potential synergy of a cotreatment with azurin. The drugs used were gefitinib or erlotinib, both EGFR inhibitors, in low concentrations. This combined treatment demonstrated an increase in cell death when compared to the sum of each agent alone, that is, a synergistic effect occurred in comparison to the single treatments [48].

In the same study, it was demonstrated by atomic force microscopy that azurin administration leads to changes in biophysical properties of the plasma membrane of cancer cells, which includes increases in cell mass, height, volume, and elasticity, thereby causing changes in signaling pathways that mediate drug resistance. These effects may be of particular interest in drug-resistant cancers, where the more rigid nature of the membrane was associated with increased resistance to the accumulation of anticancer drugs. Therefore, since azurin may disrupt lipid rafts, the effects of coadministered drugs are enhanced [48].

Another study demonstrating the above mentioned was performed by Choi *et al.* in 2011 [51]. In this study, azurin-treated oral squamous carcinoma cells showed decreased cell viability accompanied by apoptotic phenotypes, including morphological change, DNA breakage, and increases in p53 and cyclin B1 protein levels. In these cancer cells, with the combined treatment of azurin and anticancer agents (5-fluorouracil and etopside), they discovered that this protein increased the sensitivity of oral squamous carcinoma cells to these anticancer drugs [51].

9.8 Conclusions

The results of all these studies suggest that the mechanism by which azurin exerts its anticancer effects depends on its route of cancer cell entry, disrupting *caveolae* and removing from the cell membrane selective receptors that promote cell proliferation and aberrant constitutive signaling [41]. Thus, azurin, a bacterial protein secreted by *P. aeruginosa*, and its derived peptide p28 can be applied for cancer treatment, since they have such anticancer properties. They promote apoptosis and/or blocks tumor invasion, as well as inhibit angiogenesis.

References

1. Bernardes N., Seruca R., Chakrabarty A. M., Fialho A. M. Microbial-based therapy of cancer: Current progress and future prospects. *Bioengineered Bugs*, 1 (2010) 178–190.
2. Coley W. B. Contribution to the knowledge of sarcoma. *Annals of Surgery*, 14 (1891) 199–220.
3. Coley W. B. The treatment of inoperable sarcoma by bacterial toxins (the mixed toxins of the *Streptococcus erysipelatis* and *Bacillus prodigiosus*). *Journal of the Royal Society of Medicine*, 3 (1909) 1–48.
4. Karpiński T. M., Szkaradkiewicz A. K. Anticancer peptides from bacteria. *Bangladesh Journal of Pharmacology*, 8 (2013) 343–348.

5. Yamada T., Goto M., Punj V., Zaborina O., Chen M. L., Kimbara K. *et al.* Bacterial redox protein azurin, tumor supressor protein p53, and regression of cancer. *Proceedings of the National Academy of Sciences of the United States of America,* 99 (2002a) 14098–14103.
6. Morales A., Eidinger D., Bruce A. W. Intracavitary *Bacillus Calmette Guerin* in the treatment of superficial bladder tumors. *Journal of Urology,* 116 (1976) 180–183.
7. Paglia P., Arioli I., Frahm N., Chakraborty I., Colombo M. P., Guzmad C. A. The defined attenuated *Listeria monocytogenes* Δ*mpl*2 mutant is an effective oral vaccine carrier to trigger a long-lasting immune response against a mouse fibrosarcoma. *European Journal of Immunology,* 27 (1997) 1570–1575.
8. Dang L. H., Bettegowda C., Huso D. L., Kinzler K. W., Vogelstein B. Combination bacteriolytic therapy for the treatment of experimental tumors. *Proceedings of the National Academy of Sciences of the United States of America,* 98 (2001) 15155–15160.
9. Kamp M. van de, Chiara M., Brunori M., Beeumen J. Van, Hali F. C., Canters G. W. Involvement of the hydrophobic patch of azurin in the electron-transfer reactions with cytochrome c_{551} and nitrite reductase. *European Journal of Biochemistry,* 118 (1990) 109–118.
10. Rienzo F. De, Gabdoulline R. R., Menziani M. C., Wade R. C. Blue copper proteins: A comparative analysis of their molecular interaction properties. *Protein Science,* 9 (2000) 1439–1454.
11. Yamada T., Fialho A. M., Punj V., Bratescu L., Gupta T. K. Das, Chakrabarty A. M. Internalization of bacterial redox protein azurin in mammalian cells: Entry domain and specificity. *Cell Microbiology,* 7 (2005) 1418–1431.
12. Yanagisawa S., Banfield M. J., Dennison C. The role of hydrogen bonding at the active site of a cupredoxin: The Phe114Pro azurin variant. *Biochemistry,* 45 (2006) 8812–8822.
13. Fialho A. M., Salunkhe P., Manna S., Mahali S., Chakrabarty A. M. Glioblastoma multiforme: Novel therapeutic approaches. *ISRN Neurology,* 2012 (2012) 1–10.
14. Warren J. J., Lancaster K. M., Richards J. H., Gray H. B. Inner- and outer-sphere metal coordination in blue copper proteins. *Journal of Inorganic Biochemistry,* 115 (2012) 119–126.
15. Bernardes N., Ribeiro A. S., Abreu S., Mota B., Matos R. G., Arraiano C. M. *et al.* The bacterial protein azurin impairs invasion and FAK/Src signaling in P-cadherin-overexpressing breast cancer cell models. *PLOS One,* 8 (2013) e69023.

16. Yamada T., Mehta R. R., Lekmine F., Christov K., King M. L., Majumdar D. *et al.* A peptide fragment of azurin induces a p53-mediated cell cycle arrest in human breast cancer cells. *Molecular Cancer Therapeutics*, 8 (2009) 2947–2958.

17. Fialho A. M., Stevens F. J., Das Gupta T. K., Chakrabarty A. M. Beyond host-pathogen interactions: Microbial defense strategy in the host environment. *Current Opinion in Biotechnology*, 18 (2007) 279–286.

18. Fialho A. M., Bernardes N., Chakrabarty A. M. Exploring the anticancer potential of the bacterial protein azurin. *AIMS Microbiology*, 2 (2016) 292–303.

19. Quest A. F. G., Gutierrez-Pajares J. L., Torres V. A. Caveolin-1: An ambiguous partner in cell signalling and cancer. *Journal of Cellular and Molecular Medicine*, 12 (2008) 1130–50.

20. Parton R. G., Pozo M. A del. *Caveolae* as plasma membrane sensors, protectors and organizers. *Nature Reviews Molecular Cell Biology*, 14 (2013) 98–112.

21. Martinez-Outschoorn U. E., Sotgia F., Lisanti M. P. *Caveolae* and signalling in cancer. *Nature Reviews Cancer*, 15 (2015) 225–237.

22. Murai T. Cholesterol lowering: Role in cancer prevention and treatment. *Biological Chemistry*, 396 (2015) 1–11.

23. Taylor B. N., Mehta R. R., Yamada T., Lekmine F., Christov K., Chakrabarty A. M. *et al.* Noncationic peptides obtained from azurin preferentially enter cancer cells. *Cancer Research*, 69 (2009) 537–546.

24. Mehta R. R., Yamada T., Taylor B. N., Christov K., King M. L., Majumdar D., *et al.* A cell penetrating peptide derived from azurin inhibits angiogenesis and tumor growth by inhibiting phosphorylation of VEGFR-2, FAK and Akt. *Angiogenesis*, 14 (2011) 355–369.

25. Yamada T., Christov K., Shilkaitis A., Bratescu L., Green A., Santini S. *et al.* p28, a first in class peptide inhibitor of cop1 binding to p53. *British Journal of Cancer*, 108 (2013a) 2495–2504.

26. Yamada T., Gupta T. K. Das, and Beattie C. W. p28, an anionic cell-penetrating peptide, increases the activity of wild type andmutated p53 without altering its conformation. *Molecular Pharmaceutics*, 10 (2013b) 3375–3383.

27. Martin A. C. R., Facchiano A. M., Cuff A. L., Hernandez-Boussard T., Olivier M., Hainaut P., *et al.* Integrating mutation data and structural analysis of the TP53 tumor-suppressor protein. *Human Mutation*, 19 (2002) 149–164.

28. Apiyo D., Wittung-Stafshede P. Unique complex between bacterial azurin and tumor-suppressor protein p53. *Biochemical and Biophysical Research Communications*, 332 (2005) 965–968.

29. Li Y. F., Wang D. D., Zhao B. W., Wang W., Huang C. Y., Chen Y. M., *et al.* High level of COP1 expression is associated with poor prognosis in primary gastric cancer. *International Journal of Biological Sciences*, 8 (2012) 1168–1177.

30. Dornan D., Bheddah S., Newton K., Ince W., Frantz G. D., Dowd P., *et al.* COP1, the negative regulator of p53, is overexpressed in breast and ovarian adenocarcinomas. *Cancer Research*, 64 (2004) 7226–7230.

31. Signorelli S., Santini S., Yamada T., Bizzarri A. R., Beattie C. W., Cannistraro S. Binding of amphipathic cell penetrating peptide p28 to wild type and mutated p53 as studied by raman, atomic force and surface plasmon resonance spectroscopies. *Biochimica et Biophysica Acta*, 1861 (2017) 910–921.

32. Yamada T., Goto M., Punj V., Zaborina O., Kimbara K., Gupta T. K. Das, *et al.* The bacterial redox protein azurin induces apoptosis in J774 macrophages through complex formation and stabilization of the tumor suppressor protein p53 the bacterial redox protein azurin induces apoptosis in J774 macrophages through complex formation and stabilization of the tumor suppressor protein p53. *Infection and Immunity*, 70 (2002b) 7054–7062.

33. Goto M., Yamada T., Kimbara K., Horner J., Newcomb M., Gupta T. K., *et al.* Induction of apoptosis in macrophages by *Pseudomonas aeruginosa* azurin: Tumour-suppressor protein p53 and reactive oxygen species, but not redox activity, as critical elements in cytotoxicity. *Molecular Microbiology*, 47 (2002) 549–559.

34. Yamada T., Signorelli S., Cannistraro S., Beattie C. W., Bizzarri A. R. Chirality switching within an anionic cell-penetrating peptide inhibits translocation without affecting preferential entry. *Molecular Pharmacology*, 12 (2015) 140–149.

35. Zhao J., Guan J.-L. Signal transduction by focal adhesion kinase in cancer. *Cancer and Metastasis Reviews*, 28 (2009) 35–49.

36. Kessenbrock K., Plaks V., Werb Z. Matrix metalloproteinases: Regulators of the tumor microenvironment. *Cell*, 141 (2010) 52–67.

37. Paredes J., Albergaria A., Oliveira J. T., Jerónimo C., Milanezi F., Schmitt F. C. P-cadherin overexpression is an indicator of clinical outcome in invasive breast carcinomas and is associated with CDH3 promoter hypomethylation. *Clinical Cancer Research*, 11 (2005) 5869–5877.

38. Albergaria A., Ribeiro A. S., Vieira A. F., Sousa B., Nobre A. R., Seruca R. *et al.* P-cadherin role in normal breast development and cancer. *International Journal Of Developmental Biology*, 55 (2011) 811–822.
39. Ribeiro A. S., Albergaria A., Sousa B., Correia A. L., Bracke M., Seruca R., *et al.* Extracellular cleavage and shedding of P-cadherin: A mechanism underlying the invasive behaviour of breast cancer cells. *Oncogene*, 29 (2010) 392–402.
40. Van Marck V., Stove C., Van Den Bossche K., Stove V., Paredes J., Haeghen Y. V., *et al.* P-cadherin promotes cell-cell adhesion and counteracts invasion in human melanoma. *Cancer Research*, 65 (2005) 8774–8783.
41. Bernardes N., Ribeiro A. S., Abreu S., Vieira A. F., Carreto L., Santos M., *et al.* High-throughput molecular profiling of a P-cadherin overexpressing breast cancer model reveals new targets for the anti-cancer bacterial protein azurin. *International Journal of Biochemistry & Cell Biology*, 50 (2014) 1–9.
42. Luo M., Guan J. L. Focal adhesion kinase: A prominent determinant in breast cancer initiation, progression and metastasis. *Cancer Letters*, 289 (2010) 127–139.
43. Hsia D. A., Mitra S. K., Hauck C. R., Streblow D. N., Nelson J. A., Ilic D., *et al.* Differential regulation of cell motility and invasion by FAK. *Journal of Cell Biology*, 160 (2003) 753–767.
44. Guarino M. Src signaling in cancer invasion. *Journal of Cellular Physiology*, 223 (2010) 14–26.
45. Hanahan D., Weinberg R. A. Hallmarks of cancer: The next generation. *Cell*, 144 (2011) 646–674.
46. Irwin M. E., Mueller K. L., Bohin N., Ge Y., Boerner J. L. Lipid raft localization of EGFR alters the response of cancer cells to the EGFR tyrosine kinase inhibitor gefitinib. *Journal of Cellular Physiology*, 226 (2011) 2316–2328.
47. Abella J. V., Park M. Breakdown of endocytosis in the oncogenic activation of receptor tyrosine kinases. *American Journal of Physiology-Endocrinology and Metabolism*, 296 (2009) 973–984.
48. Bernardes N., Abreu S., Carvalho F. A., Fernandes F., Santos N. C., Fialho A. M. Modulation of membrane properties of lung cancer cells by azurin enhances the sensitivity to EGFR-targeted therapy and decreased β1 integrin-mediated adhesion. *Cell Cycle*, 20 (2016) 1–10.
49. Chaudhari A., Mahfouz M., Fialho A. M., Yamada T., Granja A. T., Zhu Y., *et al.* Cupredoxin-cancer interrelationship: azurin binding with

EphB2, interference in EphB2 tyrosine phosphorylation, and inhibition of cancer growth. *Biochemistry*, 46 (2007) 1799–1810.

50. Mehta R. R., Hawthorne M., Peng X., Shilkaitis A., Mehta R. G., Beattie C. W., *et al.* A 28-amino-acid peptide fragment of the cupredoxin azurin prevents carcinogen-induced mouse mammary lesions. *Cancer Prevention Research*, 3 (2010) 1351–1360.
51. Choi J.-H., Lee M.-H., Cho Y.-J., Park B.-S., Kim S., Kim G.-C. The bacterial protein azurin enhances sensitivity of oral squamous carcinoma cells to anticancer drugs. *Yonsei Medical Journal*, 52 (2011) 773–778.
52. Warso M. A., Richards J. M., Mehta D., Christov K., Schaeffer C., Rae Bressler L., *et al.* A first-in-class, first-in-human, phase I trial of p28, a non-HDM2-mediated peptide inhibitor of p53 ubiquitination in patients with advanced solid tumours. *British Journal of Cancer*, 108 (2013) 1061–1070.
53. Mehta N., Lyon J. G., Patil K., Mokarram N., Kim C., Bellamkonda R. V. Bacterial carriers for glioblastoma therapy. *Molecular Therapy: Oncolytics*, 4 (2016) 1–17.
54. Lulla R. R., Goldman S., Yamada T., Beattie C. W., Bressler L., Pacini M., *et al.* Phase 1 trial of p28 (NSC745104), a non-HDM2-mediated peptide inhibitor of p53 ubiquitination in pediatric patients with recurrent or progressive central nervous system tumors: A Pediatric Brain Tumor Consortium Study. *Neuro-Oncology*, 28 (2016) 17.
55. Fialho A. M., Chakrabarty A. M. Patent controversies and court cases. Cancer diagnosis, therapy and prevention. *Cancer Biology & Therapy*, 13 (2012) 1229–1234.
56. Chakrabarty A. M., Bernardes N., Fialho A. M. Bacterial proteins and peptides in cancer therapy. *Bioengineered*, 5 (2014) 234–242.
57. Kurz E. U., Douglas P., Lees-Miller S. P. Doxorubicin activates ATM-dependent phosphorylation of multiple downstream targets in part through the generation of reactive oxygen species. *Journal of Biological Chemistry*, 279 (2004) 53272–53281.
58. Yamada T., Gupta T. K. Das, Beattie C. W. p28-mediated activation of p53 in G_2–M phase of the cell cycle enhances the efficacy of DNA damaging and antimitotic chemotherapy. *Cancer Research*, 76 (2016) 2354–2365.
59. Kim J. H., Yoon E. K., Chung H. J., Park S. Y., Hong K. M., Lee C. H., *et al.* p53 acetylation enhances Taxol-induced apoptosis in human cancer cells. *Apoptosis*, 18 (2013) 110–120.

Chapter 10

Prospective Therapeutic Applications of Bacteriocins as Anticancer Agents

Lígia F. Coelho,[a] Nuno Bernardes,[a] and Arsénio M. Fialho[a,b]

[a]*iBB-Institute for Bioengineering and Biosciences, Biological Sciences Research Group, Av. Rovisco Pais 1, 1049-001 Lisbon, Portugal*
[b]*Department of Bioengineering, Instituto Superior Técnico, University of Lisbon, Lisbon, Portugal*

afialho@tecnico.ulisboa.pt

In the last decades the anticancer activity of some bacteriocins has been explored. These anticancer proteins/peptides have a variety of physicochemical characteristics that enable them to target effectively and selectively malignant cells yet in some cases displaying a nontoxic profile in normal cells. Indeed, the successful results of several *in vitro* studies exploring bacteriocin action against both solid and hematologic cancer cells led to *in vivo* experiments in human tumor xenografts, resulting, in most cases, in a slower tumor growth, tumor reduction, prolonged survival of the model, suppressed metastasis, improved immune response mediated by bacteriocins against the tumor cells, and tumor necrosis/apoptosis consequence of lytic effect in malignant cells' membranes. Given their novelty, the state of art for most

Microbial Infections and Cancer Therapy: Recent Advances
Edited by Ananda M. Chakrabarty and Arsénio M. Fialho

ISBN 978-981-4774-86-4 (Hardcover), 978-1-351-04190-4 (eBook)
www.panstanford.com

bacteriocins in study is the preclinical assay in murines. However, some of these peptides have surpassed this phase and are currently being tested in humans. Also, it has been proven that these molecules are also promising in other anticancer strategies, such as photodynamic therapy. In conclusion, anticancer peptides show favorable antitumor characteristics and should be further explored in cancer therapies. There are several studies unraveling bacteriocins' modes of action currently taking place, and hopefully more preclinical trials will evolve to human trials.

10.1 Introduction

Microorganisms have been among the most important sources of bioactive compounds, from antibiotics to chemotherapeutic drugs. Bacteriocins are small proteins or ribosomally synthesized peptides with significant relevance in human health, contributing as probiotics, antimicrobials, and anticancer agents, which are produced by both gram-positive and gram-negative bacteria and by *Archaea* [1, 2]. They are usually classified into peptides that endure significant post-translational modifications (class I) and unmodified peptides (class II), although other classifications have been proposed [3]. These molecules represent a subgroup of the anticancer peptides (ACPs) identified to date. ACPs have been proved to be a resourceful strategy for the molecularly targeted cancer drug discovery and development process. Peptide-based therapy has numerous advantages over small molecules, including high specificity, low production cost, high tumor penetration, and ease of synthesis and modification [4]. ACPs are reported to have efficient tissue penetration and uptake by heterogeneous cancer cells, endowed with intrinsic activity or synergized with existing therapeutics, which is of major relevance for the battle against chemotherapeutic drug resistance.

10.2 Bacteriocins, from Antimicrobial to Anticancer Agents

ACPs are small peptides with lengths reported between 5 and 40 amino acids, a molecular mass less than 10 kDa, and a positive net charge at physiological pH. Structurally, ACPs have either an α-helix (α-ACPs) or a β-sheet (β-ACPs) conformation, but some linear and extended structures have already been reported [5]. It is common to find ACPs rich in Arg, Lys, and Pro, which are hydrophobic amino acids, but His and Trp are also likely to be present. Indeed, ACPs rich in Pro, called polyproline peptides, can be classified on the basis of their membrane-internalization predisposition, depending on the specific conformation they adopt, given the amount and spatial disposition of Pro residues [6]. High amphipathicity, positive net charge, small size, and good balance between hydrophobic and polar regions are the overall physical characteristics for the greater part of both anticancer and antimicrobial peptides (AMPs) that are likely to be important for their function. However, there is immense structural diversity yet to be explored [7].

Accordingly, ACPs are often derived from AMPs, which are essentially cationic and hydrophobic in nature [4, 8]. AMPs are produced quite ubiquosly among all living creatures. There are AMPs known to be expressed in bacteria, fungi, plants, and animals, such as arthropods, fish, amphibians, and mammals [9]. ACPs and AMPs obtained either from eukaryotes or from bacteria share some common properties. They normally consist of 5–50 amino acid residues, their overall net charge is positive, they are hydrophobic and/or amphiphilic, and they are usually membrane active [10]. However, in respect to both their activity and structure they can be quite different.

Antimicrobial bacteriocins can be anionic or cationic proteinaceous substances [11] with bactericidal and bacteriolytic effects. However, the cationic bacteriocins represent anticancer proteinaceous molecules derived from prokaryotes that are ribosomally synthesized [12]. Nevertheless, some peptides derived from prokaryotes that are redesigned, modified, and unnaturally synthesized usually continue to be designated as bacteriocins that may justify a reclassification.

These microbial-origin molecules often exhibit higher target specificity and stronger potency, at least 10^2–10^3-fold, over those produced by the eukaryotes [2, 13]. Their physiological functions in bacteria seem to be the inhibition of competitive microorganisms in a specific niche. In fact, the bacteriocin producer strains are usually insensitive to their own bacteriocins. This phenomenon is related to a set of immunity genes present in the same operon on the bacteriocin gene. Indeed, cloning this set of genes in susceptible strains has proved to increase the sensitivity to the bacteriocin in comparison with the parental strain, thus proving their functionality. Additionally, the proteins involved in immunity are also cationic, like the bacteriocins themselves, but are usually bigger [10].

The anticancer potential of bacteriocins was only discovered 70 years after the detection of their antimicrobial action, which was first found almost a century ago [14, 15]. Since then tests have proved that some bacteriocins have exhibited unambiguous cytotoxic effect on different types of human cancer lines. Also *in vivo* studies in murines using natural or synthetic bacteriocins have shown antiproliferation effects in solid tumors whereas exhibiting no deleterious effects in normal tissue. The selectivity of some bacteriocins toward malignant cells can be explained on the basis of the known differences between cancer cells and normal cells.

10.3 ACPs as a Selective Oncolytic Therapy

It has been established that tumor cells are up to 50 times more sensitive to lytic peptides than normal cells [16]. Regarding selectivity, ACPs can be classified into two broad categories. One category contains the group of ACPs (ACP_{AO}) that is active against microbial cells and cancer cells while not being active against healthy mammalian cells. The other one includes ACPs (ACP_{T}) that are cytotoxic for bacteria and mammalian cells [17, 18].

The reason behind ACP_{AO} selectivity is still a controversial topic. However, some conclusions are evident. Cancer and normal mammalian cells have a number of confirmed differences that are considered responsible for this selectivity phenomenon. The most described differences are membrane based, more exclusively regarding membrane net negative charge and abnormal fluidity due to a change in the cholesterol profile that characterizes malignant cells in contrast with healthy mammalian cells [17].

Interactions between ACPs and nonmalignant mammalian cells are not favored due to the zwitterionic effect present in the membranes of these cells that confers an overall neutral nature. On the contrary, neoplastic cells carry a typical negative net charge due to an abnormal expression of anionic molecules, such as phosphatidylserine (PS, in a proportion of 1:10 of total phospholipids in the membrane), O-glycosylated mucins, sialylated gangliosides, and heparin sulfate [5, 18]. In fact, PS is a good indicator of cell neoplastic transformation since it will oddly accumulate in the outer leaflet of the membrane, unbalancing the charge asymmetric profile.

Regarding fluidity, there is evidence suggesting that cholesterol confers protection to nonmalignant cells from the action of α-ACP_{AO} by blocking its access. Indeed, it was found that the presence of lipid rafts rich in cholesterol can be a key factor in differentiating the action and effect of both ACP_{AO} and ACP_T, which can also explain their different effects on diverse cancer cell lines depending on the nature of their lipid raft constitution. In fact, it was shown that certain tumors, like breast and prostate, present a higher content of cholesterol in the cell membranes [19]. In addition, the abundant presence of microvilli in cancer cells has direct relation to their increased surface area in contrast to healthy mammalian cells. It is suggested that this feature can enhance the toxicity and selectivity of ACP_{AO} due to the possibility of its accumulation in higher levels on a bigger cell surface [17].

Consequently, these differences may be key to explain why many AMPs present ACP potential considering that microbial membranes also have a negative net charge and sterols are absent in bacteria [5].

To promote the research, education, and information exchange of bacteriocins with anticancer properties some bioinformatic tools have been developed [20, 21]. The database APD3 (AMP database) and BACTIBASE are two of these free access tools, and so, a complete list of ACPs can be accessed on http://aps.unmc.edu/AP/database/antiC.php and http://bactibase.hammamilab.org/main.php. Also, an ACP prediction algorithm has been incorporated that has been widely used as an *in silico* approach for drug design.

Usually, the algorithm of these drug design tools will give the option for the user to replace more/less hydrophilic amino acids over more/less hydrophobic ones depending on the peptides' original amphipathicity and net charge values [4, 17].

Finally, peptide-based anticancer therapy has garnered tremendous interest in the last decade due to the need for more efficient, easy-to-produce, and antichemoresistance therapy solutions. *In silico* drug design tools have improved tremendously due to this demand and allowed peptide improvement in specific aspects through manipulation of several physical and chemical properties, such as overall net charge, amphipathicity, and peptide length by alteration of point amino acid residues.

A summarizing list of the mainly best described bacteriocins that present anticancer action in the literature is presented in Table 10.1, along with information on selectivity, origin, targets, mode of action, and study progress, respectively, for each ACP.

10.4 Classification of Bacteriocins

The classification of bacteriocins has been revised on several occasions. There is no unanimity regarding the grounds for classification because of numerous existing factors that can be the bases for cataloging these substances, such as the producing strain being gram positive or gram negative, mechanism of destruction, common resistance mechanisms, genetics, chemistry, molecular weight, and method of production. In fact, some investigators consider that large molecules, such as colicins, should not be considered bacteriocins and only peptides should be included in this classification, ending with a bacteriocin list poor in molecules with a gram-negative origin. On the other hand, other investigators defend a distinction between "true bacteriocins," such as colicins, and peptides derived from lactic acid bacteria (LAB) or other gram-positive bacteria, which they consider to be only "bacteriocin-like" [3, 12]. Indeed, there are significant differences between gram-positive and gram-negative bacteriocins.

The standard bacteriocins of gram-negative bacteria are the colicins, which are large toxins 30–70 kDa in molecular mass. In parallel, bacteriocins of gram-positive bacteria are typically small peptides (2–5 kDa in mass), which may be a result of the different envelope building of gram-positive bacteria, consisting mainly of the dense peptidoglycan network that is permeable to peptides but not to proteins. The majority of bacteriocins from gram-positive bacteria are produced as unmodified peptides; however, a different group of these bacteriocins, called lantibiotics, endures post-translational side-chain modifications, resulting in unusual amino acids not known to occur in other peptides or proteins [54].

Table 10.1 Summarized list of bacteriocins, their producers, the cancer cells they affect, their action, and the progress of their study until now

Peptide	Class	Original producer	Cancer cells	Anticancer action	Study progress	Refs.
Bovicin HC5	I	*Streptococcus bovis*HJ50	Human breast and liver carcinoma	Membrane permeabilization	*In vitro* assays were performed on cell lines.	[1]
Cinnamycin	I	*Streptomyces*	Human cervix carcinoma	Membrane reorganization	*In vitro* assays were performed on cell lines.	[22]
Chaxapeptin	I	*Streptomyces leeuwenhoekii*	Human lung carcinoma	Decrease of cellular invasion capacity	*In vitro* assays were performed on cell lines.	[23]
Duramycin	I	*Streptoverticillium cinnamoneus*	Human ovarian and pancreatic cancer	Necrosis	*In vitro* assays were performed on cell lines.	[24]
Nisin A	I	*Lactococcus lactis*	Human skin, neck, head, breast, and liver cancer	Apoptosis and membrane pore formation	*In vitro* assays were performed on cell lines, and *in vivo* tests were performed on mice.	[1, 25, 26]
Nisin Z	I	*Lactococcus lactis*	Human neck and head cancer	Apoptosis	*In vivo* tests were performed on mice.	[26]
Sungsanpin	I	*Streptomyces*	Human lung cells	Cell invasion inhibition	*In vitro* assays were performed on cell lines.	[27]

(*Continued*)

Table 10.1 (*Continued*)

Peptide	Class	Original producer	Cancer cells	Anticancer action	Study progress	Refs.
Warnericin RK	I	*Staphylococcus warneri* RK	Human glioma, prostatic carcinoma, and leukemia	Membranolysis	*In vitro* assays were performed on cell lines.	[28]
KL15	II	*Lactobacillus casei* ATCC 334	Human colon adenocarcinoma	Necrosis	*In vitro* assays were performed on cell lines	[13]
Microcin E492	II	*Klebsiella pneumoniae* RYC492	Human cervix and colon carcinoma, T cell leukemia, and lymphoma	Apoptosis	*In vitro* assays were performed on cell lines, and *in vivo* tests were performed on nude mice.	[29, 30]
Pediocin K2a2-3	II	*Pediococcus acidilactici*	Human cervix and colon adenocarcinoma	NA	*In vitro* assays were performed on cell lines.	[31]
Pediocin CP2	II	*Pediococcus acidilactici*	Human breast and cervix adenocarcinoma and hepatocarcinoma	Apoptosis	*In vitro* assays were performed on cell lines.	[32]
Pep27	II	*Streptococcus pneumoniae*	Human breast adenocarcinoma, gastric cancer, and leukemia	Apoptosis	*In vitro* assays were performed on cell lines.	[33]

Peptide	Class	Original producer	Cancer cells	Anticancer action	Study progress	Refs.
Plantaricin A	II	*Lactobacillus plantarum* C11	Human T-cell leukemia and brain cancer and rat pituitary tumor	Apoptosis and necrosis	*In vitro* assays were performed on cell lines.	[34–37]
Azurin	III	*Pseudomonas aeruginosa*	Multiple human carcinomas	Apoptosis and alterations in cell membrane fluidity	*In vitro* assays were performed in cell lines, and *in vivo* assays were performed in murine models.	[38–42]
Colicin A	III	*Citrobacter freundii and Escherichia coli*	Human breast and colon carcinoma; bone, smooth muscle, and fibroblast sarcoma; and lymphoma	Membrane pore formation; apoptosis	*In vitro* assays were performed on cell lines, and *in vivo* assays were performed in murine models.	[15, 43]
Colicin E3	III	*Escherichia coli*	Human breast, colon, and cervix carcinoma and bone and fibroblastic sarcoma	RNase activity and necrosis	*In vitro* assays were performed on cell lines, and *in vivo* assays were performed in murine models.	[43–47]
Colicin E1	III	*Escherichia coli*	Human breast carcinoma and fibrosarcoma	Membrane pore formation	*In vitro* assays were performed on cell lines.	[43]

(*Continued*)

Table 10.1 (*Continued*)

Peptide	Class	Original producer	Cancer cells	Anticancer action	Study progress	Refs.
Colicin HSC 4	III	*Escherichia coli* HSC 4	Murine L cell fibroblasts	Cell cycle arrest	*In vitro* assays were performed on cell lines.	[44, 48]
Colicin HSC 10	III	*Escherichia coli* HSC 10	Murine L cell fibroblasts	Cell cycle arrest	*In vitro* assays were performed on cell lines.	[44, 48]
Laz	III	*Neisseria meningitidis*	Human breast and brain cancer	NA	*In vitro* assays were performed on cell lines.	[49, 50]
Pyocin P1	III	*Pseudomonas aeruginosa* P1	Murine L cell fibroblasts	Cell cycle arrest	*In vitro* assays were performed on cell lines.	[44, 48]
Pyocin I-4	III	*Pseudomonas aeruginosa*I-4	Murine L cell fibroblasts	Cell cycle arrest	*In vitro* assays were performed on cell lines.	[44, 48]
Pyocin S2	III	*Pseudomonas aeruginosa*	Human hepatocarcinoma and myeloma	NA	*In vitro* assays were performed on cell lines.	[51]
Smegmatocin	III	*Mycobacterium smegmatis*	Human cervix and ovarian carcinoma andrat kidney cancer	NA	*In vitro* assays were performed on cell lines.	[52, 53]
Vibriocin 41-SV	III	*Vibrio cholerae* NIH41	Murine L cell fibroblasts	Cell cycle arrest	*In vitro* assays were performed on cell lines.	[44, 48]
Vibriocin 506	III	*Vibrio eltor* T-506	Murine L cell fibroblasts	Cell cycle arrest	*In vitro* assays were performed on cell lines.	[44, 48]

Perhaps the most commonly used classification is the three-class division, where bacteriocins are grouped on the basis of their structure and physicochemical properties: class I are the lantibiotics and lasso peptides; class II are the heat-stable, unmodified bacteriocins; and class III are the larger, heat-labile bacteriocins [2, 10]. This classification started to be applied only to LAB-produced bacteriocins, although gram-negative bacteriocins, such as colicins, have been classified as class III, creating further confusion [2, 12, 55]. The most used definitions for bacteriocins are only unanimous in the following points: they are proteinaceous substances ribosomally produced by microorganism. Consequently, the objective of this work is to explore bacteriocins that are also ACPs so that class III bacteriocins, which also enclose proteins, will be less explored.

Class I bacteriocins, the lantibiotics, are small (<5 kDa), heat-stable peptides that enclose a high occurrence of post-translational modifications. These peptides contain characteristic polycyclic thioether aminoacids, such as lanthionine and methyllanthionine, and unsaturated aminoacids, such as dehydroalanine and 2-aminoisobutyric acid [54]. Lantibiotics are encoded by the structural genes lanA (the abbreviation lan is used for homologous genes of different lantibiotic gene clusters) and produced as prepeptides consisting of an N-terminal leader peptide and a C-terminal propeptide part. Together with lan genes paraphernalia regarding proteolysis and modification, they form biosynthetic gene clusters with several transcription units that can be located either on the chromosome or on mobile elements such as plasmids or transposons [56].

Due to their different forms and charge lantibiotics can be subdivided into lantibiotics A or B. Nisins (Table 10.1) are typical lantibiotics A, which are more flexible, elongated, and cationic. ACPs' positive net charge is related to targeting cancer cell specifically, given that the net charge of the outer leaflet of cancer cells' membranes is usually negative [18]. In contrast, duramycin and cinnamycin are examples of lantibiotics B, which are globular and have either no net charge or a net negative charge. These bacteriocins are reported to interfere with cellular enzymatic reactions, such as cell wall synthesis [54].

Lasso peptides are also included in this division. What distinguishes lasso peptides from other ribosomally produced peptides is their unique topology. At the most basic structural level, they consist of a macrolactam ring comprised of seven to nine residues and a linear C-terminal peptide tail [57]. The peptides chaxapeptin and sungsanpin are lasso bacteriocins with reported anticancer properties [23, 27].

Class II bacteriocins are heat-stable peptides with a molecular mass usually not higher than 10 kDa. In contrast with lantibiotics, these bacteriocins have no lanthionine content or other post-translational modification beyond the removal of the signal peptide and the formation of a conserved N-terminal disulfide bridge. They have an amphiphilic helical structure, which allows them to enter into the membrane of the target cell, leading to depolarization and necrosis. Indeed, the different biophysical structures that ACPs are reported to assume are crucial for cancer cell membranes' attachment and pore formation [9]. Class II bacteriocins have at least three subclasses (a, b, and c), and most standard class II bacteriocins with anticancer properties are pediocins and plantaricins. However, the growing interest in LAB bacteriocins for therapeutic purposes has required new classifications for emerging bacteriocins. As examples, new peptides such as the template peptides of KL15 have been proposed to be included in a new branch called class IId bacteriocins [10, 13], and other literature also refers to a subclass IIe [3].

Finally, class III bacteriocins include a great amount of gram-negative bacteriocins. This class includes heavy, heat-labile (>20 kDa) proteinaceous molecules. Some of these peptides or proteins are presented in Table 10.1, such as colicins and azurin (from *Pseudomonas aeruginosa*). Although the least employed, a fourth class has been proposed, comprising complex bacteriocins carrying lipid or carbohydrate moieties or circular peptides [55, 58].

10.5 Action against Cancer Cells

There have been continuous difficulties in empirically confirming ACPs' modes of action against malignant cells and the nature of their interactions. As previously shown in Table 10.1, the most frequently registered ACP targets were the malignant cell membranes.

Indeed, some bacteriocins were registered to be able to cause membrane disturbance, inducing in some cases cell necrosis or apoptosis. In addition, many of these peptides have had promising results both *in vitro* and *in vivo*. Regardless of their clinical success, other modes of action are described but not yet completely explained and this information would be vital for drug design purposes [4, 18].

Some bacteriocins' anticancer effect on hematological malignancies have been reported *in vitro* and *in vivo*, such as the effect of plantaricin A, microcins, and pep27 on leukemia and lymphoma cell lines or murine xenografts [30, 33, 34]. However, a large number of studies were performed on solid tumors, in particular *in vitro* tests on carcinoma cell lines of various types. Solid tumors are masses composed of malignant cells *per se* and the stroma surrounding them. In carcinomas a third compartment—the basement membrane—often punctuates the space between the malignant cells and the stroma. The carcinoma cells have also the ability to change the nature of this basement membrane in order to easily invade healthy new tissues [59]. Currently, the most common solid cancers in adults are carcinomas, such as cancer of the colon, breast, lung, and prostate [60]. Indeed, it is estimated that breast and prostate cancers account for, respectively, 23% and 14% of the total new cancer cases in the last decade [61].

These tumor masses may contain heterogeneous populations of cells with variable phenotypes that express aberrant differentiation markers that replicate the tissue of origin, as well as cancer cells that have an undeveloped morphology and do not express these markers [60].

This phenotypic heterogeneity may be another cause for anticancer therapy failure. If only a portion of the malignant cells present in the solid tumor is capable of proliferating indefinitely and invading the organism, then the goal of anticancer therapy should be to specifically target these actively tumorigenic malignant cells in the whole tumor mass [62]. Given that metastases are the principal cause of death for patients with solid tumors, it is not unusual for patients to have a relapse years later, getting distant metastases as a residual number of cancer stem cells persisted after chemotherapy [59, 60]. ACPs may be a solution against tumorigenic untargeted cells due to their high efficiency in killing tumor cells in very low concentration doses (Fig. 10.1).

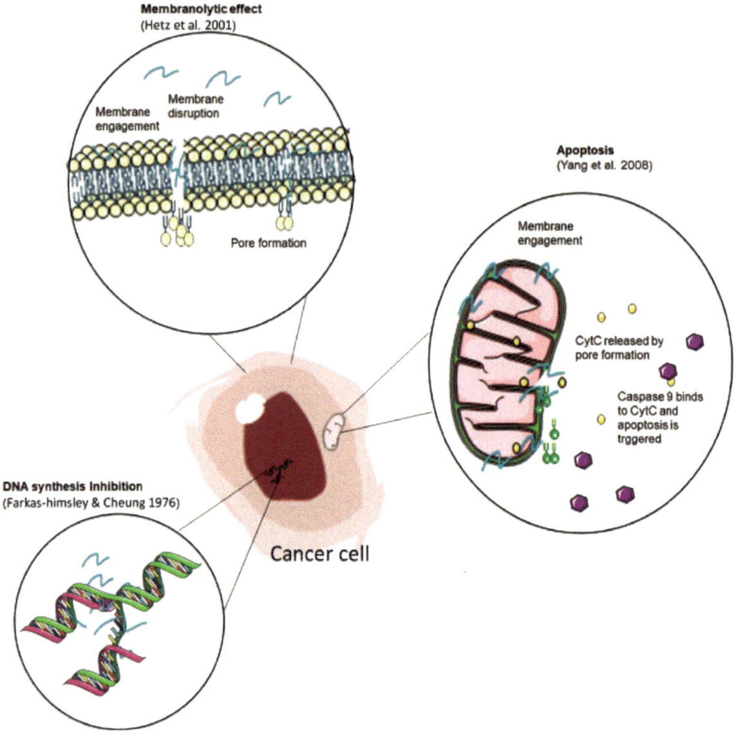

Figure 10.1 The modes of action of anticancer peptides (ACPs) may include disruption of plasma/mitochondrial membranes, necrosis, and apoptosis. **Membranolytic effect:** The peptide targets the membrane components and attaches. This interaction creates pores or completely disrupts the membrane [29]. **Apoptosis:** The mitochondrial membrane can also suffer the lytic effect of these peptides, resulting in the releasing of cytochrome C (CytC), which will be available to bind to caspase-9. This complex triggers the apoptotic intrinsic signaling cascade [29]. **DNA synthesis inhibition:** During DNA replication, some ACPs have the ability of interlacing with the newly synthesized chain, obstructing the whole mechanism [44].

10.5.1 Class I: Lantibiotics and Lasso Peptides

Some evidence of anticancer activity has been described in assays where HeLa cells were treated with cinnamycin. In 2003, a study reported that this globular lantibiotic specifically targeted the phospholipid phosphatidylethanolamine (PE) in these cells, disturbing their membranes [22]. Nevertheless, the anticancer potential of duramycin, another PE-binding globular lantibiotic, has been more exhaustively investigated. Duramycin is a 19-residue peptide produced by *Streptoverticillium cinnamoneus*, and it is one of the very few known small peptides to have a defined and stable 3D structure, being resistant to both thermal and proteolytic degradation [63]. Adding to its antimicrobial potential, duramycin is the object of studies related to antitumor therapies as a solo agent or in conjugation with other drugs or drug-release vehicles [24, 64]. In 2016, in a study executed by Broughton *et al.*, two ovarian cancer cell lines and two pancreatic cancer cell lines were assessed for cell viability by flow cytometry after treatment with a series of duramycin concentrations [24]. Increasing levels of necrosis were observed in all four cell lines in a duramycin concentration–dependent manner. At concentrations as low as 5 μmol/L, cell death was induced in these cell lines and at concentrations above 500 μmol/L, duramycin wielded its highest cytotoxic effect, where around 90% of all cells were necrotic. In the same study, duramycin induced calcium ion (Ca^{2+}) release from the cancer cell lines and confocal microscopy showed duramycin-induced morphological changes, all in a concentration-dependent and time-dependent fashion. These results suggest it is possible that duramycin-induced cell death may be a result of a combination of both loss of intracellular components through membrane pores and membrane destabilization [24].

In 2005, a heat-stable anti-*Alicyclobacilli* substance produced by *Staphylococcus warneri* RB4 was isolated and named warnericin RB4. In the same study, resemblances between warnericin RK and nukacin ISK-1, a lantibiotic, were pointed out, suggesting that warnericin too is a lantibiotic. Soon after, warnericin RK's unique anti-*Legionella* potential was discovered and explored [65, 66]. Later, in 2016, this AMP and its derivates were tested against solid and hematological tumor cells. These peptides showed cytotoxic activity on prostatic tumor, glioma, and leukemia cell lines, the latter being the most sensitive. The results of chemical Raman imaging suggested that the mode of action of the peptide is membrane lysis. Despite apparent warnericin RB4 low cytotoxicity against mononuclear cells, its derivates were even less hemolytic, though maintaining good levels of activity against leukemia cell lines. Consequently, the authors suggest they could be good candidates for leukemia treatment [28].

Nisin is a low-molecular-weight pentacyclic antibacterial peptide produced by *Lactococcus lactis* (Table 10.1). As a lantibiotic, this ACP has uncommon post-translational amino acids, such as lanthionine, methyllanthionine, and didehydroalanine. Although studies on nisin antibacterial potential have been performed since the 1950s, specifically on the basis of oral health and food preservation, its anticancer potential was not documented until 2012 [67, 68]. The work of Joo *et al.* demonstrated *in vitro* and *in vivo* that nisin A is cytotoxic to head and neck squamous cell carcinoma (HNSCC) [69]. In this work, nisin was added in different concentrations to three human HNSCC cell cultures, increasing the levels of DNA fragmentations and apoptosis on the basis of changes in the calcium influx, all in concentrations ranging from 20 to 80 μg/ml. By blocking CHAC1, a cation transporter regulator, apoptosis effect is suppressed, which suggests that nisin's effect against HNSCC cells is mediated by these transporters. Accordingly, the same results were observed *in vivo*. The HNSCC cells were injected into the floor of the mouth in mice, after which nisin was administrated, resulting in a significant reduction in the tumor burden. No adverse effects in mice resulted from nisin administration. Indeed, nisin was already known to be nontoxic toward animals. In 2015, another study from the same team proved that alternative forms of nisin at 95% purity (nisin AP and ZP with point mutations on residue 27) had a superior cytotoxic effect against the same *in vitro* and *in vivo* HNSCC models in comparison with a solution of low-content nisin. In fact, in this study, Nisin ZP increased apoptosis levels *in vitro* in cancer cells and reduced tumorigenesis *in vivo* and long-term treatment with nisin ZP extended survival. In addition, nisin did not seem to be cytotoxic either to nonmalignant oral keratinocytes or to the mice [26]. Indeed, the World Health Organization, in 1969, and the Food and Drug administration (FDA), in 1988, approved the consumption of nisin by humans, saying itis safe. It interacts with lipid II, a membrane-bound precursor involved in cell-wall biosynthesis, and generates pores in the target bacterial cells but not in their host [2, 69].

Also in 2012, in another study, this time performed by Paiva *et al.*, nisin and bovicin HC5, another lantibiotic, proved to be cytotoxic against breast and liver cancer cell lines. The IC_{50} was reached at concentrations near 110 μM and 290 μM for both cell lines after treatment with nisin and bovicin HC5, respectively. At this concentration, shrinkage and vacuolization of the cytoplasm, condensation and lateralization of the nucleus, and detachment of the cell mat were also observed [1].

Synergy between nisin and chemotherapeutic agents has also been explored. In 2015, an animal bioassay was performed on mice with DMBA-induced skin tumors. Nisin and doxorubicin (DOX) reduced the mean tumor burden by 14% and 51.3%, respectively, after four weeks of treatment. However, the combination effect of nisin and DOX was confirmed by a larger reduction in the tumor burden (more than 66%). Synergy in the effect on tumor volumes was also observed where nisin appeared to potentially increase the anticancer therapeutic potential of DOX by approximately one and half times just after four weeks of chemotherapy. Consequently, histological observations suggested that nisin-DOX therapy causes significant chromatin condensation and marginalization of nuclear material in skin cells of treated mice, which validated the increased apoptosis levels also referred to in the study [25].

Finally, the anticancer potential of antimicrobial lasso peptides was also investigated in the last few years. Genome mining has allowed the exploration of sea microbial diversity, leading to the finding of new substances with therapeutic potential. Especially, deep-sea *Streptomyces* are known to produce several compounds of interest, such as antibiotics and antivirals. Sungsanpin is a lasso peptide that is ribosomally synthesized and has an N-terminal eight- or nine-residue ring with a linear C-terminal tail threaded through the ring. This peptide has shown to inhibit lung A549 adenocarcinoma cell invasion by near 50% at a concentration of 50 μM, which inhibits matrix metalloproteinases' (MMPs') degradation of the extracellular matrix [27, 57]. Additionally, a very similar lasso peptide isolated from *Streptomyces leeuwenhoekii*, called chaxapeptin, has shown to reduce A549 cells' invasive capacity by 50% at concentrations near 50 μM [23].

10.5.2 Class II: Microcin, Pediocins, and Plantaricin A

Microcins are produced by *Enterobacteriaceae*, and just like colicins they are secreted under conditions of lack of nutrients compelling antibacterial activity against closely related species. Microcin E492 (Table 10.1), expressed by *Klebsiella pneumoniae* RYC492, was suggested in 2002 by Hetz *et al.*, to exert toxicity against solid and hematological malignant cell lines, such as human cervix adenocarcinoma, T cell leukemia, lymphoma, and colorectal carcinoma cell [29]. The effects appeared to be typical of apoptosis in HeLa cells, although in higher concentrations microcin caused necrosis. Indeed, regulatory apoptosis proteins, such as the Bcl-2 family, are controlled by mitochondrial permeability. ACPs that are able to enter malignant cells and cause membrane pores in the mitochondria trigger the release of its components and liberate Bcl-2. Usually, the recently released cytochrome c forms a complex with caspase-9, initiating a cascade of signals related to apoptosis intrinsic pathway, leading to cell death [17, 70, 71]. In situations where the plasmatic and/or mitochondrial membrane is too disrupted, the necrosis mechanism is triggered. Dual-action ACPs are very valuable, given the fact that apoptosis is a preferred mode of cell death in comparison with necrosis because it is not known to induce an inflammatory response. Also, in this study other effects, including cell shrinkage, DNA fragmentation, and extracellular exposure of PS, were observed in cancer cells treated with microcin E492. Finally, microcin did not appear to be cytotoxic against nonmalignant bone marrow cells and mice [29, 72]. Lastly, there is also registration of antitumoral activity of microcin E492 fibrils administered in a human colorectal carcinoma xenograft in nude mice [30].

Pediocins are heat-stable small molecules considered in the class II bacteriocins category. These molecules are produced by species of the LAB bacteria genera *Pediococcus*, and they are encoded in plasmids. Pediocins PA-1, K2a2-3, and CP2 are produced by different strains of *Pediococcus acidilactici*, which have been reported to have anticancer activity. Tests in human lung A549 and human colon adenocarcinoma cell lines showed viability decrease on treatment with pediocin PA-1 at very low concentrations. Likewise, pediocin K2a2-3, isolated from *Pediococcus acidilactici* K2a2-3, also displayed toxic bioactivity against human colon and cervical adenocarcinoma cell lines, inhibiting these cells by 50%, although no mechanism of action is suggested. Pediocin CP2, produced by *Pediococcus acidilactici* CP2 MTCC5101, decreased viability of human breast, cervical, and liver carcinoma cells as also of murine spleen lymphoblast cell line. And rec-pediocin CP2 decreased cell viability by 100% of the murine spleen lymphoblast cell line. Finally, the authors also described that rec-pediocin caused apoptosis of the cancer cells after 48h of incubation, as studied by the DNA fragmentation method [2, 31, 32].

10.5.3 Class III: Anticancer Proteins

Colicins are AMPs found in *Enterobacteriaceae.* Functionally, these molecules will confer to the producer organism some type of competitive advantage against other *Enterobacteriaceae* strains. Beside the antimicrobial activities colicins are known to have anticancer activities against a selection of human tumor cell lines *in vitro*, such as leukemia, breast cancer, colon cancer, bone cancer, and cervix cancer [15, 45]. Colicins A and E1 have been demonstrated to be cytotoxic against 11 different tumor cell lines with defined mutations of suppressor gene p53, with variations between 17% and 60% depending on the cell line and on the colicin used. Colicin A appeared also to be cytotoxic against the fibroblast normal cell line in contrast with colicin E1, which proved to be less cytotoxic against this normal cell line, giving preliminary confirmation of some type of selectivity. Colicin E1 showed 50% inhibition in fibrosarcoma and breast carcinoma cell lines, with inhibition ranges varying from 15% to 25% depending on the colicin used [43].

Produced by more than 90% of *Pseudomonas aeruginosa* strains, pyocins were first isolated in 1962 [2]. Although proof of pyocins' anticancer potential was first observed 40 years ago, in a more recent study, pyocin S2 was observed to inhibit tumor cell lines whereas both pyocin S2 and partially purified protein were totally nontoxic to the noncancer cell line HFFF [44, 51].

Proteins with anticancer potential, such as smegmatocin and azurin, are also considered bacteriocins [73]. From *Mycobacterium smegmatis*, smegmatocin is not secreted by the bacteria in the culture supernatant. Therefore, to purify smegmatocin, the cells are ultrasonicated to release the bacteriocin in the culture supernatant, just like *Pseudomonas aeruginosa*'s azurin. Both these proteins are proven to have anticancer activity against solid tumors [52, 74].

10.6 Clinical Applications and Patents

Bacteriocins have characteristics of great interest, such as great affinity to some malignant cells, low synthesis cost, and short size, and their usage in conjugation with other drugs or as vehicles for improvement of anticancer technologies has been consequently explored. In fact, there have been significant efforts to innovate on the subject of controlled formulation of new anticancer molecules in combination with nanomedicines.

The 19-residue bacteriocin duramycin has an incredibly stable 3D structure, given the presence of four covalent bridges formed from characteristic amino acids, such as lanthionine. Thus, this peptide presents itself as a unique molecule resistant to proteolysis and heat degradation. In addition, this bacteriocin has high affinity to the phospholipid PE, present in the outer leaflets of cancer cells. Upon binding to PE, duramycin will induce calcium release in cancer cells, more likely by creating pores [24]. Lately, this selective interaction between duramycin and PE has been used in other anticancer strategies. Photodynamic therapy (PDT) is an anticancer approach that takes advantage of photoactive drugs called photosensitizers (PSs). Upon attaching to cancer cells and the emission of light, PSs will generate reactive oxygen species (ROS) and degrade cells [75]. However, one of the main problems of this technique is the lack of specificity of PS molecules to exclusively attach to cancer cells. Thus, a study has shown that conjugation of duramycin and PS ensured the retention of good binding affinity of the conjugate for the target and, following irradiation, reduced cell proliferation of pancreatic and ovarian cancer cell lines [76].

Duramycin's high affinity to PE in cancer cells has also been explored to formulate a new validated biomarker for anticancer treatment response evaluation. Early detection of the treatment response is vital for therapy readjustment and to prevent undesired toxicity. In a study, duramycin was radiolabeled with technetium

(Tc-duramycin) and was proved to be able to image induction of cell death early after chemotherapy and radiotherapy [77].

Consequently, several patents have been proposed to protect duramycin's anticancer potential [78], but this is not the only bacteriocin for which patents have been filed to protect its anticancer activity. US patents to protect the anticancer potential of some apoptogenic bacteriocins, such as microcins, have been filed in July of 2005 [79].

10.7 Future Perspectives of Bacteriocins as Anticancer Agents

ACPs from more distant organisms have several advantages. Problems related to instability in human serum and proteolysis are less associated with bacteriocins in comparison with peptides of eukaryotic origin. In addition, ACPs in general are easy to synthesize and *in silico* improve. Subsequently, ACP drug development is now substantially depending on drug design software's. These bioinformatic tools allow the improvement or *de novo* construction of potential ACPs by predicting their antitumor competence and are expected to have a more powerful significance in the future of peptide optimization. To complement, during the last 30 years, drug delivery has been one of the fields where peptides have caused a high impact, as proven by the design and development of cell penetrating peptides (CPPs), homing peptides, and blood–brain barrier (BBB)-shuttles, among others. Some of these new vectors have even reached clinical trials. Consequently, many groups are dedicated to peptide drug designing for anticancer cancer drug delivery and researching new appealing qualities, such as resistance to protease degradation [6].

Also for the future, the fusion of nanotechnology, materials science, and biotechnology is bringing progress in the medical technologies used for the diagnosis and treatment of cancer, as well as the monitoring of drug delivery. Lipid-based or organometallic nanoconjugations with ACPs clearly represent new options in the management of this critically important disease. For the success of nanoconjugates, further combinations should be studied and further tests are required to access their viability and bioactivity. Most importantly, the long-term safety of nanomaterials for *in vivo* applications should be confirmed. It is also necessary to devise a means of mass producing nanoparticles, as well as optimizing their dose or concentration, flow rate, size of the microfluidic channel reactor, and so forth.

Finally, further studies into the emerging field of ACPs need to be embraced. More *in vitro* studies need to be conducted correlating with the effects reported on numerous cancer cell lines. Understanding the detailed and precise mechanisms of this class of agents and structure-activity relationship will provide a knowledge platform to respond to some unanswered questions about both ACPs and AMPs, which will most possibly allow the design of superior agents. The target and mode of action of these peptides need to be further studied in order for these agents to exert their full therapeutic potentials and perhaps to help us decipher some activities unknown in the present days.

References

1. Paiva A. D., *et al.* Toxicity of bovicin HC5 against mammalian cell lines and the role of cholesterol in bacteriocin activity. *Microbiology*, 158 (2012) 2851–2858.
2. Kaur S., Kaur S. Bacteriocins as potential anticancer agents. *Frontiers in Pharmacology*, 6(272) (2015) 1–11.
3. Cotter P. D., Ross R. P., Hill C. Bacteriocins—a viable alternative to antibiotics? *Nature Reviews Microbiology*, 11(2) (2013) 95–105.
4. Tyagi A., *et al. In silico* models for designing and discovering novel anticancer peptides. *Scientific Reports*, 3 (2013) 1–8.
5. Hoskin D. W., Ramamoorthy A., Studies on anticancer activities of antimicrobial peptides. *Biochimica et Biophysica Acta–Biomembranes*, 1778(2) (2008) 357–375.
6. Sanchez-Navarro M., Teixido M., Giralt E. Jumping hurdles: Peptides able to overcome biological barriers. *Accounts of Chemical Research*, 50 (2017) 1847–1854.
7. Rodrigues E. G., *et al.* Antifungal and antitumor models of bioactive protective peptides. *Anais da Academia Brasileira de Ciencias*, 81(3) (2009) 503–520.

8. Teixeira V., Feio M. J., Bastos M. Role of lipids in the interaction of antimicrobial peptides with membranes. *Progress in Lipid Research*, 51(2) (2012) 149–177.
9. Mader J. S., Hoskin D. W. Cationic antimicrobial peptides as novel cytotoxic agents for cancer treatment. *Expert Opinion on Investigational Drugs*, 15(8) (2006) 933–946.
10. Nes I., Holo H., Class II antimicrobial peptides from lactic acid bacteria. *Peptide Science* 55(1) (2000) 50–61.
11. Kuijk S. Van, Noll K. S., Chikindas M. L., The species-specific mode of action of the antimicrobial peptide subtilosin against Listeria monocytogenes Scott A. *Letters in Applied Microbiology*, 52 (2011) 52–58.
12. Chikindas M. L., *et al.* Functions and emerging applications of bacteriocins. *Current Opinion in Biotechnology*, 49 (2017) 23–28.
13. Chen Y. C., *et al.* Anti-proliferative effect on a colon adenocarcinoma cell line exerted by a membrane disrupting antimicrobial peptide KL15. *Cancer Biology and Therapy*, 16(8) (2015) 1172–1183.
14. Gratia A. *Sur un remarquable exemple d'antagonisme entre deux souches de colibacille. Compt. Rend. Soc. Biol.*, 93 (1925) 1040–1042.
15. Šmarda J., Ovarec C. Cytocidal effect of bacteriocins toward lymphatic cells. *Aktual.Klin.Onkol*, 21 (1989) 209–212.
16. Leuschner C. Targeting breast and prostate cancers through their hormone receptors. *Biology of Reproduction*, 73(5) (2005) 860–865.
17. Harris F., *et al.* On the selectivity and efficacy of defense peptides with respect to cancer cells. *Medicinal Research Reviews*, 29(6) (2011) 1292–1327.
18. Gaspar D., Salomé Veiga A., Castanho M. A. R. B. From antimicrobial to anticancer peptides. A review. *Frontiers in Microbiology*, 4 (2013) 1–16.
19. Li Y. C., *et al.* Elevated levels of cholesterol-rich lipid rafts in cancer cells are correlated with apoptosis sensitivity induced by cholesterol-depleting agents. *The American Journal of Pathology*, 168(4) (2006) 1107–1118.
20. Wang G., Li X., Wang Z. APD2: The updated antimicrobial peptide database and its application in peptide design. *Nucleic Acids Research*, 37 (2009) 933–937.
21. Hammami R., *et al.* BACTIBASE second release: A database and tool platform for bacteriocin characterization. *BMC Microbiology*, 10(22) (2010) 1–5.

22. Makino A., *et al.* Cinnamycin (Ro 09-0198) Promotes cell binding and toxicity by inducing transbilayer lipid movement. *Journal of Biological Chesmistry*, 278(5) (2003) 3204–3209.

23. Elsayed S. S., *et al.* Chaxapeptin, a lasso peptide from extremotolerant *Streptomyces leeuwenhoekii* strain C58 from the hyperarid atacama desert. *Journal of Organic Chemistry*, 80 (2015) 10252–10260.

24. Broughton L. J., Crow C., *et al.* Duramycin-induced calcium release in cancer cells. *Anticancer Drugs*, 27(3) (2016) 173–182.

25. Preet S., *et al.* Effect of nisin and doxorubicin on DMBA-induced skin carcinogenesis—a possible adjunct therapy. *Tumor Biology*, 36(11) (2015) 8301–8308.

26. Kamarajan P., *et al.* Nisin ZP, a bacteriocin and food preservative, inhibits head and neck cancer tumorigenesis and prolongs survival. *PLOS One*, 10(7) (2015) 1–20.

27. Park S., Shin J., Oh D. Sungsanpin, a lasso peptide from a deep-sea streptomycete. *Journal of Naural Products*, 76 (2013) 873–879.

28. Loiseau C., *et al.* Specific anti-leukemic activity of the peptide warnericin RK and analogues and visualization of their effect on cancer cells by chemical raman imaging. *PLOS one*, 11(9) (2016) 1–15.

29. Hetz C., *et al.* Microcin E492, a channel-forming bacteriocin from *Klebsiella pneumoniae*, induces apoptosis in some human cell lines. *Proceedings of the National Academy of Sciences of the United States of America*, 99(5) (2002) 2696–2701.

30. Lagos R., *et al.* Antibacterial and antitumorigenic properties of microcin E492, a pore-forming bacteriocin. *Current Pharmaceutical Biotechnology*, 10 (2009) 74–85.

31. Villarante K. I., *et al.* Purification, characterization and in vitro cytotoxicity of the bacteriocin from Pediococcus acidilactici K2a2-3 against human colon adenocarcinoma (HT29) and human cervical carcinoma (HeLa) cells. *World Journal of Microbiology and Biotechnology*, 27 (2011) 975–980.

32. Kumar B., *et al.* In vitro cytotoxicity of native and rec-pediocin CP2 against cancer cell lines: A comparative study. *Pharmaceutica Analytica Acta*, 3(8) (2012) 1–4.

33. Lee D. G., *et al.* Functional and structural characteristics of anticancer peptide Pep27 analogues. *Cancer Cell International*, 5(21) (2005) 1–14.

34. Zhao H., *et al.* Interaction of the antimicrobial peptide pheromone Plantaricin A with model membranes: Implications for a novel mechanism of action. *Biochimica et Biophysica Acta*, 1758 (2006) 1461–1474.

35. Sand S. L., Haug T. M., *et al.* The bacterial peptide pheromone plantaricin a permeabilizes cancerous, but not normal, rat pituitary cells and differentiates between the outer and inner membrane leaflet. *Journal of Membrane Biology*, 216 (2007) 61–71.

36. Sand S. L., *et al.* Peptides Plantaricin A, a peptide pheromone produced by *Lactobacillus plantarum*, permeabilizes the cell membrane of both normal and cancerous lymphocytes and neuronal cells. *Peptides*, 31 (2010) 1237–1244.

37. Sand S. L., *et al.* Plantaricin A, a cationic peptide produced by *Lactobacillus plantarum*, permeabilizes eukaryotic cell membranes by a mechanism dependent on negative surface charge linked to glycosylated membrane proteins. *Biochimica et Biophysica Acta*, 1828(2) (2013) 249–259.

38. Punj V., *et al.* Bacterial cupredoxin azurin as an inducer of apoptosis and regression in human breast cancer. *Oncogene*, 23(13) (2004) 2367–2378.

39. Yamada T., *et al.* A peptide fragment of azurin induces a p53-mediated cell cycle arrest in human breast cancer cells. *Molecular Cancer Therapeutics*, 8(10) (2009) 2947–2958.

40. Ramachandran S., Mandal M. Induction of apoptosis of azurin synthesized from *P. aeruginosa* MTCC 2453 against Dalton's lymphoma ascites model. *Biomedicine et Pharmacotherapy*, 65(7) (2011) 461–466.

41. Bernardes N., *et al.* The bacterial protein azurin impairs invasion and FAK/Src signaling in P-cadherin-overexpressing breast cancer cell models. *PLOS One*, 8(7) (2013) e69023.

42. Bernardes N., *et al.* Modulation of membrane properties of lung cancer cells by azurin enhances the sensitivity to EGFR-targeted therapy and decreased β1 integrin-mediated adhesion. *Cell Cycle*, 15(11) (2016) 1415–1424.

43. Chumchalová J., Smarda J. Human tumor cells are selectively inhibited by colicins. *Folia Microbiologica*, 48(1) (2003) 111–115.

44. Farkas-Himsley H., Cheung R. Bacterial proteinaceous products (bacteriocins) as cytotoxic agents of Neoplasia1. *Cancer Research*, 36 (1976) 3561–3567.

45. Šmarda J., *et al.* The cytotoxic and cytocidal effect of colicin E3 on mammalian tissue cells. *Folia Microbiologica*, 23 (1978) 272–277.

46. Fuska J. Effect of colicin E3 on leukemia cells P 388 in vitro. *Experientia*, 1 (1978) 406–407.

47. Smarda J., Fialová, M., Smarda J. Cytotoxic effects of colicins E1 and E3 on v-myb-transformed chicken monoblasts. *Folia Biologica*, 47 (2001) 11–13.

48. Picker D. H., Serino A. J., Henson G. W. Bacteriocin-targeted compunds for cancer therapy. (1987) (EP 0213811 A2).

49. Hong C. S., *et al.* Disrupting the entry barrier and attacking brain tumors: The role of the *Neisseria* lipobox-containing H.8 epitope and the laz protein chang. *Cell Cycle*, 5(15) (2006) 1633–1641.

50. Hong C., *et al.* Transport agents for crossing the blood-brain barrier and into brain cancer cells, and methods of use thereof. (2010) (US Patent No. 7,807,183, 2010.).

51. Abdi-Ali A., Worobec E. A., *et al.* Cytotoxic effects of pyocin S2 produced by *Pseudomonas aeruginosa* on the growth of three human cell lines. *Canadian Journal of Microbiology*, 50 (2004) 375–381.

52. Saito H., Watanabe T. A., Tomioka H. Purification, properties, and cytotoxic effect of a bacteriocin from mycobacterium smegmatis. *Antimicrobial Agents and Chemotherapy*, 15(4) (1979) 504–509.

53. Saito H., Watanabe T. Effect of a bacteriocin produced by mycobacterium smegmatis on growth of cultured tumor and normal cells. *Cancer Research*, 39 (1979) 5114–5117.

54. Guder A., Wiedemann I., Sahl H. Posttranslationally modified bacteriocins—the lantibiotics. *Biopolymers*, 55(1) (2000) 62–73.

55. Gillor O., Etzion A., Riley M. A. The dual role of bacteriocins as anti- and probiotics. *Applied Microbiology and Biotechnology*, 81(4) (2009) 591–606.

56. Jack R. W., Bierbaum G. *Lantibiotics and Related Peptides*, (1998) Springer-Verlag Berlin Heidelberg GmbH.

57. Hegemann J. D., *et al.* Lasso peptides: An intriguing class of bacterial natural products. *Accounts of Chemical Research*, 48(7) (2015) 1909–1919.

58. Gabrielsen C., *et al.* Circular bacteriocins: Biosynthesis and mode of action. *Applied and Environmental Microbiology*, 80(22) (2014) 6854–6862.

59. Liotta, L. A. Tumor invasion and metastases: Role of the basement membrane. *American Journal of Pathology*, 117(3) (1984) 339–348.

60. Al-Hajj M., Clarke M. F. Self-renewal and solid tumor stem cells. *Oncogene*, 23 (2004) 7274–7282.

61. Ferlay J., *et al.* Cancer incidence and mortality patterns in Europe: Estimates for 40 countries in 2012. *European Journal of Cancer*, 49(6) (2013) 1374–1403.

62. Tannishtha R., *et al.* Stem cells, cancer, and cancer stem cells. *Nature*, 414 (2001) 105–111.

63. Huo L., *et al.* Insights into the biosynthesis of duramycin. *Applied and Environmental Microbiology*, 83(3) (2017) 1–12.

64. Steiner I., *et al.* Pulmonary pharmacokinetics and safety of nebulized duramycin in healthy male volunteers. *Naunyn-Schmiedeberg's Arch Pharmacol*, 378 (2008) 323–333.

65. Minamikawa M., *et al.* Purification and characterization of warnericin RB4, anti-alicyclobacillus bacteriocin, produced by *Staphylococcus warneri* RB4. *Current Microbiology*, 51 (2005) 22–26.

66. Verdon J., *et al.* Characterization of anti-*Legionella* activity of warnericin RK and delta-lysin I from *Staphylococcus warneri. Peptides*, 29 (2008) 978–984.

67. Delves-Broughton J. Nisin and its application as a food preservative. *Journal of the Society of Dairy Technology*, 43(3) (1990) 73–76.

68. Shin J. M., *et al.* Biomedical applications of nisin. *Journal of Applied Microbiology*, 120 (2015) 1449–1465.

69. Joo N. E., *et al.* Nisin, an apoptogenic bacteriocin and food preservative, attenuates HNSCC tumorigenesis via CHAC1. *Cancer Medicine*, 1(3) (2012) 295–305.

70. Huang Z. Bcl-2 family proteins as targets for anticancer drug design. *Oncogene*, 19(56) (2000) 6627–6631.

71. Ausbacher D., *et al.* Anticancer mechanisms of action of two small amphipathic β 2,2-amino acid derivatives derived from antimicrobial peptides. *Biochimica et Biophysica Acta-Biomembranes*, 1818(11) (2012) 2917–2925.

72. Xu H., *et al.* Dual modes of antitumor action of an amphiphilic peptide A9K. *Biomaterials*, 34(11) (2013) 2731–2737.

73. Nguyen C., Nguyen V. D., Discovery of azurin-like anticancer bacteriocins from human gut microbiome through homology modeling and molecular docking against the tumor suppressor p53. *BioMed Research International*, 2016 (2016) 1–12.

74. Fialho A. M., Bernardes N., Chakrabarty A. Exploring the anticancer potential of the bacterial protein azurin. *AIMS Microbiology*, 2(3) (2016) 292–303.

75. Ferreira D. P., *et al.* Characterization of a squaraine/chitosan system for photodynamic therapy of cancer. *Journal of Physical Chemistry B*, 120(7) (2016) 1212–1220.

76. Broughton L. J., Giuntini F., *et al.* Duramycin-porphyrin conjugates for targeting of tumour cells using photodynamic therapy. *Journal of Photochemistry & Photobiology, B: Biology*, 163 (2016) 374–384.

77. Elvas F., *et al.* Early prediction of tumor response to treatment: Preclinical validation of 99mTc-duramycin. *Journal of Nuclear Medicine*, 57(5) (2016) 805–812.

78. Thorpe P., Ran S., Huang X. Selected antibodies and duramycin peptides binding to anionic phospholipids and aminophospholipids and their use in treating viral infections and cancer. (2003) 1–4 (WO 2004006847 A2).

79. Soto C., Lagos R. Apoptogenic-bacteriocins combining broad spectrum antibiotic and selective anti-tumoral activities, and compositions and uses thereof. (2005) 1–31 (US 2005/0159349 A1).

Chapter 11

Bacteriocins as Anticancer Peptides: A Biophysical Approach

Filipa D. Oliveira, Miguel A.R.B. Castanho, and Diana Gaspar

Instituto de Medicina Molecular, Faculdade de Medicina, Universidade de Lisboa, Av. Prof. Egas Moniz, 1649-028 Lisbon, Portugal

dianagaspar@medicina.ulisboa.pt

Cancer remains a class of diseases with a significant detrimental impact on society. Even though many cancer patients survive, new therapies are essential for increasing survival rate and improving their life quality. Anticancer peptides (ACPs) have appealing features for industrial drug development. However, few molecules have reached clinical studies. Several disadvantages related mainly to selectivity and high production costs account for this low success rate of clinical approvals. Researchers thus seek to develop new tools that allow a better understanding of ACPs' mechanisms of action and how these mechanisms can be related to their structure to feed the pharmaceutical pipelines

Microbial Infections and Cancer Therapy: Recent Advances
Edited by Ananda M. Chakrabarty and Arsénio M. Fialho

ISBN 978-981-4774-86-4 (Hardcover), 978-1-351-04190-4 (eBook)
www.panstanford.com

with better alternatives. Peptides produced by bacteria represent an interesting pool of molecules that should be explored as a source of anticancer agents or as templates for new molecules. In this chapter, we will review different biophysical studies performed with bacteriocins and also reveal their importance in the process of developing an effective and selective ACP.

11.1 Introduction

Cancer is a group of diseases characterized by the uncontrolled growth and spreading of abnormal cells [1, 2]. As a major cause of death worldwide, there are several factors that may influence the development of a cancer and they can be generally classified as intrinsic genetic mutations or environmentally induced mutations [1, 3]. The fact that cancer cells exhibit characteristics such as replicative immortality and the ability to escape immunosurveillance and invade distant or surrounding tissues and organs immediately reveals the challenging effort that cancer treatment requires [4, 5]. Conventional therapies for cancer treatment include chemotherapy, radiotherapy, and surgery. Despite the ability of transforming many malignancies into chronic diseases and consequently extending the life expectancy of patients, these therapeutic strategies are often associated with a broad spectrum of severe side effects and development of resistance mechanisms [2, 4, 6, 7]. Radiotherapy requires the use of large doses of radiation, which may lead to injuries in healthy tissues since the radiosensitivity of the neoplasm is often similar to that observed in healthy tissues [8]. Moreover, radiotherapy-induced changes in the tumor microenvironment (TME) associated with hypoxia, fibrotic responses, and immune activation may grant initial resistance to the treatment and eventually promote tumor invasion and spread, as already suggested by preclinical studies in some tumor models [9]. Chemotherapeutical drugs used to treat cancer, such as DNA alkylating agents, hormone agonists, and antagonists and antimetabolites, are designed to attack cancer cells on the basis of the fact that these are rapidly dividing cells [2]. As a consequence, chemotherapeutic drugs will also act on normal cells with an increased dividing rate, such as cells from the bone marrow, the gastrointestinal (GI) tract, and hair follicles, explaining why secondary effects usually include decreased production of blood cells, inflammation of the GI tract, and hair loss [2, 10]. Additionally, tumor cells with slower doubling times or in a growth-arrested state are less susceptible to conventional chemotherapeutic drugs [6, 11]. Together with this lack of selectivity, chemotherapy is also associated with the development of resistance events, since cancer cells may adopt several mechanisms that confer them multiple drug resistance (MDR) [2, 12]. These mechanisms include the activation of detoxification mechanisms and transport proteins for drug efflux, alterations in the drug-target interaction, and alteration of different factors that influence the cellular response, affecting cell survival [12].

All shortfalls and drawbacks of current therapies make it urgent to create and develop new treatment options that will decrease the economic burden of oncological treatments and improve patients' life. In this context, the use of bioactive peptides as templates in drug design has been regarded as an innovative and resourceful approach for anticancer drug development. These peptides show low toxicity, low molecular weight, high bioavailability, strong specificity, tumor-penetrating ability, small size, easy manufacturing, and low-cost production [5, 13, 14]. Consequently, the research on anticancer peptides (ACPs) is a very active field [14], with studies on structure-activity relationship (SAR) as well as on cytotoxic activities and mechanisms of action being regularly revealed to the scientific community [15–18]. From all the possible natural sources of peptides, bacteria stand out as a promising one. The human microbiome can be considered a reservoir of novel molecules that may constitute a new line of investigation for the development of new ACPs [19], and therefore in this chapter we will discuss and briefly review peptides obtained from bacterial sources studied in an anticancer drug development perspective as well as the contribution of several biophysical techniques to the characterization of these peptides' mode of action.

11.2 Antimicrobial Peptides with Anticancer Activity: An Innovative Anticancer Treatment

The discovery of peptides in the lymph of insects and granules of human neutrophils and on the skin of frogs with the ability of killing bacteria in culture [20, 21] led to the identification of a new class of antimicrobial agents, the antimicrobial peptides (AMPs), a form of defense against microbial infections or competing microorganisms [22, 23]. These peptides are usually small molecules, with 11 to 50 amino acid residues, which adopt an amphipathic conformation since they present a hydrophilic face with polar and positively charged amino acid residues and a hydrophobic face containing nonpolar amino acid residues' sidechains [20, 23]. AMPs have also a positive net charge conferred by the high level of arginine (Arg) and lysine (Lys) residues in their structure [20, 23]. AMPs' action toward bacteria relies on the electrostatic interaction between the positively charged peptides and the membrane of bacteria, which exhibits an overall negative charge [20, 24]. Following electrostatic interaction, AMPs can act on the bacterial membrane, causing membrane disruption, integrity loss, and bacterial death, or they may cross the membrane and act on intracellular targets [24]. The advantage of this peculiar mode of action relies on the short timeframe of interaction, which culminates in the microbe's rapid death and naturally reduces the probability of resistance development [25].

Similarly to the bacterial membrane, a cancer cell's membrane is endowed with an overall negative surface charge due to high levels of anionic molecules, such as phosphatidylserine (PS), O-glycosylated mucins, sialylated gangliosides, and heparan sulfate [2, 26–28] (Fig. 11.1). This common feature of bacterial and cancer cells' membranes led to the question of whether AMPs were also able to affect cancer cells' viability and whether they could be classified as ACPs.

The additional activity toward cancer cells of several natural and synthetic AMPs can vary in terms of selectivity for this type of cells, and this is a topic revised in the literature [1, 2, 4, 29–31]. Although the exact mechanisms of specificity toward cancer cells have not been described in detail, there are many factors influencing the selective behavior of ACPs, and these have been associated with differences between cancer and healthy cells' membrane surface [22]. In addition to the overall negative surface charge, cancer cells exhibit an increased surface area when compared to normal cells due to an elevated number of microvilli (small projections of the cell membrane), which appear also more irregular in size and shape [1, 32, 33]. The high number of microvilli contributes to an increase in the number of ACP molecules interacting with the cell membrane, while the irregularities in their size and shape can influence the access to receptors, cell adhesion, and cell-to-cell and TME communication [1]. Moreover, cancer cells have an increased membrane fluidity when compared to normal cells, which promotes membrane destabilization by the ACPs, enhancing their lytic activity on this type of cell [1, 34, 35]. Peptides' selectivity toward cancer cells results also from typical features observed on normal cells. The membrane of normal mammalian cells exhibits an overall neutral charge due to the presence of zwitterionic phospholipids, such as phosphatidylethanolamine (PE), phosphatidylcholine (PC), and sphingomyelin (SM) [1, 2, 24, 36]. A normal mammalian cell's membrane has a typical asymmetry characterized by the exclusive presence of PS in the inner leaflet of the membrane [36, 37]. Since PS exposure on the outer leaflet of the cell membrane may be associated with its recognition by phagocytes, the maintenance of this asymmetry is a homeostatic process that contributes to the differentiation between cancer and normal cells [37]. A healthy cell's membrane also has high levels of cholesterol, which may alter membrane fluidity and hamper membrane insertion of lytic peptides, protecting these cells from cytolytic effects [2, 27]. Interestingly, there is also evidence of tumors with higher levels of cholesterol in the cell's membrane, such as breast and prostate, which confers them an additional resistance to ACPs lytic activity [2, 34, 38].

The use of peptides in anticancer therapy has many pharmaceutical advantages, such as low toxicity and strong specificity. ACPs that are not directed to extracellular/intracellular receptors can be associated with the impairment of resistance development [39, 40], while peptides able to recognize and bind to specific proteins and receptors on the cancer cells' membranes can further contribute to surpass the low tissue penetration and cellular uptake, typical for other molecules used in anticancer therapy, increasing tumor penetrating ability and selectivity [4, 5, 14, 15]. On the negative side, the low selectivity observed in many cases, low proteolytic resistance, poor stability, and high cost of production on a large scale limit the application of these peptides in oncology [41, 42]. Many strategies have been designed to overcome these limitations [2], including the conjugation of peptides with chemotherapeutic drugs [43].

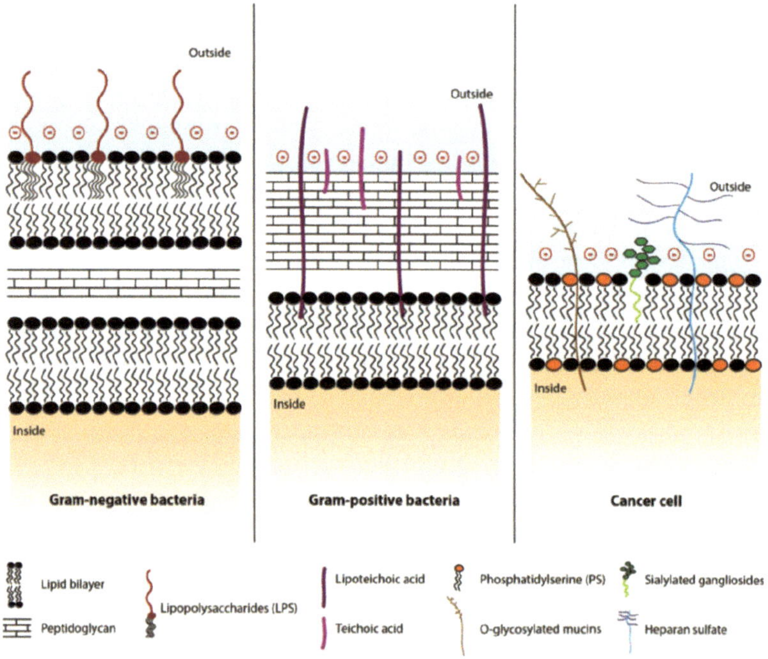

Figure 11.1 Schematic view of bacterial and cancer cell membranes. The negative surface charge of bacterial membranes is a characteristic shared by the cancer cells, leading to the hypothesis that AMPs and ACPs might share molecular principles for selectivity and activity.

11.3 Bacteria as a Source of Anticancer Peptides: Bacteriocins

The human microbiome contains trillions of eukaryotes, archaea, bacteria, and viruses [19]. The relationship between the human microbiome and health or disease is currently a subject of interest and has been reviewed in the literature [19, 44, 45]. With a remarkable metabolic capacity, the human microbiome has been mentioned as the "second liver," and several pieces of evidence point to its influence on human health and disease [44, 46]. A practical example is the fact that changes in our microbiome can contribute to the propagation of deadly microorganisms, such as *Clostridium difficile* and methicillin-resistant *Staphylococcus aureus* [47, 48]. This effect is not surprising since one of the main roles of an intact microbiome is to prevent invasions by pathogenic microorganisms [49]. The microbiome has influence on other diseases, such as cancer, from its prevention, in the earliest stages, to the response to chemotherapy, in the later stages [44]. However, the application of antibiotics in oncology needs deep examination and understanding of the benefits and disadvantages that are included in this practice. The use of antibiotics as chemotherapeutic agents or adjuvants in the clinic would aggravate the development of antibiotic-resistant bacterial strains and also destroy part of the commensal bacteria responsible for promoting homeostasis and protection from carcinogenesis [44]. In fact, eradication of *Helicobacter pylori* in western countries led to a decrease in gastric cancer but an increase in esophageal cancer [44, 49]. It is believed that these bacteria can alter acid reflux in the stomach, inducing protection against Barrett's esophagus and esophageal cancer [44, 49]. Also, commensal microbes from the intestinal tract make a major contribution toward estrogen metabolism and it is known that high levels of this hormone constitute a risk factor for the development of endometrial and breast cancer [50]. The microbiome also influences pharmaceutical agents' metabolism, including the ones used in cancer treatment [50, 51]. Additionally, a link between a chemotherapeutic drug and specific microbiome metabolic activities from the gut has been established [50, 52].

Bacteriocins are AMPs produced by several types of bacteria, synthesized at the ribosome level [22, 53]. In 1925 Gratia identified the first bacteriocin from *Escherichia coli*, colicin [54]. After this discovery, several other bacteriocins from different bacterial strains have been identified, such as nisin, plantaricin A (PlnA), bovicin, and smegmatocin [22]. Within bacteria, these peptides' physiological function consists in inhibiting the development of competing microorganisms by destroying them, without any effect on the producer bacteria [22, 55, 56]. Bacteriocins are generally cationic, exhibit an amphipathic character due to the presence of high levels of Arg and Lys amino acid residues, and have a low molecular weight, typically below 10kDa [57–59]. Since the GI tract contains proteolytic enzymes with the ability to easily degrade bacteriocins, these peptides are considered safe for human consumption [59]. Bacteriocins' classification has been discussed over time [22], and in 2015, Kaur and Kaur reviewed a classification based on structural and physicochemical properties, considering three different classes of bacteriocins [59].

Class I bacteriocins, known as lantibiotics or lanthionine-containing antibiotics, are small and low-weighted peptides, usually less than 5 kDa, and have 19 to 38 amino acid residues [22, 56]. These peptides are heat stable and exhibit post-translation modifications, such as the substitution of D-alanine for L-serine amino acid residues [22, 56]. They also contain polycyclic thioether amino acids, such as lanthionine and β-methyllanthionine, which promote the formation of disulfide bonds between amino acid residues, resulting in internal "rings" that confer lantibiotics their unique structure with specific features [22, 56]. Lantibiotics also contain unsaturated amino acids, namely dehydroalanine and 2-aminoisobutyric acid [22, 56]. This complex structure limits a subdivision of the class of lantibiotics, and there are several different proposed subclassifications [56, 60, 61]. A subclassification is based on peptide charge, structure, and target. Type A lantibiotics, such as nisin and lacticin 3147, are screw shaped, elongated, and flexible and exhibit a positive net charge [22, 56]. Such lantibiotics act on the cell membrane, inducing pore formation and leading to the depolarization of the cytoplasmic membrane [22]. Type B lantibiotics exhibit either a neutral or a negative net charge and a globular shape. These lantibiotics' action consists in disturbing enzymatic reactions occurring within the target cell, interfering with cell wall synthesis, for example [22]. Mersacidin is representative of type B lantibiotics [61].

Class II bacteriocins are the most common bacteriocins without lanthionine in their structure, and they are also heat stable and small, usually less than 10 kDa [22, 56]. Contrary to what is described for lantibiotics, these peptides are not extensively modified after translation, and in this case post-translation modifications simply include the removal of the leader peptide and the formation of a conserved disulfide bridge in the N-terminus [22, 56]. These bacteriocins display an amphiphilic helical structure, and their activity is mainly due to the ability to induce membrane permeabilization, leading to depolarization of this structure and the death of the target cell [22, 56]. Since this is a very heterogeneous class, various systems have been proposed to subdivide the class II bacteriocins [55, 56, 59, 62, 63]. Bacteriocins from the subclass IIa or pediocin-like bacteriocins are monomeric and exhibit a highly specific activity toward *Listeria monocytogenes*, a food pathogen. These bacteriocins, such as pediocin PA-1 and sakacin A, usually consist of a sequence with 37 to 48 amino acid residues and one or two disulfide bridges [56]. This subclass exhibits a consensus sequence, located in the N-terminus, which may be responsible for promoting nonspecific binding to the surface of the target cell [22, 56, 64, 65]. Despite the absence of a well-described physical interaction between a subclass IIa bacteriocin and the mannose permease, there is evidence pointing to the fact that this could be a receptor of this bacteriocins' subclass [56]. Subclass IIb bacteriocins, such as lactacin F and lactococcin G, are composed of two peptides working synergistically to produce an antimicrobial effect [22]. This bacteriocins' mode of action consists in the dissipation of the membrane potential, leading to the loss of ions and a decrease of the intracellular concentrations of ATP [56]. Subclass IIc, also known as class V, contains the cyclic bacteriocins, and few bacteriocins from this class have been identified [22, 56]. Gassericin A, circularin A, and carnocyclin A are three examples of subclass IIc [22]. The structure of these peptides exhibits two transmembrane segments with the ability to enhance pore formation on the target cells [22, 66].

Class III bacteriocins can also be referred to as bacteriolysins, and they are large and heat-labile proteins, with high molecular weights, often above 30 kDa [22, 56]. Their structure is organized by domains, each one associated with functions such as translocation, receptor binding, and lethal activity [56]. These bacteriocins may have a different action mechanism when compared to the other subclasses since their action includes the lysis of target cells through the catalysis of the cell wall's hydrolysis [56]. Klebicin, helveticin I, enterolysin, and some colicins and megacins are examples of subclass III bacteriocins [22].

Several bacteriocins from all the three aforementioned classes have shown selective activity toward cancer cells [22, 67–70]. Despite being a promising feature of these peptides, this additional activity is not surprising since bacteriocins are AMPs and the interplay between AMPs and ACPs has already been debated in the literature [1, 2]. Since bacteriocins are generally cationic peptides, they will preferentially interact with the negatively charged cancer cell's membrane, while interaction with the normal cell's membrane is not favored because of the overall neutral charge and different membrane components [1, 2, 22, 26]. As the interest in the clinical application of peptides keeps rising, the exploitation of bacteriocins as templates for anticancer agents has also been a focus of research [22]. The selective activity against cancer cells of several bacteriocins has been recently revised [22], and a summary of bacteriocins with cytotoxic and/or antiproliferative activity is shown in Table 11.1.

Table 11.1 Bacteriocins with anticancer and/or antiproliferative activities against different cell lines

Bacteriocins	Producer organism	Cell lines	Refs.
Nisin	*Lactococcus lactis*	MCF-7, HepG2, Jurkat, HT29, Caco-2, UM-SCC-17B, UM-SCC-14A, and HSC-3 cells	[67, 71–73]
Nisin ZP	Synthetic high content form of nisin Z from *Lactococcus lactis*	UM-SCC-17B, UM-SCC-14A, HSC-3, and OSCC-3	[74]
Bovicin HC5	*Streptococcus bovis* HC5	MCF-7 and HepG2	[67]
Azurin	*Pseudomonas aeruginosa*	MCF-7, MDA-MB-157, MDD2, MDA-MB-231, UISO-Mel-2, UISO-Mel-6, U2OS, and MG63	[75–78]
p28	*Pseudomonas aeruginosa* (synthetic derivative)	MCF-7, MDA-MB-231, ZR-75-1, UISO-Mel-2, UISO-Mel-23, UISO-Mel-29, LNCaP, DU145, IMR-32, SK-N-BE2, U87, and LN229	[79–81]

Bacteriocins	Producer organism	Cell lines	Refs.
Pediocin-PA1	*Pediococcus acidilactici* PAC1.0	A-549 and DLD-1	[22]
Pediocin K2a2-3	*Pediococcus acidilactici* K2a2-3	HeLa and HT29	[68]
Pediocin CP2	*Pediococcus acidilactici*	HeLa, MCF-7, and HepG2	[82]
Colicin A	*Escherichia coli*	MCF-7, ZR75, BT549, BT474, MDA-MB-231, SKBR3, T47D, HT29, HOS, SKUT-1, and HS913T	[69]
Colicin E1	*Escherichia coli*	MCF-7, ZR75, BT549, BT474, MDA-MB-231, SKBR3, T47D, HOS, SKUT-1, and HS913T	[69]
Colicin E3	*Escherichia coli*	P388 and HeLa	[83, 84]
Colicin U	*Shigella boydii*	HS913T	[69]
Microcin E492	*Klebsiella pneumoniae*	HeLa, Jurkat, Ramos, and RJ2.25	[70]
Pyocin S2	*Pseudomonas aeruginosa* 42A	XC, TSV-5, HepG2, Im9, HeLa-S3, AS-II, and mKS-A TU-7	[85, 86]
Smegmatocin	*Mycobacterium smegmatis* 14468	HeLa-S3, mKS-A TU-7, AS-II, HGC-27, XC, TSV-5, and 155-4 T2	[87, 88]
Plantaricin A	*Lactobacillus plantarum* C11	Jurkat, GH_4C_1, Reh, PC12, and N2A	[89–92]
Duramycin	*Streptoverticillium* sp.	CFPAC-1, $ASPC_1$, MIA PaCa-2, and Colo320	[93]
Halocin H6	*Haloferaxgibbonsii* SH7	Jurkat E6-1	[94]
m2163 m2386	*Lactobacillus casei* ATCC 334	SW480, Caco-2, and BFTC 905	[95]
KL15	*Lactobacillus casei ATCC* 334 (synthetic derivative)	SW480 and Caco-2	[96]

11.4 Biophysical Techniques: A Key to Unravelling Bacteriocins' Modes of Action

Despite all the information brought to light on what concerns peptide-based therapeutics, it is still a challenge to design a selective and effective ACP. SAR studies point to the importance of several biophysical properties, such as the peptides' secondary structure, overall net charge, size and balance between hydrophobic and polar region, and even hydrophobicity and amphipathicity, for determining their ability to permeabilize cellular membranes [97, 98]. Cellular and molecular targets, mechanisms of action, and possible collateral damages within human physiology must be investigated with molecular detail during the drug development process [4]. By understanding the molecular mechanism(s) supporting the mode of action of anticancer drugs it is possible to obtain information that may be used to develop new and innovative strategies for cancer treatment [4, 99]. In this field, biophysical techniques are a powerful tool to characterize a peptide's structure and expected activity, to unravel its mode of action in the target cells, and to understand selectivity requirements. Circular dichroism (CD), fluorescence, and nuclear magnetic resonance (NMR) are examples of biophysical spectroscopies that inform us on the secondary structure, membrane interaction, and 3D structure of the peptides, respectively [100, 101]. Other techniques, such as atomic force microscopy (AFM), light scattering, and flow cytometry, have been used to determine the effects and mode(s) of action of several peptides against cancer and normal cells [15–17, 69, 81, 101–103]. The increasing application of biophysical methodologies to the study of molecular events on bacteria and cancer cells has allowed the important development of knowledge about a cell's biophysics, which without a doubt will positively influence the clinical application of bacteriocins in cancer treatment. A summary of several biophysical techniques applied in the study of different bacteriocins is presented in Fig. 11.2 and Table 11.2.

Table 11.2 Biophysical techniques used for the study of the effect of bacteriocins in several cell lines

Technique	Bacteriocin	Producer bacteria	Cell lines	Short description	Refs.
MTT assay (cell viability), **UV-Vis. absorbance spectroscopy** (hemoglobin release assay), and **fluorescence spectroscopy** (carboxyfluorescein leakage)	Bovicin HC5	*Streptococcus bovis*	Vero, MCF-7, and HepG2	A parallel study with bovicin HC5 and nisin revealed that these bacteriocins induced a concentration-dependent decrease in cell viability. Both bacteriocins exhibited low hemolytic activity. The presence of cholesterol in liposomes didn't alter the rate of carboxyfluorescein (CF) release induced by bovicin HC5.	[67]
Fluorescence spectroscopy (carboxyfluorescein leakage, effect on lipid dynamics through Ie/Im, lipid-induced Trp fluorescence alteration, quenching of Trp emission by acrylamide or brominated PC, and light scattering), and **fluorescence/ confocal microscopy** (intracellular caspase-3 activity, morphology and viability, and amyloid fiber formation)	Plantaricin A-26L	*Lactobacillus plantarum* C11	Jurkat	CF release from liposomes induced by PlnA depends on vesicles' lipid composition. Cell viability decreased significantly in the presence of PlnA, in a concentration- and temperature-dependent manner. PlnA induced cancer cell death by necrosis and apoptosis, leading to nuclear fragmentation and plasma membrane blebbing. Caspase-3 activity was enhanced in the presence of PlnA. Amyloid-like fibers were observed after the binding between PlnA with membranes with negatively charged phospholipids.	[92]
Flow cytometry (cytotoxicity, loss of mitochondrial membrane potential, and PS exposure), **confocal microscopy** (lactate	Microcin E492	*Klebsiella pneumoniae* RYC492	HeLa, KG-1, RJ2,25, Jurkat, Ramos, and AMG-3	HeLa, RJ2.25, and Jurkat cells were sensitive to microcin E492 in different degrees. The cytotoxic effect of the bacteriocin was characterized on HeLa cells. Flow cytometry revealed cell shrinkage	

(*Continued*)

Table 11.2 (*Continued*)

Technique	Bacteriocin	Producer bacteria	Cell lines	Short description	Refs.
dehydrogenase activity and intracellular Ca^{2+} levels), and **UV-Vis absorbance spectroscopy** (caspase-1 and -3 release assay)				and decrease of mitochondrial membrane potential induced by microcin E492. Apoptosis induction by microcin E492 is related with caspases' activation.	[70]
Flow cytometry (morphological changes and cell viability) and **epifluorescence microscopy** (intracellular Ca^{2+} levels)	Plantaricin A-22	*Lactobacillus plantarum* C11	Lymphocytes B and T, Reh, Jurkat, rat cortical neurons, PC12, and N2A	Flow cytometry revealed decreased particle size and increased granularity in cells treated with PlnA. Ca^{2+} imaging with the fluorophores fura-red and fluo-4 showed the rapid increase of Ca^{2+}intracellular levels, and the gradual leakage of the fluorophore indicated membrane disruption or cell lysis.	[89]
MTT assay (cell viability) and **flow cytometry** (effect on cells' cycle)	Colicin A, E1, E3, and U	*Escherichia coli* 185M4 (Colicin E3), *Shigella boydii* M592 (Colicin U), and *Escherichia coli* (Colicin E1 and A)	MRC5, MCF-7, ZR75, BT549, MT474, MDA-MB-231, SKBR3, T47D, HT29, HOS, SKUT-1, and HS913T	The cytotoxic effect of these colicins was evaluated by a MTT assay, and it revealed that colicins E3 and U weren't capable of a significant effect on the cell lines. Colicins A and E1 exhibited a cytotoxic effect, and flow cytometry pointed out alterations in the cell cycle and apoptosis induction.	[69]
MTT assay (cell viability), **fluo-rescence microscopy** (effect on cells' morphology), **transmission electron microscopy (TEM)** (effect on cells' morphology), and **flow cytometry** (PS exposure, apoptotic/necrotic cells, and effect on cells' cycle)	Azurin	*Pseudomonas aeruginosa*	U2OS, MG63, and L02	A MTT assay revealed specific cytotoxic activity of azurin against U2OS cells. Morphology alterations related with apoptosis were observed in treated U2OS cells, through fluorescence microscopy and TEM. Flow cytometry showed that azurin induces apoptosis and cell cycle alterations in U2OS cells.	[78]

Technique	Bacteriocin	Producer bacteria	Cell lines	Short description	Refs.
MTT assay (cell viability), **confocal microscopy** (cellular uptake and distribution), **flow cytometry** (cellular uptake, effect of entry inhibitors, and entry kinetics), **fluorescence spectroscopy** (LDH leakage), and **UV-Vis absorbance spectroscopy** (hemolysis assay)	Azurin, p18, and p28	*Pseudomonas aeruginosa* (azurin and synthetic derivatives of azurin: p18 and p28)	A549, NCI-H23, CCD-13Lu, DU145, LN-CAP, CRL11611, MCF-7, MCF 10A, HCT116, CCD33Co, HT1080, SK-OV3, normal fibroblast, HOSE6-3, UISO-Mel-2, UISO-Mel-23, and UISO-Mel-29	Confocal microscopy and flow cytometry showed that p18 and p28 preferentially enter cancer cells. The study of LDH release in UISO-Mel-2 through fluorescence spectroscopy pointed out the maintenance of membrane integrity. The hemolytic assay confirmed the lack of membrane disruption. Azurin and p28 significantly reduced UISO-Mel-2, -23, and -29 survival. p18 did not inhibit cell proliferation.	[79]
Flow cytometry (PE expression, tissue factor expression, and cell viability), **UV-Vis absorbance spectroscopy** (cell proliferation), **TEM** (effect on cells' morphology), and **confocal microscopy** (effect on cell's morphology)	Duramycin	*Streptoverticillium* sp.	Colo320, $ASPC_1$, CFPAC-1, and MIA-PaCa-2	Flow cytometry showed increased expression of PE and decreased tissue factor expression in treated CFPAC-1 and $ASPC_1$. The effect of duramycin on $ASPC_1$, CFPAC-1, and MIA-PaCa-2 cells was assessed by flow cytometry and resulted in apoptosis induction. Duramycin has a lower effect of Colo320 cell proliferation when compared to other cell lines. Treated and untreated $ASPC_1$ cells were imaged by TEM and imaged live by confocal microscopy.	[93]

(*Continued*)

Table 11.2 (*Continued*)

Technique	Bacteriocin	Producer bacteria	Cell lines	Short description	Refs.
MTT assay (cell viability), **flow cytometry** (apoptotic/necrotic cells, cell membrane permeability tests, and peptide distribution), and **confocal microscopy** (peptide distribution)	m2163 and m2386	*Lactobacillus casei* ATCC 334	SW480, H184B5F5/M10, Caco-2, BFTC 905, and CHO-k1	A MTT assay indicates that both peptides are selective toward cancer cells. Flow cytometry indicated that the treatment of SW480 cells with m2163 or m2386 may induce apoptosis or necrosis. Membrane permeability was studied using PI and flow cytometry in the presence of m2163. Confocal microscopy revealed that both peptides preferentially entered SW480 cells with increased treatment time, over normal H184B5F5/M10 cells.	[95]
CD spectroscopy (peptides' secondary structure), **MTT assay** (cell viability), trypan **blue dye exclusion** (cell viability), **UV-Vis. absorbance spectroscopy** (LDH release), **flow cytometry** (cell cycle analysis and apoptotic/necrotic cells), **scanning electron microscopy (SEM)** (effect on cells' morphology), and **confocal microscopy** (peptide's distribution)	KL15	Synthetic derivative from m2163 and m2386	SW480, H184B5F5/M10, and Caco-2	KL15 acts preferentially on cancer cells SW480 and Caco-2 over the normal H184B5F5/M10 cells. Flow cytometry and confocal microscopy of SW480-treated cells revealed enhanced cell membrane permeability. SEM images showed significant changes in SW480 cell morphology, and several porous structures were observed. Confocal microscopy and SEM images are in accordance, indicating that KL15 may damage SW480 cells by penetrating the membrane and entering these cells.	[96]

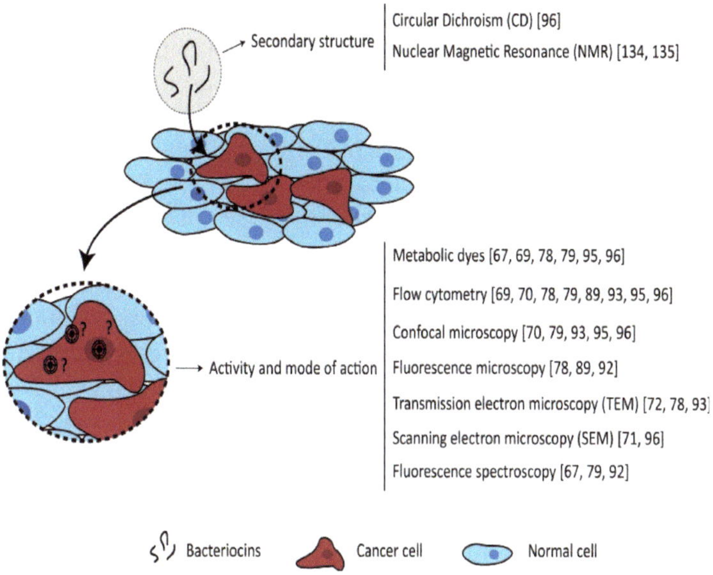

Figure 11.2 Different biophysical techniques can be applied to study the action of bacteriocins. Predictions of peptides' secondary structure can be made using CD and NMR, and mechanisms of action can be depicted through flow cytometry and confocal microscopy, among other techniques.

11.4.1 Cellular Viability: Metabolic Dyes

For assessing the cytotoxic activity of a drug, cell viability assays must be performed. These methods can be broadly divided into two different groups: methods to analyze a whole population and methods that analyze individual cells [104]. Although the population analysis delivers results more promptly, it may provide less detailed information compared with viability measurements obtained at the single-cell level. Colorimetric assays for living cells must use colorless substrates that are processed by any viable cell but not by dead cells or tissue culture medium, resulting in a colored product [105]. Tetrazolium salts thus constitute a promising tool for assessing cell viability, fitting in with the description of an ideal colorimetric assay for living cells [105]. The reduction of these salts, colorless or poorly colored in aqueous solution, to strongly colored products has been used in redox histochemistry and in biochemical applications for more than half a century [106]. 3-(4,5-dimethylthiazol-2-yl)-2,5-diphenyltetrazolium bromide (MTT) was the first known metabolic dye [104] and is the most widely used monotetrazolium salt [106]. The principle of this assay remains based on MTT reduction catalyzed by NAD(P)H-dependent oxidoreductases and dehydrogenases on metabolically active cells, resulting in formazan (dark purple) crystals in direct proportion to viable cells [106–108]. The use of this dye in a 96-well assay and the fact that the final measurement can be carried out in a plate reader simply by using absorption spectroscopy facilitate the screening of different treatment groups, and this represents a major advantage [105]. The MTT assay is versatile and quantitative, and it constitutes a breakthrough when compared to other assays applied to assess the proliferative and cytotoxic activity of many molecules [105]. In fact, this assay has been widely used for evaluating the dose-dependent cytotoxic effect of bacteriocins against several different cancer cell lines and for the determination of the peptide concentration required for achieving 50% of cell death (IC_{50}). This assay was already used for evaluating the cytotoxic effect of bacteriocins, such as nisin [67, 71, 72], bovicin HC5 [67], azurin [75, 77], p28 [79, 80], pediocin K2a2-3 [68], pediocin CP2 [82], colicins E1, A and U [69], pyocin S2 [86], and KL15 [96], on several cancer cell lines, including human breast cancer cells (MCF-7, ZR75, BT549, BT474, MDA-MB-231, SKBR3, and T47D), melanoma cells (UISO-Mel-2, -6, -23, and -29), colon carcinoma cells (HT29, Caco-2, and SW480), osteosarcoma cells (U2OS, MG63, and HOS), leukemia cells (Jurkat and MOLT-4), hepatocarcinoma cells (HepG2), fibrosarcoma cells (HS913T), leiomyosarcoma cells (SKUT-1), and cervical carcinoma cells (HeLa). Many of the IC_{50} values found for these bacteriocins are in the micromolar range, as for the cytotoxic effect of nisin and bovicin HC5 against cancer cell lines MCF-7 and HepG2 [67], nisin towards human colon carcinoma cells HT29 and Caco-2 [72] and leukemia cells Jurkat and MOLT-4 [71] and also the peptide KL15 tested against colon adenocarcinoma cells SW480 and Caco-2 [96]. Chen and coworkers [96] identified several *loci* for bacteriocins from the *Lactobacillus casei* ATCC 334 genomic sequence. DNA sequences corresponding to putative bacteriocins, such as m2163 and m2386, were expressed, and these AMPs revealed cytotoxic activity against SW480 and Caco-2 cells and human bladder papillary transitional cells carcinoma BFTC 905 [95]. Tsai *et al.* reported on the m2163 and m2386 cytotoxic effect on the previously mentioned cell lines using the MTT assay, and the obtained IC_{50} values ranged from 40 to 54 μg/mL [95]. A normal mammary epithelial cell line was also included in this study, and the IC_{50} values obtained for m2163 and m2386 were 96 and 104 μg/mL [95], indicating that these bacteriocins preferentially attack cancer cells. The sequences of these bacteriocins have been modified and characterized in terms of hydrophobicity, positive net charge, and predicted secondary structure [96]. One of the modifications resulted in the peptide KL15, which exhibited an anticancer activity toward SW480 and Caco-2 cells. H184B5F5/M10 normal cells were also included in this study in order to evaluate the selectivity of this bacteriocin to cancer cells [96]. The MTT assay was used to determine the IC_{50} for KL15 on these cell lines, and the values obtained were close to 50 μg/mL (26.3 μM) for the cancer cell lines and 150 μg/mL for the normal cell line H184B5F5/M10 [96].

11.4.2 Flow Cytometry

Flow cytometry is based on the movement of cells or micrometric particles through a channel subjected to a laser beam [109]. This technique measures the light absorbed, scattered, or emitted by a single particle or cell as a result of its physical properties [109], providing information on cell size, granularity, intracellular complexity, and protein composition [110]. In flow cytometry technique cells are usually stained with fluorescent dyes [109]. The evolution of flow cytometry associated with the use of new fluorochromes or probes emphasized this technique's applicability in the evaluation of cell viability, membrane structure integrity, and membrane potential in individualized cells [109]. In fact, the use of fluorescence probes in flow cytometry allows us to measure the fluorescence intensity as a result of the metabolic activity of the cells [17]. Overall, the probes used in flow cytometry can be organized into nucleic acid binding and metabolic, cellular, or protein binding probes [109]. Since flow cytometry allows its users to assess different parameters, such as membrane integrity and potential, at a single-cell level it may represent a more accurate method to report on the cells' function than the traditional cell viability- or cell growth-based methods [109].

Flow cytometry was used in combination with confocal microscopy by Chen *et al.* to demonstrate the membrane permeability of SW480 cells induced by KL15 [96]. The formation of pores promoted by KL15 was confirmed by scanning electron microscopy (SEM) [96]. In this study, the authors used propidium iodide (PI) to identify cells in different cell cycle phases, namely G1, S, and G2/M [96]. PI is a DNA-staining dye that intercalates with DNA molecules, and it is used for distinguishing live from dead cells [109]. PI does not enter cells without permeabilized membranes when applied isolated and therefore allows the detection and quantification of dying and dead cells [111]. The authors reported that by increasing the exposure time of SW480 cells to KL15, there is a consequent increase in the percentage of the sub-G1 cell population. A similar effect was obtained when the cells were exposed to increasing concentrations of KL15 for 24 h, resulting in an increase in the cell number within the sub-G1 population [96]. Chen and coworkers also used PI and Annexin V-fluorescein isothiocyanate (FITC) in flow cytometry to distinguish early apoptotic, late apoptotic-necrotic, and primary necrotic cells as a result of cell damage induced by KL15 [96]. Annexin V-FITC is a powerful fluorochrome that binds to PS, a marker of the early stages of apoptosis [36, 95, 112]. In fact, a correlation was observed between increased KL15 concentrations and the increase of late apoptotic-necrotic cells. Moreover, when in the presence of KL15 in concentrations between 80 and 120 μg/mL, the existence of significant shifts in PI fluorescence intensities indicated a dose-dependent damaged cell membrane as an effect of KL15 on cancer cells [96].

Similar to the work performed by Chen and coworkers [96], the effect of microcin E492 on HeLa cell cycle was also studied by Hetz *et al.* using flow cytometry with PI and Annexin V-FITC [70]. In this study, the stain 3,3′-dihexyloxacarbocyanine ($DiOC_6$) was used to detect the loss of the mitochondrial membrane's potential in the presence of the bacteriocin. Additionally, with this technique it was possible to observe that cell death and DNA fragmentation were dose-dependent effects and side-scatter-versus-forward-scatter plots allowed the evaluation of microcin E492 on HeLa cells' light scattering characteristics [70]. The effect of the bacteriocin duramycin on $ASPC_1$ cells was also evaluated by Yates and coworkers [93] using this technique, and it was demonstrated that the increase in the number of apoptotic and necrotic cells as well as the decrease in tumor proliferation were dose-dependent effects [93]. Sand *et al.* used flow cytometry to analyze the cytotoxic effect and morphological changes in Jurkat and Reh cancer cells and normal lymphocytes B and T cells in the presence of PlnA [89]. Morphological changes were also evaluated through the study of the forward and side light scattered, indicating a decrease in particle size and increase in granularity [89]. Both analyses revealed that PlnA bacteriocin was slightly more active toward cancerous lymphocytes (Jurkat and Reh) [89]. The potential anticancer activity of three different nisin variants against UM-SCC-17B, UM-SCC-14A, HSC-3, and OSCC-3 cells was evaluated by Kamarajan and coworkers [74]. In this study, flow cytometry and the stain Annexin V were applied in order to assess the apoptotic effects induced by the peptides [74]. Chumchalová and Šmarda [69] reported on the effect of colicins A, E1, and U on the cell cycles of five different cancer cell lines. While colicin U did not change significantly the cell cycle of any cell line, colicin A increased the population of cells in the G1 phase of the normal fibroblast cell line MRC5 and the cancer cells HS913T [69]. In the presence of colicin A, a decreased number of MDA-MB-231 cancer cells undergoing phase G1 was registered [69]. For cancer cells treated with colicin E1, cell cycle alterations were registered only for the MCF-7 cells, and an increase of the number of cells undergoing phase G1 was observed [69]. In the same study, the effect of the bacteriocin on the number of apoptotic cells was also evaluated. When all five cancer cell lines are treated with colicin A, there was an increase in the number of apoptotic cells, except for HS913T cancer cells. For HS913T and MCF-7 cancer cells treated with colicin E1, an increased cell number undergoing apoptosis was observed [69]. Interestingly, flow cytometry was used by Lequerica and coworkers [94] to demonstrate the effect of halocin H6 on the Na^+/H^+ exchanger (NHE) in mammalian cells. This bacteriocin inhibited NHE in Jurkat E6-1, exhibiting a dose-dependent effect. In fact, halocin H6 appears to be the first biological compound with the ability to inhibit NHE, in eukaryotic cells [94].

11.4.3 Microscopy Techniques

Different studies show the importance of microscopy techniques for detailing bacteriocins' mechanism(s) of action. Chen *et al.* relied on confocal microscopy to investigate the distribution of KL15 in SW480 cells [96]. Confocal microscopy allows imaging fixed or living cells and tissues previously labeled with fluorescent probes, with an increased lateral and axial resolution when compared to epifluorescence microscopy [113]. In this study, the bacteriocin-derived peptide KL15 was labeled with *N*-hydroxysuccinimide (NHS)-fluorescein, a green fluorescent dye, while the cell membrane was labeled with the red fluorescent dye di-8-ANEPPS and the blue fluorescent dye 4,6-diamidino-2-phenylindole (DAPI) was applied to label the cell nucleus [96]. Evaluating the colocalization of the dyes it was possible to infer KL15 localization inside the cell. Confocal microscopy images indicated that KL15 enters the cells and causes significant changes in their morphology [96]. Nonetheless, red fluorescence was detected and found to be colocalized with DAPI, used for nuclei staining. This observation was in agreement with the results obtained from SEM, as it was demonstrated that KL15 may damage treated cells by cell membrane penetration and consequent intrusion into the cells [96].

Confocal microscopy was also used by Yamada and coworkers [75] to study the localization of the bacteriocin azurin in UISO-Mel-2 and UISO-Mel-6 cell lines, p53 positive ($p53^+$) and negative ($p53^-$), respectively [75]. p53 is a tumor-suppressor protein that may be involved in azurin's nuclear transportation. It is proposed that the azurin-receptor binding may constitute a key step in azurin's trafficking toward the nucleus [75]. This step of receptor binding is probably mediated by an association with p53. This protein has the ability to traffic freely between the cytoplasm and the nucleus [114], and it may, therefore, participate in azurin's transport to the cell nucleus. In this study, azurin was labeled with Alexa Fluor 568 and further microinjected into the cells' cytoplasm [75]. DNA was stained with DAPI [75]. After the microinjection of labeled azurin in $p53^+$-UISO-Mel-2 cells, this bacteriocin was found in the cytosol and later in the cell nucleus, which apparently suffers morphological changes, probably due to apoptosis [75]. In $p53^-$-UISO-Mel-6 cells, after azurin's microinjection, the bacteriocin is localized in the cytoplasm of the cells and 3 h later remains in the cytoplasm surrounding the nucleus, even though it does not colocalize with the nuclear area [75]. Other similar study was performed by Yamada *et al.*, where the uptake of azurin and one mutant azurin by MCF-7 cell line was investigated [77]. Both bacteriocins had the ability to enter the cells [77]. Punj and coworkers also used microinjection of labeled azurin to investigate the localization of this bacteriocin in MCF-7 cells, a $p53^+$ cell line, and MDA-MB-157, a $p53^-$ cell line [76]. Confocal images obtained 4 h after microinjection show a colocalization of the labeled azurin and the nucleus in the MCF-7 cancer cells, while for MDA-MB-157 cells azurin is accumulated in the surrounding areas of the nucleus but not colocalized with the nucleus [76]. An additional example of confocal microscopy application is the investigation of the ability of p28 and azurin derivatives to penetrate cancer cells UISO-Mel-2, DU145, SKOV-3, A549, and MCF-7 by Taylor *et al.* [79]. From the obtained images it was possible to observe that p28 was capable of internalizing the cancer cells but it did not penetrate histologically matched normal cells with the same efficacy [79]. Taylor and coworkers also relied on the use of kits for the detection of mitochondria and lysosomes and revealed that azurin colocalizes with mitochondria and lysosomes while p28 colocalizes with lysosomes alone [79]. Yamada *et al.* studied p28's ability to penetrate human breast cancer cell lines and the obtained confocal images report that this azurin derivative enters MCF-7, T47D, and ZR-75-1 cancer cells preferentially over the normal cells MCF 10A [81].

Yates *et al.* used confocal microscopy for live cell imaging of $ASPC_1$ in the presence of duramycin [93]. In this study, the plasma membrane dye CellMask was used, allowing the observation of small cell membrane projections but not a significant effect of duramycin in the overall cell morphology/physiology (82). Hetz *et al.* reported DNA fragmentation induced by microcin E492 on HeLa cells, using the apoptotic detection system [70]. Moreover, in this same study, confocal microscopy was applied to determine the level of intracellular Ca^{2+} in HeLa cells. It was demonstrated that in the presence of microcin E492, there is the release of intracellular Ca^{2+} stores, which leads to an increase of the Ca^{2+} intracellular levels [70]. Therefore, it was proposed that the depletion of Ca^{2+} intracellular levels leads to the overload of mitochondria with Ca^{2+}, which results in an alteration in the regular mitochondrial metabolism, resulting in apoptosis activation [70, 115]. Changes in Ca^{2+} levels were also evaluated by Sand and coworkers but in this case by using conventional fluorescence microscopy to study the effect of PlnA on the intracellular levels of Ca^{2+} in PC12 cells [89, 91]. In these studies, it was demonstrated that in the presence of PlnA there is an immediate increase in the intracellular levels of Ca^{2+} [89, 91]. Sand *et al.* proposed that the Ca^{2+} levels increase is a result of rapidly induced membrane permeability caused by PlnA [89, 91]. Finally, Zhao *et al.* used fluorescence microscopy to obtain images of amyloid-like fibers formed after the binding between PlnA and membranes with negatively charged phospholipids [92]. In this study, fluorescence microscopy was also applied for evaluating the cytotoxic effect of PlnA on Jurkat cells through the use of the stain sytox green and cell counting from the fluorescence images obtained with a confocal scanner [92]. The intracellular caspase-3 activity was also investigated with the PhiPhiLux™ assay, which reports on the caspase-3 activity with green fluorescence, as a result of the cleavage of a synthetic peptide by caspase-3 [92]. Additionally, Jurkat cells were stained with PhiPhiLux, PI, and Hoechst 33342 to evaluate the relation between caspase-3 activity, cell viability, and nuclear morphology, respectively [92]. In the presence of PlnA, there is a significant decrease in Jurkat cells' viability and this cytotoxic effect depends on concentration and temperature [92]. The fluorescence images obtained revealed that PlnA induced cell death by necrosis and apoptosis, leading to plasma membrane blebbing and nuclear fragmentation, typical of apoptosis, and caspase-3 activity was higher in PlnA-treated cells when compared with the control [92].

Transmission electron microscopy (TEM) has been used by several authors for evaluating bacteriocin-induced morphological alterations in cancer cells [72, 78, 93]. Yang *et al.* evaluated the morphological changes in human osteosarcoma cells U2OS induced by azurin using TEM [78]. In this study, the obtained images revealed that after azurin treatment, U2OS cells displayed reduced cell volume and shrunk cytoplasm while the plasma membrane remained intact [78]. In the presence of the bacteriocin, it was also possible to observe condensed chromatin close to the nuclear envelope, nuclear membrane irregularities, and several vacuoles across the cytoplasm [78]. In this case, TEM images of U2OS cells in the presence of azurin allowed the authors to propose an induced apoptosis, leading to the investigation of the mechanism behind this phenomenon [78]. In a different example, TEM application shows the effect of duramycin on pancreatic cancer cells $ASPC_1$ [93]. In this study, Yates and coworkers observed cell lysis, which may point to an increase in cell fragility promoted by necrosis [93]. Also, Maher and McClean [72] used TEM images to confirm that nisin had no potential to disturb intestinal epithelial integrity, using Caco-2 cells as a GI cell model. The obtained images displayed Caco-2 cells treated with nisin with typical characteristics from polarized Caco-2 cells, exhibiting cell–cell adhesion, tight junctions, and microvilli at the apical membrane surface, making it impossible to distinguish between treated and untreated cells [72].

SEM has also been used in several studies in order to evaluate the effect of different bacteriocins on cancer cells as well as on the innate immune system response [71, 96]. Chen *et al.* used several biophysical techniques to describe the effect of KL15 on colon adenocarcinoma cells [96]. In this work, SEM was used to examine the morphology of the cells SW480 in the presence of KL15 [96]. SEM images revealed that untreated SW480 cells exhibited an intact structure with surrounding cilia, while cells treated with KL15 had significant changes in their morphology, which became more notorious with passage of time [96]. SW480 cells treated for longer periods of time with KL15 displayed several pores on their membranes, and the absence of cilia around the cells was noticed [96]. The morphological evaluation with SEM was consistent with the results obtained from the use of other techniques, such as confocal microscopy and flow cytometry, which pointed toward cell membrane damage [96]. This technique was also applied by Begde *et al.* along with fluorescence microscopy in order to evaluate the effect of nisin on neutrophil extracellular trap (NET) formation by polymorphonuclear neutrophils (PMNs) [71]. In this case, the use of SEM confirmed that nisin induced NET formation by PMNs, providing information concerning the effect of nisin on the innate immune system [71].

The inherent versatility of cancer cells allows them to constantly adapt and adjust their characteristics, such as deformability, in accordance with the surrounding environment. This has direct consequences on the cellular behavior concerning adherence, migration, invasion, and metastization [116]. Therefore, studying the mechanical properties of cancer cells in the presence of bacteria-derived peptides is relevant as it may report the ability to hamper the formation of metastasis. Not only is AFM a reference for obtaining high-resolution images of human cells, it also assumes an important position for the study of cells' biomechanical properties [17, 117, 118]. AFM technique allow us to obtain information regarding cells' ultrastructure on the nanometer scale [17, 119]. With a very broad spectrum of application in the field of oncology, AFM has been used to investigate interactions between molecules [120], details of membrane structure [121–123], and elasticity and cellular morphology [122, 123]. The principle of AFM relies on the measurement of very small forces between atoms or molecules when they come close together, enabling the detection of forces as small as 10^{-7} and 10^{-12} N [124]. Recently, AFM has been used along with a bioinformatics tool to investigate protein–protein interactions between azurin and the tumoral protein p53 [125]. This technique was also used to analyze the effect of bacteriocins on bacteria [126]. The use of AFM for the study of bacteriocins' effects on cancer cells' morphology and mechanical properties is a promising work that may provide information on cells' biophysics, as demonstrated in previous works using this technique [17].

11.4.4 Fluorescence Spectroscopy

The use of fluorescent probes is not limited to their application in fluorescence microscopy. These molecules have also been applied in fluorescence spectroscopy, and they may constitute a valuable source of information on the effect of peptides in lipid bilayers [67, 92]. Paiva *et al.* used fluorescence spectroscopy to study carboxyfluorescein (CF) leakage from large unilamellar vesicles (LUVs) with different lipid composition, induced by bovicin HC5 and nisin [67]. Different models were used: liposomes made of pure 1,2-dioleoyl-sn-glycero-3-phosphocholine ($C_{18:1}$, DOPC) or 1,2-dipal-mitoleoyl-sn-glycero-3-phosphocholine ($C_{16:1}$, DPoPC) and liposomes containing DOPC or DPoPC and cholesterol [67]. The use of phospholipids containing 16 and 18 carbon atoms is due to the fact that these are the most common lipids found in eukaryotic cell membranes [67]. The model membrane systems used in this study didn't include lipid II, the target of both bacteriocins, since the goal was the mimicking of eukaryotic cell membrane, which lacks this lipid [67]. Both bacteriocins led to a residual CF leakage from DOPC-composed liposomes, and no leakage was detected in cholesterol-containing DOPC liposomes [67]. Bovicin HC5 and nisin induced significant efflux of CF from DPoPC liposomes, and in the presence of cholesterol- and DPoPC-containing liposomes, CF release caused by bovicin HC5 was not influenced while release caused by nisin was significantly reduced [67]. Therefore, this study points out that the presence of cholesterol may hamper membrane permeabilization by nisin [67].

In another study, Zhao and coworkers used fluorescence spectroscopy to report on the effect of PlnA on liposomes' permeability and to evaluate the effect of this bacteriocin on lipid dynamics in bilayers [92].

11.4.5 Circular Dichroism and Nuclear Magnetic Resonance Spectroscopy

There are several proofs resulting from studies with different biophysical techniques revealing that AMPs are disordered in aqueous solutions and they instantly assume an organized conformation when in membrane mimetic solutions or when in interaction with phospholipid bilayers [24]. Many of these peptides require the presence of a bilayer with an overall negative charge in order to adopt such a conformation [24]. Studies with ACPs also indicate that the amphipathic structures adopted by these peptides next to the cell membrane can play a key role in their mode of action [16, 127, 128]. Therefore, the study of bacteriocins' secondary structure may provide valuable information that may support the characterization of these peptides' mode of action.

CD provides a rapid analysis of peptides' and proteins' secondary structures [129]. This technique allows one to perform structural analysis under particular conditions/environments experienced by proteins and to measure the rates of structural changes in proteins, essential for their biological function [130]. When the chromophores of amides in the polypeptide backbones of proteins happen to be aligned in arrays, there occurs a shift or split in their optical transitions into multiple transitions and different structural elements result in different CD spectra [129]. Therefore, a protein with an α-helical structure exhibits typical negative bands at 222 and 208 nm and a positive band at 193 nm, a protein with a β-pleated sheet displays a negative band at 218 nm and a positive one at 195 nm, and a disordered protein exhibits a characteristic low ellipticity above 210 nm and negative bands close to 195 nm [129]. Since proteins' spectra deeply rely on their conformation, CD can be applied to unravel an unknown protein's structure and to evaluate the effect of temperature, mutations, heat, denaturants, or binding interactions on the protein's conformation [129]. Nonetheless, CD provides low-resolution structural information on the overall molecular structure, contrasting with X-ray crystallography and NMR, both providing information at the atomic level of resolution [130]. However, CD requires less sample quantity and time and it is a nondestructive technique [130]. On the other hand, diffracting crystals of proteins are a requirement for X-ray crystallography and NMR requires highly concentrated samples [130]. Additionally, CD can be applied in conditions similar to those used in NMR [130]. NMR relies on the fact that magnetic nuclei, such as those in ^{1}H, ^{13}C, and ^{15}N, may form nuclear-spin states of different energies and can alternate between these states when exposed to radiofrequency radiation [131]. The NMR properties of a molecule's magnetic nucleus depend on its chemical environment [131]. Through the interaction of the magnetic nuclei with each other and with the applied field it is possible to associate resonance signals to specific nuclei from a molecular structure, providing information on the distance between them [131].

Chen *et al.* used CD to assess the secondary structure of KL15 and five other peptides, derived from the bacteriocins m2163 and m2386, in three different solutions: doubly deionized water (ddw), phosphate-buffered saline (PBS), and a membrane-mimicking solution with 2,2,2-trifluoroethanol (TFE) at 50% [96]. The obtained spectra revealed that all the peptides exhibit a random coil conformation in ddw or PBS and an α-helical conformation in 50% TFE [96]. In this study the CD spectra in sodium dodecyl sulfate (SDS) or with LUVs made from dodecyl phosphocholine (DPC) were also performed for KL15, revealing an α-helical structure. SDS and DPC are used as a membrane-mimicking environment [132, 133]. These results indicate that KL15 can act as an amphipathic AMP and it may penetrate the cell's lipid bilayer, which is in accordance with the results obtained with other biophysical techniques, such as SEM, flow cytometry, and confocal microscopy, also used in this study [96].

Fregeau and coworkers relied on CD and NMR to evaluate the secondary structure of leucocin A (LeuA), a type IIa bacteriocin from *Leuconostoc gelidum* [134]. In this study, CD spectra for this bacteriocin were performed in different TFE concentrations and in an aqueous solution of DPC [134]. CD spectra with increasing concentrations of TFE revealed the transition to an α-helical conformation, and similar changes in conformation were obtained with the DPC:LeuA in the water system [134]. In this case NMR was also applied to TFE and DPC, and it provided detailed information regarding the bacteriocin's secondary structure [134]. It was possible to conclude that in TFE and DPC, LeuA displays a β-sheet structure from the amino acid residues 6 to 16 and within this region there is a disulfide bridge, with an interruption between residues 11 and 12 forming a turn [134]. After this β-sheet loop there's an α-helix, comprising the amino acid residues 18–30 [134]. NMR provided very detailed information about LeuA at the atomic level of resolution [134].

Wang *et al.* reanalyzed the NMR spectra obtained by Frageau and coworkers, namely the total correlation spectroscopy spectra (TOCSY) and 2D nuclear Overhauser effect spectroscopy (NOESY) [134], and they applied NMR to unravel the secondary structure of carnobacteriocin B2 (CbnB2), a type IIa bacteriocin from *Carnobacterium piscicola* LV17B [135]. With this study it was possible to obtain detailed information about CbnB2's secondary structure [135]. Also, a comparative study between LeuA and CbnB2 structures revealed that, despite these bacteriocins exhibiting a high degree of similarity in their sequences, the conformation adopted by the N-terminus differs when in TFE [135]. While the N-terminus of LeuA adopts a three-stranded antiparallel β-sheet in TFE, the N-terminus of CbnB2 is disordered

[135]. This difference in both structures may be a result of different secondary structural propensities and different effect of TFE on both amphipathic structures [135]. Additionally, this variation in the N-terminus structure points out that the β-sheet structure present in the N-terminus of LeuA may not be a requirement for type IIa bacteriocins' function [135].

Additional and similar studies have been relying on CD and NMR to unravel the secondary structures of several bacteriocins [61, 136, 137], such as curvacin A [138], sakacin P and one sakacin P variant [139], nisin A [140–142], duramycin B and C [143], lactococcin G [144, 145], mersacidin [146] plantaricin E/F and plantaricin J/K [147], and plantaricin C [148].

11.5 Final Remarks

As novel peptide sequences enter the process of drug development, more extensive details on activity, selectivity, and efficacy are needed. Bacteriocins are potential important sources of anticancer drugs, but their successful application in chemotherapy requires further and thorough examination of their effects on normal and cancer cells and how these can be related with human physiology. Biophysics plays an important role in this process, allowing researchers to engage in a multidisciplinary approach involving studies on different cells, from bacterial to eukaryotic. Future research on bacteriocins might benefit from the inclusion of other biophysical techniques, such as dynamic light scattering. Zeta potential can be used to report on interactions between peptides and biological membranes by the detection of variations in the cell surface electrostatic potential [15–17]. Considering that most of the bacteriocins shown in the literature exhibit a positive net charge [59] and considering the composition of cancer and normal cell membranes [1, 2], the use of zeta potential is thus feasible and will deliver important information for progressing in SAR studies. Studies of bacteriocins' effects on cell morphology and biomechanical properties should also account for a wider range of human cell types, tumor and normal. Since different cells might carry specific molecules on their membranes in accordance with their tumor origin, it is important to include in the overall analysis cells from different organs. A better comprehension of the selectivity determinants is expected during these studies, and consequently improved peptide sequences can be expected to reach clinical stages.

Acknowledgment

The authors thank Fundação para a Ciência e a Tecnologia (FCT I.P., Portugal) for funding—PTDC/BBB-BQB/1693/2014. Filipa D. Oliveira also acknowledges FCT I.P. for fellowship PD/BD/135046/2017. Diana Gaspar also acknowledges FCT I.P. for fellowship SFRH/BPD/109010/2015. Marie Skłodowska-Curie Research and Innovation Staff Exchange (RISE) is also acknowledged for funding: call H2020-MSCA-RISE-2014, Grant Agreement 644167, 2015–2019.

References

1. Hoskin D. W., Ramamoorthy A. Studies on anticancer activities of antimicrobial peptides. *Biochimica et Biophysica Acta–Biomembranes*, 1778 (2008) 357–375.
2. Gaspar D., Veiga A. S., Castanho M. A. R. B. From antimicrobial to anticancer peptides. A review. *Frontiers in Microbiology*, 4 (2013) 1–16.
3. Vineis P., Wild C. P. Global cancer patterns: Causes and prevention. *The Lancet*, 383 (2014) 549–557.
4. Gaspar D., Castanho M. A. R. B. Anticancer peptides: Prospective innovation in cancer therapy, In *Host Defense Peptides and Their Potential as Therapeutic Agents* (2016) pp. 95–109, Springer International Publishing.
5. Wu D., Gao Y., Qi Y., Chen L., Ma Y., Li Y. Peptide-based cancer therapy: Opportunity and challenge. *Cancer Letters*, 351 (2014) 13–22.
6. Harris F., Dennison S. R., Singh J., Phoenix D. A. On the selectivity and efficacy of defense peptides with respect to cancer cells. *Medicinal Research Reviews*, 33 (2011) 190–234.
7. Savarese D. M. F., Savy G., Vahdat L., Wischmeyer P. E., Corey B. Prevention of chemotheraphy and radiation toxicity with glutamine. *Cancer Treatment Reviews*, 29 (2003) 501–513.

8. Berthrong M. Pathologic changes secondary to radiation. *World Journal of Surgery*, 10 (1986) 155–170.
9. Barker H. E., Paget J. T. E., Khan A. A., Harrington K. J. The tumour microenvironment after radiotherapy: Mechanisms of resistance and recurrence. *Nature Reviews Cancer*, 15 (2015) 409–425.
10. Riedl S., Zweytick D., Lohner K. Membrane-active host defense peptides—Challenges and perspectives for the development of novel anticancer drugs. *Chemistry and Physics of Lipids*, 164 (2011) 766–781.
11. Naumov G. N., Townson J. L., MacDonald I. C., Wilson S. M., Bramwell V. H. C., Groom A. C., *et al.* Ineffectiveness of doxorubicin treatment on solitary dormant mammary carcinoma cells or late-developing metastases. *Breast Cancer Research and Treatment*, 82 (2003) 199–206.
12. Gatti L., Zunino F. Overview of tumor cell chemoresistance mechanisms, In *Methods in Molecular Medicine* Vol. 111 (2005) pp. 127–148, Humana Press, New Jersey.
13. Sah B. N. P., Vasiljevic T., Mckechnie S., Donkor O. N. Identification of anticancer peptides from bovine milk proteins and their potential roles in management of cancer: A critical review. *Comprehensive Reviews in Food Science and Food Safety*, 14 (2015) 123–138.
14. Barras D., Widmann C. Promises of apoptosis-inducing peptides in cancer therapeutics. *Current Pharmaceutical Biotechnology*, 12 (2011) 1153–1165.
15. Sinthuvanich C., Veiga A. S., Gupta K., Gaspar D., Blumenthal R., Schneider J. P. Anticancer β-hairpin peptides: Membrane-induced folding triggers activity. *Journal of the American Chemical Society*, 134 (2012) 6210–6217.
16. Gaspar D., Veiga A. S., Sinthuvanich C., Schneider J. P., Castanho M. A. R. B. Anticancer peptide SVS-1: Efficacy precedes membrane neutralization. *Biochemistry*, 51 (2012) 6263–6265.
17. Gaspar D., Freire J. M., Pacheco T. R., Barata J. T., Castanho M. A. R. B. Apoptotic human neutrophil peptide-1 anti-tumor activity revealed by cellular biomechanics. *Biochimica et Biophysica Acta–Molecular Cell Research*, 1853 (2015) 308–316.
18. Falcao C. B., Pérez-Peinado C., de la Torre B. G., Mayol X., Zamora-Carreras H., Jiménez M. Á., *et al.* Structural dissection of crotalicidin, a rattlesnake venom cathelicidin, retrieves a fragment with antimicrobial and antitumor activity. *Journal of Medicinal Chemistry*, 58 (2015) 8553–8563.

19. M. Fialho A., Bernardes N., M Chakrabarty A. Exploring the anticancer potential of the bacterial protein azurin. *AIMS Microbiology*, 2 (2016) 292–303.
20. Hancock R. E. Cationic peptides: Effectors in innate immunity and novel antimicrobials. *The Lancet Infectious Diseases*, 1 (2001) 156–164.
21. Phoenix D. A., Dennison S. R., Harris F. Antimicrobial peptides: Their history, evolution, and functional promiscuity, In *Antimicrobial Peptides* (2013) pp. 1–37, Wiley-VCH Verlag GmbH & Co. KGaA, Weinheim, Germany.
22. Kaur S., Kaur S. Bacteriocins as potential anticancer agents, In *Frontiers in Pharmacology*, 6 (2015) 1–11.
23. Hancock R. E. Peptide antibiotics. *The Lancet*, 349 (1997) 418–422.
24. Yeaman M. R., Yount N. Y. Mechanisms of antimicrobial peptide action and resistance. *Pharmacological Reviews*, 55 (2003) 27–55.
25. Fernebro J. Fighting bacterial infections—Future treatment options. *Drug Resistance Updates*, 14 (2011) 125–139.
26. Dobrzynska I., Szachowicz-Petelska B., Sulkowski S., Figaszewski Z. Changes in electric charge and phospholipids composition in human colorectal cancer cells. *Molecular and Cellular Biochemistry*, 276 (2005) 113–119.
27. Schweizer F. Cationic amphiphilic peptides with cancer-selective toxicity. *European Journal of Pharmacology*, 625 (2009) 190–194.
28. Lee H. S., Park C. B., Kim J. M., Jang S. A., Park I. Y., Kim M. S., *et al.* Mechanism of anticancer activity of buforin IIb, a histone H2A-derived peptide. *Cancer Letters*, 271 (2008) 47–55.
29. Papo N., Shai Y. Host defense peptides as new weapons in cancer treatment. *Cellular and Molecular Life Sciences*, 62 (2005) 784–790.
30. Zasloff M. Antimicrobial peptides of multicellular organisms. *Nature*, 415 (2002) 389–395.
31. Simmaco M., Mignogna G., Barra D. Antimicrobial peptides from amphibian skin: What do they tell us? *Biopolymers*, 47 (1998) 435–450.
32. Chaudhary J., Munshi M. Scanning electron microscopic analysis of breast aspirates. *Cytopathology*, 6 (1995) 162–167.
33. Domagala W., Koss L. G. Surface configuration of human tumor cells obtained by fine needle aspiration biopsy. *Scanning Electron Microscopy*, (1980) 101–108.

34. Sok M., Sentjurc M., Schara M. Membrane fluidity characteristics of human lung cancer. *Cancer Letters*, 139 (1999) 215–220.
35. Kozłowska K., Nowak J., Kwiatkowski B., Cichorek M. ESR study of plasmatic membrane of the transplantable melanoma cells in relation to their biological properties. *Experimental and Toxicologic Pathology*, 51 (1999) 89–92.
36. Cooper G. M., Hausman R. E. *The Cell. A Molecular Approach* (5th ed.), (2009) Sinauer Associates, Inc.
37. Utsugi T., Schroit A. J., Connor J., Bucana C. D., Fidler I. J. Elevated expression of phosphatidylserine in the outer membrane leaflet of human tumor cells and recognition by activated human blood monocytes. *Cancer research*, 51 (1991) 3062–3066.
38. Li Y. C., Park M. J., Ye S.-K, Kim C.-W, Kim Y.-N. Elevated levels of cholesterol-rich lipid rafts in cancer cells are correlated with apoptosis sensitivity induced by cholesterol-depleting agents. *The American Journal of Pathology*, 168 (2006) 1107–1118.
39. Giuliani A., Pirri G., Nicoletto S. Antimicrobial peptides: An overview of a promising class of therapeutics. *Open Life Sciences*, 2 (2007) 1–33.
40. Tørfoss V., Isaksson J., Ausbacher D., Brandsdal B.-O., Flaten G. E., Anderssen T., *et al.* Improved anticancer potency by head-to-tail cyclization of short cationic anticancer peptides containing a lipophilic β(2,2)-amino acid. *Journal of Peptide Science*, 18 (2012) 609–619.
41. Hu J., Chen C., Zhang S., Zhao X., Xu H., Zhao X., *et al.* Designed antimicrobial and antitumor peptides with high selectivity. *Biomacromolecules*, 12 (2011) 3839–3843.
42. Torcato I. M., Huang Y.-H., Franquelim H. G., Gaspar D., Craik D. J., Castanho M. A. R. B., *et al.* Design and characterization of novel antimicrobial peptides, R-BP100 and RW-BP100, with activity against Gram-negative and Gram-positive bacteria. *Biochimica et Biophysica Acta–Biomembranes*, 1828 (2013) 944–955.
43. Zhao B-X, Zhao Y., Huang Y., Luo L.-M., Song P., Wang X., *et al.* The efficiency of tumor-specific pH-responsive peptide-modified polymeric micelles containing paclitaxel. *Biomaterials*, 33 (2012) 2508–2520.
44. Bultman S. J. Emerging roles of the microbiome in cancer. *Carcinogenesis*, 35 (2014) 249–255.
45. Cho I., Blaser M. J. The human microbiome: At the interface of health and disease. *Nature Reviews Genetics*, 13 (2012) 260–270.

46. Nicholson J. K., Holmes E., Kinross J., Burcelin R., Gibson G., Jia W., *et al.* Host-gut microbiota metabolic interactions. *Science*, 336 (2012) 1262–1267.

47. Chang J. Y., Antonopoulos D. A., Kalra A., Tonelli A., Khalife W. T., Schmidt T. M., *et al.* Decreased diversity of the fecal microbiome in recurrent *Clostridium difficile*-associated diarrhea. *The Journal of Infectious Diseases*, 197 (2008) 435–438.

48. Blaser M. J., Falkow S. What are the consequences of the disappearing human microbiota? *Nature Reviews Microbiology*, 7 (2009) 887–894.

49. Blaser M. Stop the killing of beneficial bacteria. *Nature*, 476 (2011) 393–394.

50. Plottel C. S., Blaser M. J. Microbiome and malignancy. *Cell Host & Microbe*, 10 (2011) 324–335.

51. Clayton T. A., Baker D., Lindon J. C., Everett J. R., Nicholson J. K. Pharmacometabonomic identification of a significant host-microbiome metabolic interaction affecting human drug metabolism. *Proceedings of the National Academy of Sciences*, 106 (2009) 14728–14733.

52. Wallace B. D., Wang H., Lane K. T., Scott J. E., Orans J., Koo J. S., *et al.* Alleviating cancer drug toxicity by inhibiting a bacterial enzyme. *Science*, 330 (2010) 831–835.

53. Parisien A., Allain B., Zhang J., Mandeville R., Lan C. Q. Novel alternatives to antibiotics: Bacteriophages, bacterial cell wall hydrolases, and antimicrobial peptides. *Journal of Applied Microbiology*, 104 (2007) 1–13.

54. Gratia A. Sur un remarquable exemple d'antagonisme entre deux souches de colibacille. *Comptes Rendus des Seances de la Societe de Biologie*, 93 (1925) 1040–1041.

55. Nes I. F., Holo H. Class II antimicrobial peptides from lactic acid bacteria. *Biopolymers*, 55 (2000) 50–61.

56. Cotter P. D., Hill C., Ross R. P. Bacteriocins: Developing innate immunity for food. *Nature Reviews Microbiology*, 3 (2005) 777–788.

57. Rodríguez E., González B., Gaya P., Nuñez M., Medina M. Diversity of bacteriocins produced by lactic acid bacteria isolated from raw milk. *International Dairy Journal*, 10 (2000) 7–15.

58. Rodríguez J., Martínez M. I., Horn N., Dodd H. M. Heterologous production of bacteriocins by lactic acid bacteria. *International Journal of Food Microbiology*, 80 (2003) 101–116.

59. Zacharof M. P., Lovitt R. W. Bacteriocins produced by lactic acid bacteria a review article. *APCBEE Procedia*, 2 (2012) 50–56.

60. Cotter P., Hill C., Ross R. Bacterial lantibiotics: Strategies to improve therapeutic potential. *Current Protein & Peptide Science*, 6 (2005) 61–75.

61. Sahl H.-G., Bierbaum G. Lantibiotics: Biosynthesis and biological activities of uniquely modified peptides from gram-positive bacteria. *Annual Review of Microbiology*, 52 (1998) 41–79.

62. Diep D., Nes I. Ribosomally synthesized antibacterial peptides in gram positive bacteria. *Current Drug Targets*, 3 (2002) 107–122.

63. van Belkum M. J., Stiles M. E. Nonlantibiotic antibacterial peptides from lactic acid bacteria. *Natural Product Reports*, 17 (2000) 323–335.

64. Kazazic M., Nissen-Meyer J., Fimland G. Mutational analysis of the role of charged residues in target-cell binding, potency and specificity of the pediocin-like bacteriocin sakacin P. *Microbiology*, 148 (2002) 2019–2027.

65. Lozano J. C. N., Meyer J. N., Sletten K., Pelaz C., Nes I. F. Purification and amino acid sequence of a bacteriocin produced by *Pediococcus acidilactici*. *Journal of General Microbiology*, 138 (1992) 1985–1990.

66. Kawai Y., Kemperman R., Kok J., Saito T. The circular bacteriocins gassericin A and circularin A. *Current Protein & Peptide Science*, 5 (2004) 393–398.

67. Paiva A. D., de Oliveira M. D., de Paula S. O., Baracat-Pereira M. C., Breukink E., Mantovani H. C. Toxicity of bovicin HC5 against mammalian cell lines and the role of cholesterol in bacteriocin activity. *Microbiology*, 158 (2012) 2851–2858.

68. Villarante K. I., Elegado F. B., Iwatani S., Zendo T., Sonomoto K., de Guzman E. E. Purification, characterization and in vitro cytotoxicity of the bacteriocin from *Pediococcus acidilactici* K2a2-3 against human colon adenocarcinoma (HT29) and human cervical carcinoma (HeLa) cells. *World Journal of Microbiology and Biotechnology*, 27 (2011) 975–980.

69. Chumchalová J., Šmarda J. Human tumor cells are selectively inhibited by colicins. *Folia Microbiologica*, 48 (2003) 111–115.

70. Hetz C., Bono M. R., Barros L. F., Lagos R. Microcin E492, a channel-forming bacteriocin from *Klebsiella pneumoniae*, induces apoptosis in some human cell lines. *Proceedings of the National Academy of Sciences*, 99 (2002) 2696–2701.

71. Begde D., Bundale S., Mashitha P., Rudra J., Nashikkar N., Upadhyay A. Immunomodulatory efficacy of nisin—a bacterial lantibiotic peptide. *Journal of Peptide Science*, 17 (2011) 438–444.

72. Maher S., McClean S. Investigation of the cytotoxicity of eukaryotic and prokaryotic antimicrobial peptides in intestinal epithelial cells in vitro. *Biochemical Pharmacology*, 71 (2006) 1289–1298.

73. Joo N. E., Ritchie K., Kamarajan P., Miao D., Kapila Y. L. Nisin, an apoptogenic bacteriocin and food preservative, attenuates HNSCC tumorigenesis via CHAC1. *Cancer Medicine*, 1 (2012) 295–305.

74. Kamarajan P., Hayami T., Matte B., Liu Y., Danciu T., Ramamoorthy A., *et al.* Nisin ZP, a bacteriocin and food preservative, inhibits head and neck cancer tumorigenesis and prolongs survival. *PLOS One*, 10 (2015) e0131008.

75. Yamada T., Goto M., Punj V., Zaborina O., Chen M. L., Kimbara K., *et al.* Bacterial redox protein azurin, tumor suppressor protein p53, and regression of cancer. *Proceedings of the National Academy of Sciences*, 99 (2002) 14098–14103.

76. Punj V., Bhattacharyya S., Saint-Dic D., Vasu C., Cunningham E. A., Graves J., *et al.* Bacterial cupredoxin azurin as an inducer of apoptosis and regression in human breast cancer. *Oncogene*, 23 (2004) 2367–2378.

77. Yamada T., Hiraoka Y., Ikehata M., Kimbara K., Avner B. S., Das Gupta T. K., *et al.* Apoptosis or growth arrest: Modulation of tumor suppressor p53's specificity by bacterial redox protein azurin. *Proceedings of the National Academy of Sciences*, 101 (2004) 4770–4775.

78. Yang D., Miao X., Ye Z., Feng J., Xu R., Huang X., *et al.* Bacterial redox protein azurin induce apoptosis in human osteosarcoma U2OS cells. *Pharmacological Research*, 52 (2005) 413–421.

79. Taylor B. N., Mehta R. R., Yamada T., Lekmine F., Christov K., Chakrabarty A. M., *et al.* Noncationic peptides obtained from azurin preferentially enter cancer cells. *Cancer Research*, 69 (2009) 537–546.

80. Yamada T., Das Gupta T. K., Beattie C. W. P28-Mediated activation of p53 in G2-M phase of the cell cycle enhances the efficacy of DNA damaging and antimitotic chemotherapy. *Cancer Research*, 76 (2016) 2354–2365.

81. Yamada T., Mehta R. R., Lekmine F., Christov K., King M. L., Majumdar D., *et al.* A peptide fragment of azurin induces a p53-mediated cell cycle arrest in human breast cancer cells. *Molecular Cancer Therapeutics*, 8 (2009) 2947–2958.

82. Kumar B., Balgir P. P., Kaur B., Mittu B., Chaunhan A. In Vitro cytotoxicity of native and rec-pediocin CP2 against cancer cell lines: A comparative study. *Pharmaceutica Analytica Acta*, 3 (2012) 8–11.

83. Fuska J., Fusková A, Šmarda J., Mach J. Effect of colicin E3 on leukemia cells P 388 in vitro. *Experientia*, 35 (1979) 406–407.

84. Šmarda J., Obdržálek V. I., Táborský I, Mach J. The cytotoxic and cytocidal effect of colicin E3 on mammalian tissue cells. *Folia Microbiologica*, 23 (1978) 272–277.

85. Watanabe T., Saito H. Cytotoxicity of pyocin S2 to tumor and normal cells and its interaction with cell surfaces. *Biochimica et Biophysica Acta–General Subjects*, 633 (1980) 77–86.

86. Abdi-Ali A., Worobec E. A., Deezagi A., Malekzadeh F. Cytotoxic effects of pyocin S2 produced by *Pseudomonas aeruginosa* on the growth of three human cell lines. *Canadian Journal of Microbiology*, 50 (2004) 375–381.

87. Saito H., Watanabe T., Tomioka H. Purification, properties, and cytotoxic effect of a bacteriocin from *Mycobacterium smegmatis*. *Antimicrobial Agents and Chemotherapy*, 15 (1979) 504–509.

88. Saito H., Watanabe T. Effect of a bacteriocin produced by *Mycobacterium smegmatis* on growth of cultured tumor and normal cells. *Cancer Research*, 39 (1979) 5114–5117.

89. Sand S. L., Oppegård C., Ohara S., Iijima T., Naderi S., Blomhoff H. K., *et al.* A peptide pheromone produced by *Lactobacillus plantarum*, permeabilizes the cell membrane of both normal and cancerous lymphocytes and neuronal cells. *Peptides*, 31 (2010) 1237–1244.

90. Sand S. L., Nissen-Meyer J., Sand O., Haug T. M. Plantaricin A. A cationic peptide produced by *Lactobacillus plantarum*, permeabilizes eukaryotic cell membranes by a mechanism dependent on negative surface charge linked to glycosylated membrane proteins. *Biochimica et Biophysica Acta–Biomembranes*, 1828 (2013) 249–259.

91. Sand S. L., Haug T. M., Nissen-Meyer J., Sand O. The bacterial peptide pheromone plantaricin A permeabilizes cancerous, but not normal, rat pituitary cells and differentiates between the outer and inner membrane leaflet. *Journal of Membrane Biology*, 216 (2007) 61–71.

92. Zhao H., Sood R., Jutila A., Bose S., Fimland G., Nissen-Meyer J., *et al.* Interaction of the antimicrobial peptide pheromone Plantaricin A with model membranes: Implications for a novel mechanism of action. *Biochimica et Biophysica Acta–Biomembranes*, 1758 (2006) 1461–1474.

93. Yates K. R., Welsh J., Udegbunam N. O., Greenman J., Maraveyas A., Madden L. A. Duramycin exhibits antiproliferative properties and induces apoptosis in tumour cells. *Blood Coagulation & Fibrinolysis*, 23 (2012) 396–401.

94. Lequerica J. L., O'Connor J. E., Such L., Alberola A., Meseguer I., Dolz M., *et al.* A halocin acting on Na^+/H^+ exchanger of Haloarchaea as a new type of inhibitor in NHE of mammals. *Journal of Physiology and Biochemistry*, 62 (2006) 253–262.

95. Tsai T. L., Li A. C., Chen Y. C., Liao Y. S., Lin T. H. Antimicrobial peptide m2163 or m2386 identified from *Lactobacillus casei* ATCC 334 can trigger apoptosis in the human colorectal cancer cell line SW480. *Tumor Biology*, 36 (2015) 3775–3789.

96. Chen Y.-C., Tsai T.-L., Ye X.-H., Lin T.-H. Anti-proliferative effect on a colon adenocarcinoma cell line exerted by a membrane disrupting antimicrobial peptide KL15. *Cancer Biology & Therapy*, 16 (2015) 1172–1183.

97. Reddy K. V. R., Yedery R. D., Aranha C. Antimicrobial peptides: Premises and promises. *International Journal of Antimicrobial Agents*, 24 (2004) 536–547.

98. Teixeira V., Feio M. J., Bastos M. Role of lipids in the interaction of antimicrobial peptides with membranes. *Progress in Lipid Research*, 51 (2012) 149–177.

99. Medina S. H., Schneider J. P. Cancer cell surface induced peptide folding allows intracellular translocation of drug. *Journal of Controlled Release*, 209 (2015) 317–326.

100. Madani F., Lindberg S., Langel Ü., Futaki S., Gräslund A. Mechanisms of cellular uptake of cell-penetrating peptides. *Journal of Biophysics*, 2011 (2011) 1–10.

101. Freire J. M., Veiga A. S., Rego de Figueiredo I., de la Torre B. G., Santos N. C., Andreu D., *et al.* Nucleic acid delivery by cell penetrating peptides derived from dengue virus capsid protein: Design and mechanism of action. *FEBS Journal*, 281 (2014) 191–215.

102. Freire J. M., Gaspar D., Veiga A. S., Castanho M. A. R. B. Shifting gear in antimicrobial and anticancer peptides biophysical studies: From vesicles to cells. *Journal of Peptide Science*, 21 (2015) 178–185.

103. Kao F.-S., Pan Y.-R., Hsu R.-Q., Chen H.-M. Efficacy verification and microscopic observations of an anticancer peptide, CB1a, on single lung cancer cell. *Biochimica et Biophysica Acta–Biomembranes*, 1818 (2012) 2927–2935.

104. Stoddart M. J. Cell Viability Assays: Introduction, In *Methods in Molecular Biology* Vol. 740 (2011) pp. 1–6, Humana Press, New York City, USA.

105. Mosmann T. Rapid colorimetric assay for cellular growth and survival: Application to proliferation and cytotoxicity assays. *Journal of Immunological Methods*, 65 (1983) 55–63.

106. Berridge M. V., Herst P. M., Tan A. S. Tetrazolium dyes as tools in cell biology: New insights into their cellular reduction. *Biotechnology Annual Review* Vol. 11 (2005) pp. 127–152, Elsevier, Oxford, UK.

107. van Meerloo J., Kaspers G. J. L., Cloos J. Cell Sensitivity Assays: The MTT Assay, In *Methods in Molecular Biology* Vol. 731, 237–245, Humana Press. New York City, USA.

108. Stockert J. C., Blázquez-Castro A., Cañete M., Horobin R. W., Villanueva Á. MTT assay for cell viability: Intracellular localization of the formazan product is in lipid droplets. *Acta Histochemica*, 114 (2012) 785–796.

109. Mathur H., C Rea M. Flow cytometry as a tool to study the effects of bacteriocins on prokaryotic and eukaryotic cells. *Journal of Molecular Biomarkers & Diagnosis*, (2016) doi:10.4172/2155-9929.S8-013.

110. Shapiro H. M. *Practical Flow Cytometry*, (2003) John Wiley & Sons, Inc. Hoboken, NJ, USA.

111. Sand S. L., Oppegård C., Ohara S., Iijima T., Naderi S., Blomhoff H. K., *et al.* A peptide pheromone produced by *Lactobacillus plantarum*, permeabilizes the cell membrane of both normal and cancerous lymphocytes and neuronal cells. *Peptides*, 31 (2010) 1237–1244.

112. Leuschner C., Hansel W. Membrane disrupting lytic peptides for cancer treatments. *Current Pharmaceutical Design*, 10 (2004) 2299–2310.

113. Paddock S. W. Principles and practices of laser scanning confocal microscopy. *Molecular Biotechnology*, 16 (2000) 127–150.

114. Vogelstein B., Lane D., Levine A. J. Surfing the p53 network. *Nature*, 408 (2000) 307–310.

115. Berridge M. J., Bootman M. D., Lipp P. Calcium—a life and death signal. *Nature*, 395 (1998) 645–648.

116. Suresh S. Biomechanics and biophysics of cancer cells. *Acta Materialia*, 55 (2007) 3989–4014.

117. Bastatas L., Martinez-Marin D., Matthews J., Hashem J., Lee Y. J., Sennoune S., *et al.* AFM nano-mechanics and calcium dynamics of prostate cancer cells with distinct metastatic potential. *Biochimica et Biophysica Acta*, 1820 (2012) 1111–1120.

118. Zhou Z., Zheng C., Li S., Zhou X., Liu Z., He Q., *et al.* AFM nanoindentation detection of the elastic modulus of tongue squamous carcinoma cells with different metastatic potentials. *Nanomedicine: Nanotechnology, Biology and Medicine*, 9 (2013) 864–874.

119. Davies J., Dawkes A. C., Haymes A. G., Sunderland R. F., Edwards J. C. Scanning tunnelling microscopy and dynamic contact angle studies of the effects of partial denaturation on immunoassay solid phase antibody. *Journal of Immunological Methods*, 186 (1995) 111–123.

120. Francis L. W., Gonzalez D., Ryder T., Baer K., Rees M., White J. O., *et al.* Optimized sample preparation for high-resolution AFM characterization of fixed human cells. *Journal of Microscopy*, 240 (2010) 111–121.

121. Canetta E., Riches A., Borger E., Herrington S., Dholakia K., Adya A. K. Discrimination of bladder cancer cells from normal urothelial cells with high specificity and sensitivity: Combined application of atomic force microscopy and modulated Raman spectroscopy. *Acta Biomaterialia*, 10 (2014) 2043–2055.

122. Docheva D., Padula D., Schieker M., Clausen-Schaumann H. Effect of collagen I and fibronectin on the adhesion, elasticity and cytoskeletal organization of prostate cancer cells. *Biochemical and Biophysical Research Communications*, 402 (2010) 361–366.

123. Eaton P., Zuzarte-Luis V., Mota M. M., Santos N. C., Prudêncio M. Infection by Plasmodium changes shape and stiffness of hepatic cells. *Nanomedicine: Nanotechnology, Biology and Medicine*, 8 (2012) 17–19.

124. Santos N. C., Castanho M. A. R. B. An overview of the biophysical applications of atomic force microscopy. *Biophysical Chemistry*, 107 (2004) 133–149.

125. Nguyen C., Nguyen V. D. Discovery of azurin-like anticancer bacteriocins from human gut microbiome through homology modeling and molecular docking against the tumor suppressor p53. *BioMed Research International*, 2016 (2016) 1–12.

126. Meincken M., Todorov S. Atomic force microscopy on the effect of bacteriocins on target cells: a new method for visualising its mode of action. *Trakia Journal of Sciences*, 7 (2009) 28–32.

127. Zhang W., Li J., Liu L. W., Wang K. R., Song J. J., Yan J. X., *et al.* A novel analog of antimicrobial peptide Polybia-MPI, with thioamide bond substitution, exhibits increased therapeutic efficacy against cancer and diminished toxicity in mice. *Peptides*, 31 (2010) 1832–1838.

128. Wang K., Zhang B., Zhang W., Yan J., Li J., Wang R. Antitumor effects, cell selectivity and structure-activity relationship of a novel antimicrobial peptide polybia-MPI. *Peptides*, 29 (2008) 963–968.

129. Greenfield N. J. Using circular dichroism spectra to estimate protein secondary structure. *Nature Protocols*, 1 (2006) 2876–2890.

130. Kelly S. M., Jess T. J., Price N. C. How to study proteins by circular dichroism. *Biochimica et Biophysica Acta–Proteins and Proteomics*, 1751 (2005) 119–139.

131. Pellecchia M., Sem D. S., Wüthrich K. NMR in drug discovery. *Nature Reviews Drug Discovery*, 1 (2002) 211–219.

132. Rizo J., Blanco F. J., Kobe B., Bruch M. D., Gierasch L. M. Conformational behavior of *Escherichia coli* OmpA signal peptides in membrane mimetic environments. *Biochemistry*, 32 (1993) 4881–4894.

133. García-Mayoral M. F., Moussaoui M., De La Torre B. G., Andreu D., Boix E., Nogués M. V., *et al.* NMR structural determinants of eosinophil cationic protein binding to membrane and heparin mimetics. *Biophysical Journal*, 98 (2010) 2702–2711.

134. Fregeau Gallagher N. L., Sailer M., Niemczura W. P., Nakashima T. T., Stiles M. E., Vederas J. C. Three-dimensional structure of leucocin a in trifluoroethanol and dodecylphosphocholine micelles: Spatial location of residues critical for biological activity in type IIa bacteriocins from lactic acid bacteria. *Biochemistry*, 36 (1997) 15062–15072.

135. Wang Y., Henz M. E., Fregeau Gallagher N. L., Chai S., Gibbs A. C., Yan L. Z., *et al.* Solution structure of carnobacteriocin B2 and implications for structure—Activity relationships among type IIa bacteriocins from lactic acid bacteria. *Biochemistry*, 38 (1999) 15438–15447.

136. Nissen-Meyer J., Rogne P., Oppegård C., Haugen H. S., Kristiansen P. E. Structure-function relationships of the non-lanthionine-containing peptide (class II) bacteriocins produced by gram-positive bacteria. *Current Pharmaceutical Biotechnology*, 10 (2009) 19–37.

137. Twomey D., Ross R. P., Ryan M., Meaney B., Hill C. Lantibiotics produced by lactic acid bacteria: Structure, function and applications. *Antonie van Leeuwenhoek*, 82 (2002) 165–185.

138. Haugen H. S., Fimland G., Nissen-Meyer J., Kristiansen P. E. Three-dimensional structure in lipid micelles of the pediocin-like antimicrobial peptide curvacin A. *Biochemistry*, 44 (2005) 16149–16157.

139. Uteng M., Hauge H. H., Markwick P. R. L., Fimland G., Mantzilas D., Nissen-Meyer J., *et al.* Three-dimensional structure in lipid micelles of the pediocin-like antimicrobial peptide sakacin P and a sakacin P variant that is structurally stabilized by an inserted C-terminal disulfide bridge. *Biochemistry*, 42 (2003) 11417–11426.

140. Hooven H. W., Fogolari F., Rollema H. S., Konings R. N. H., Hilbers C. W., Ven F. J. M. NMR and circular dichroism studies of the lantibiotic nisin in non-aqueous environments. *FEBS Letters*, 319 (1993) 189–194.

141. Ven F. J. M., Hooven H. W., Konings R. N. H., Hilbers C. W. NMR studies of lantibiotics. The structure of nisin in aqueous solution. *European Journal of Biochemistry*, 202 (1991) 1181–1188.

142. Hooven H. W., Doeland C. C. M., Kamp M., Konings R. N. H., Hilbers C. W., Ven F. J. M. Three-dimensional structure of the lantibiotic nisin in the presence of membrane-mimetic micelles of dodecylphosphocholine and of sodium dodecylsulphate. *European Journal of Biochemistry*, 235 (1996) 382–393.

143. Zimmermann N., Freund S., Fredenhagen A., Jung G. Solution structures of the lantibiotics duramycin B and C. *European Journal of Biochemistry*, 216 (1993) 419–428.

144. Hauge H. H., Nissen-Meyer J., Nes I. F., Eijsink V. G. H. Amphiphilic alpha-helices are important structural motifs in the alpha and beta peptides that constitute the bacteriocin lactococcin G. Enhancement of helix formation upon alpha-beta interaction. *European Journal of Biochemistry*, 251 (1998) 565–572.

145. Rogne P., Fimland G., Nissen-Meyer J., Kristiansen P. E. Three-dimensional structure of the two peptides that constitute the two-peptide lactococcin G. *Biochimica et Biophysica Acta–Proteins and Proteomics*, 1784 (2008) 1711–1719.

146. Prasch T., Naumann T., Marker R. L. M., Sattler M., Schubert W., Schaal S., *et al.* Constitution and solution conformation of the antibiotic mersacidin determined by NMR and molecular dynamics. *European Journal of Biochemistry*, 244 (1997) 501–512.

147. Hauge H. H., Mantzilas D., Eijsink V. G. H., Nissen-Meyer J. Membrane-mimicking entities induce structuring of the two-peptide bacteriocins plantaricin E/F and plantaricin J/K. *Journal of Bacteriology*, 181 (1999) 740–747.

148. Turner D. L., Brennan L., Meyer H. E., Lohaus C., Siethoff C., Costa H. S., *et al.* Solution structure of plantaricin C., a novel lantibiotic. *European Journal of Biochemistry*, 264 (1999) 833–839.

Chapter 12

Where Cancer and Bacteria Meet

Alexandra Merlos,[a,b] Ricardo Perez-Tomás,[c] José López-López,[b] and Miguel Viñas[a]

[a]*Laboratory of Molecular Microbiology & Antimicrobials, Department of Pathology and Experimental Therapeutics Medical School, Campus Bellvitge, University of Barcelona, Feixa Llarga s/n. Pavelló de Govern, Hospitalet, Barcelona, Spain*
[b]*Oral Medicine Section, Medical School, Campus Bellvitge, University of Barcelona, Feixa Llarga s/n. Pavelló de Govern, Hospitalet, Barcelona, Spain*
[c]*Cancer Cell Biology Research Group (CCBRG), Department of Pathology & Experimental Therapeutics, Medical School, Campus Bellvitge, University of Barcelona, Feixa Llarga s/n. Pavelló de Govern, Hospitalet, Barcelona, Spain*

mvinyas@ub.edu

12.1 Introduction

More than 10 years ago, the Australian microbiologists Barry J. Marshall and J. Robin Warren became Nobel laureates for their work demonstrating that infection by the bacterium *Helicobacter pylori* is closely related to several gastric pathologies, specifically gastritis, peptic ulcer, and gastric carcinoma. In fact, the two researchers succeeded in demonstrating that *H. pylori* is the etiologic agent of these diseases. *H. pylori* is a gram-negative microaerophilic bacterium that induces a chronic infectious state

Microbial Infections and Cancer Therapy: Recent Advances
Edited by Ananda M. Chakrabarty and Arsénio M. Fialho

ISBN 978-981-4774-86-4 (Hardcover), 978-1-351-04190-4 (eBook)
www.panstanford.com

as a precursor of chronic gastritis, peptic ulcer, gastric and duodenal cancer, and mucosa-associated lymphoid tissue lymphoma [1]. Furthermore, a role for *H. pylori* in other diseases, including cardiovascular disease, liver and biliary tract diseases, and colorectal cancer, has been studied and reported. In these cases, *H. pylori* is not the etiological agent but seems to act synergistically to significantly contribute to the development of the pathology. Roughly half of the human population, at some point, becomes infected with *H. pylori*, but only a relatively small number of individuals will develop gastric ulcer and even fewer will develop gastric cancer or one of the other aforementioned diseases. This has been attributed to the genetic diversity of *H. pylori*, such that the risk of disease depends on the colonizing strain of the bacterium [2–5].

The well-established relationship between cancer and infection has given rise to new perspectives on antimicrobials, which are now being used to prevent cancer, and also to a closer examination of the relationship between bacterial infection and cancer in general. However, despite intensive research, *H. pylori* is the only bacterium currently considered by the WHO as a class I human carcinogen, that is, as an etiologic agent of a specific form of cancer. Moreover, the relationship between cancer and infection is complex, since bacteria may contribute to or even be the main cause of cancer, but they and their products are also being effectively used in cancer treatment. This diverse and contradictory relationship is discussed in this review.

12.2 Infection and Neoplasia

Infection-mediated carcinogenesis has been confirmed through a series of long and complex epidemiological studies and meta-analyses. Indeed, ~20% of the worldwide cancer burden can be attributed to microbial-mediated oncogenesis. The recognition of the potential relationship between microbial prevalence and the incidence of cancer has revealed several previously hidden associations besides *H. pylori* and gastric cancer, some of which were later also determined to be causative. The most well-known examples include hepatitis B and C viruses, schistosomiasis, and Epstein–Barr virus, causing liver, bladder, and nasopharyngeal cancer, respectively (Table 12.1) [6]. However, most of the work linking cancer and infection has been based on epidemiological studies, some of which have become outdated. New studies, especially those concerning mechanisms of carcinogenesis, are therefore needed.

Table 12.1 The main bacterial species, viruses, chemical agents, and predisposing conditions involved in oncogenesis

Infectious/Inflammatory agent	Cancer type
Schistosomiasis	Bladder cancer
***Helicobacter pylori*-induced gastritis**	Gastric cancer
H. pylori	Mucosa-associated lymphoid tissue lymphoma
H. pylori	Pancreatic cancer
Porphyromonas gingivalis	Pancreatic cancer
P. gingivalis	Oral cancer
Fusobacterium nucleatum	Oral, pancreatic, and colorectal cancer
Bacteroides species	Colon cancer
Hepatitis virus (B and C)	Hepatocellular carcinoma
HHV8	Kaposi's sarcoma
Silica/Cigarette smoke	Bronchial carcinoma
Inflammatory bowel disease	Colorectal cancer
Barrett's metaplasia	Esophageal cancer
Prostatitis	Prostate cancer
Thyroiditis	Papillary thyroid carcinoma
Asbestos	Mesothelioma
Salpingitis/talc/ovulation/endometriosis Pelvic inflammatory disease/tissue remodeling	Ovarian cancer
Papillomavirus	Cervical cancer

Note: Approximately 20% of the total cancer burden may be mediated by microorganisms, with inflammation as the initial and main process involved in oncogenesis [7]. Chronic inflammation caused by chemical and physical agents [8] as well as by autoimmune and inflammatory reactions of uncertain etiology [7–10] also increase the risk of malignancy.

The classical division of bacteria into gram-positive and gram-negative is mostly based on the strong differences in the bacterial wall. Gram-negative bacteria are surrounded by a double membrane: a plasma membrane that is very similar to the plasma membranes of all cell systems and an additional outer membrane. This external lipid bilayer is atypical because its external leaflet is mostly (if not exclusively) formed by lipopolysaccharides (LPSs) instead of phospholipids. Nevertheless, from a physiological point of view, the permeability barrier formed by the outer membrane is similar to that of other lipid bilayers. However, unlike the plasma membrane, the outer membrane lacks biological energy because energetic metabolism is restricted to the cytoplasm, with which the outer membrane does not have contact. These differences have conditioned the evolution of bacterial strategies of infection. Thus, whereas the pathogenicity mechanisms of gram-negative bacteria are generally based on invasive processes, those of gram-positive species involve virulence factors, which in most cases are secreted proteins that include a wide variety of toxins and enzymes with broad-ranging effects on cell integrity and metabolism. Both gram-negative and gram-positive bacteria have been linked, directly or indirectly, to cancer.

12.2.1 Gram-Negative Bacteria

In addition to *H. pylori*, several other species of gram-negative bacteria are associated with cancer. *Salmonella*, like *H. pylori*, is a gram-negative facultative anaerobe with the epidemiologically demonstrated ability to promote chronic inflammation. For example, after episodes of active *Salmonella* infection the gallbladder frequently remains colonized by the bacterium. Thus, individuals carrying *Salmonella* in the gallbladder become *Salmonella* carriers. While the carrier state is nonsymptomatic, the persisting infection produces chronic inflammation, which has been shown to directly influence the emergence of gallbladder cancer [11, 12].

The healthy human stomach contains several bacterial genera, among them *Haemophilus, Prevotella, Streptococcus, Veillonella,* and *Rothia*. Nevertheless, the composition of the gastric microbial populations is diverse and mutable and is strongly influenced by factors such as antibiotic use, alcohol ingestion, diet, and disease state. The interaction between the "normal" microbiota and *H. pylori* infection may play a key role in determining the risk of gastric diseases and, subsequently, cancer. This would imply relevant roles in carcinogenicity for several other facultative gram-negative bacteria [13].

Among aerobic gram-negative bacteria, only one species, *Neisseria gonorrhoeae*, has thus far been epidemiologically related to a specific cancer, namely prostate cancer, demonstrated in a population of Mexican males [14]. The authors of that study inferred a key etiological role for sexually transmitted diseases, particularly gonorrhea, in prostate cancer, consistent with previous publications. The main mechanism was suggested to involve the direct action of either the bacterium or its products on host DNA and the subsequent deregulation of oncogenic proteins, such as p21, p27, and p53.

Anaerobic gram-negative bacteria have also been implicated in several forms of cancer. One of the best studied species is *Fusobacterium nucleatum,* representative of the genus *Fusobacterium*. This spindle-shaped strict anaerobe is commonly found both in the oral cavity and in the gut. *F. nucleatum* induces permanent chronic inflammation in the colon and has thus been associated with colorectal cancer. However, the mechanism is still unclear. Rubinstein *et al.* [15] showed that *F. nucleatum* adheres to and invades tissues, which activates inflammatory responses and stimulates the growth of colorectal cells. The underlying mechanism involves the interaction of colonic cells with the bacterial adhesin FadA, which binds to E-cadherin. The same authors showed 100 times higher *fadA* gene levels in the colon tissue from patients with adenomas and adenocarcinomas than in healthy individuals, thus identifying FadA as a potential diagnostic and therapeutic target for colorectal cancer.

Another strictly anaerobic gram-negative bacterium associated with cancer is *Bacteroides fragilis*. Carbohydrate metabolism by *B. fragilis* produces numerous organic acids as metabolic waste. A relationship between *B. fragilis* and colorectal cancer has been suggested on the basis of the induced production of reactive oxygen species (ROS), which in turn causes DNA damage, although there is also evidence of direct activation [12]. Consistent with these observations, in an animal model antibiotic treatment was shown to reduce colon tumorigenesis [16].

Among the anaerobic gram-negative bacteria associated with cancer, those in the oral microbiota merit special mention. They include some whose existence is known only from molecular data as they have not yet been cultured. Other species, such as *Porphyromonas gingivalis*, have been very well described, mainly because they cause periodontal diseases. Bacteriologically, *P. gingivalis*is closely related to *Bacteroides*, with which it shares many physiological features, but *P. gingivalis* is an oral microbe whereas *Bacteroides* is not. Epidemiological studies have established an association between *P. gingivalis* and both oral cancer and squamous carcinoma of the esophagus. Thus, while *P. gingivalis* is an oral microbe, its presence in the esophagus is common; it is also found in the gut. The carcinogenicity of *P. gingivalis* in the esophagus is thought to involve the microbe's direct inhibition of apoptosis and the modification of cyclins and cyclin-dependent kinases (CDKs), with the latter inducing drastic changes in the cell cycle and therefore in cell progression [17].

In addition, a growing number of studies suggest an underlying infectious component to pancreatic cancer [6] involving two of the usual suspects in infection-mediated carcinogenesis, *H. pylori* and *P. gingivalis*.

LPS produced by gram-negative bacteria can be inhaled through cigarette smoke. In an animal model, it plays a key role in the development of lung carcinoma [18]. The triggering of innate immunity and the mounting of an acute response are generally followed by a late phase, in which regulatory mechanisms, tissue repair, and remodeling prevail. Lung tumorigenesis in response to 4-(methylnitrosamino)-1-(3-pyridyl)-1-butanone had a more significant outcome in mice when LPS was also administered; both a higher number of and more histologically advanced tumors were observed, as was observed evidence of inflammation, including macrophage recruitment and cell proliferation [18]. Acute inflammation triggered by the exogenous administration of tumor necrosis factor (TNF)-α, interleukin (IL)-1, and LPS may, under certain conditions, promote malignancy and metastasis [9]. In mice, inflammatory mechanisms account for the tumor-promoting effect of tobacco smoke on lung cancer [19], but in humans most neoplastic conditions are provoked by chronic local inflammatory reactions, with few systemic manifestations [20].

12.2.2 Gram-Positive Bacteria

Two examples of the association of gram-positive bacteria and cancer are briefly described as following:

Propionibacterium acnes is an anaerobic rod-shaped species and a common inhabitant of human skin. It produces propionic acid as a normal metabolite. However, its presence in the prostate causes inflammation that has been linked to prostate cancer [21], although direct evidence is lacking.

Bacillus is a highly diverse, heterogeneous, and complex genus. Its virulence and pathogenic characteristics account for the ability of member species to easily colonize, grow, and develop in any tissue. Spore formation, a biofilm life style, and toxin production are three of the most relevant characteristics by which *Bacillus* causes sustained chronic irritation and/or inflammation that gradually gives way to oncogenesis. *Bacillus* species are recognized as the causative agent of several infections, but the number of isolates in cancers, wounds, or infections has probably been underestimated. This is because in clinical specimens *Bacillus* is often considered as a contaminant colony rather than as a contributing etiologic agent.

Most members of this genus and related taxa form stable biofilms, which in combination with sporulation ensure cell survival within the tissue confines. Moreover, cytotoxic molecules produced by *Bacillus* cells and secreted into the extracellular space are taken up by erythrocytes and fibroblasts and in some host species by cells of the colon, causing partial or total lysis. The pore-forming proteins of *Bacillus* enable the entry of surrounding molecules and play a key role in necrosis, inflammation, and possibly cancer development, by inducing the synthesis of ROS and other carcinogenic compounds.

The *Bacillus* species isolated from different tobacco brands include *B. amyloliquefaciens, B. cereus, B. subtilis, B. methylotrophicus, B. pumilus, Oceanobacillus chungangensis*, and *B. licheniformis*, whereas *B. subtilis, B. pumilus, B. methylotrophicus*, and *B. licheniformis* have been identified in lung cancer biopsies. Tobacco flakes carrying bacteria and trapped within the cigarette filters provide the main entrance for the pathogen into the pulmonary airways [22]. The powerful colonization ability of the isolates has been demonstrated in adhesion assays, as has the secretion of pore-forming toxins with high cytotoxicity in cytotoxicity assays using planar lipid bilayers and cell cultures [23]. Molecular pathways involving mycobacteria in carcinogenesis have been identified as well [24].

12.3 Head and Neck Cancers and Bacterial Oral Microbiota

Over 700 bacterial species inhabit the oral cavity, with most living in a more or less symbiotic relationship with host cells and the host immune system [25, 26]. However, there is increasing evidence of a link between the oral microbiota and several systemic pathologies, including cancer and especially oral squamous cell carcinoma (OSCC). Between 350,000 and 400,000 new cases of head and neck cancer are diagnosed every year throughout the world, and the incidence is rising as tobacco and alcohol consumption is increasing, particularly among young populations [27]. Nonetheless, although smoking and alcohol are the main factors contributing to the development of carcinoma in the oral cavity, their effects do not suffice to explain "field cancerization" [28, 29]. Furthermore, oral cancer is frequently diagnosed in non-smoking, non-alcohol-consuming individuals [30].

At the molecular level, the pathogenesis of oral cancer has been attributed to the deregulation of cellular pathways such that carcinogenesis is promoted and to the expression of tumor suppressors, such as p53 and CDKN2A. The cancer-provoking molecules in head and neck cancers include carcinogenic substances and their metabolites, via a chronic inflammatory process [31, 32] involving myeloid and nonmyeloid cells (polymorphonuclear neutrophils, oral keratinocytes, macrophages, osteoclasts, osteoblasts, and dendritic cells). The membrane-associated receptors, secreted pattern recognition receptors, nucleotide-binding oligomerization domain-like receptors, toll-like receptors, RIG-I-like receptors, and C-type lectin receptors on these cells interact with periodontal microbial components that include microbe-associated molecular patterns (MAMPs), such as fimbriae, BspA (*Bacteroides* surface protein A), lipoproteins, LPS, and nucleic acids. These interactions may stimulate the production of damage/danger-associated molecules, such as fibrinogen, heat-shock proteins, and nucleic acids [33].

In this context, infectious agents, mostly bacteria, influence cancer emergence and progression [34] but do not induce cancer directly. For example, long-term infection of oral cancer cells by *P. gingivalis* leads to the increased expression of the malignant stem cell markers CD44 and CD133 and exacerbates the tumorigenic properties of infected versus noninfected cancer cells [35]. Moreover, *P. gingivalis* is a noncanonical activator of β-catenin, inducing the disassociation of the β-catenin destruction complex by gingipain-dependent proteolytic processing. β-Catenin activation in epithelial cells by *P. gingivalis* may thus contribute to a proliferative phenotype [36]. A relationship between other oral bacteria, such as the above-mentioned *F. nucleatum*, and cancer has also been proposed on the basis of the observed stimulation of human OSCC proliferation and the expression of key molecules involved in tumorigenesis [37].

Several periodontal pathogens, particularly *P. gingivalis*, *F. nucleatum*, and *Prevotella intermedia*, are associated with OSCC, as per a model similar to that of gastric cancer and *H. pylori* [37]. For example, as shown in Fig. 12.1, *F. nucleatum* activates p38, leading to the secretion of MMP-9 and MMP-13 (collagenase 3). The effects of *F. nucleatum* LPS are similar to those of *P. gingivalis* LPS on epithelial cells. *F. nucleatum* LPS activates inflammatory cytokines, such as TNF-α, IL-1b, and IL-6. These events become cyclic, leading to periodontal attachment and tissue damage. However, *F. nucleatum* LPS differs from the LPS of *Escherichia coli* because of its higher content of 2-keto-3-deoxyoctonate and heptoses, both of which play a relevant role in inducing cell injury and in cytokine-mediated inflammation, through the modulation of several apoptotic pathways [37–39].

Other suspected culprit bacterial species are *Prevotella melaninogenica, Streptococcus mitis*, and *Capnocytophaga gingivalis*, high levels of which have been proposed as OSCC markers [40] on the basis of the following capabilities of different serotypes (Fig. 12.2): (i) epithelial colonization; (ii) carcinogen production (nitrosamines, acetaldehyde, and 4-nitroquinoline-1-oxide, among others) [41, 42]; (iii) their ability to metabolize procarcinogens, such as acetaldehyde and hydroethyl radicals, ethoxy radicals, and tobacco, to acetaldehyde; and (iv) their modification of chronic inflammation, for example, by suppressing the activation of activator protein-1. Periodontal pathogenic species may also induce anticardiolipin antibodies in periodontitis patients in response to the antigenically similar bacterial proteins glycoprotein I and serum protein β-2. Because the induction of antiphospholipid antibodies is closely related to the infectious process and thus to chronic inflammation [43], chronic periodontal disease and the presence of subgingival plaques containing anaerobic bacteria have been implicated in head-and-neck squamous cell carcinoma.

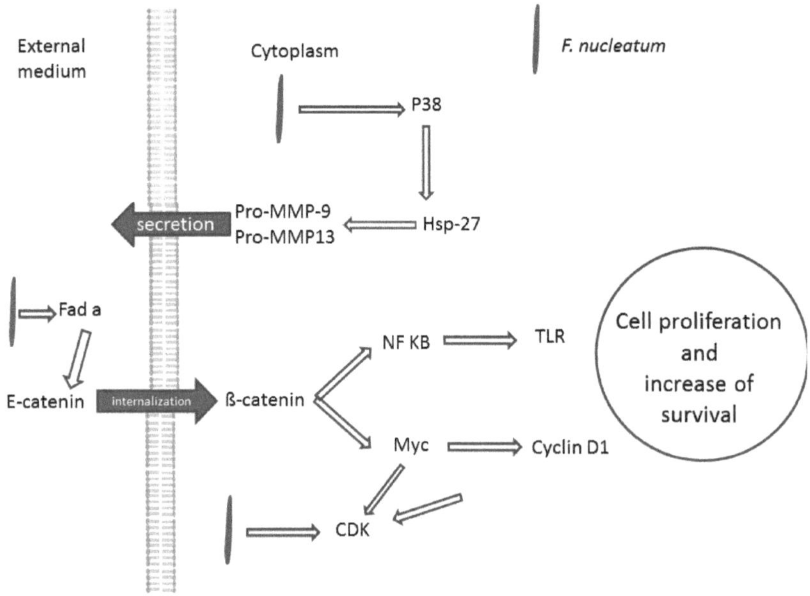

Figure 12.1 The possible role of *F. nucleatum* in the transformation of an epithelial cell into an oncogenic phenotype involves FadA (encoding a critical host colonization factor), which promotes the internalization of *β*-catenin and therefore cell survival and proliferation. Intracellular *Fusobacterium* activates P38, leading to the secretion of MMP-9 and MMP-13, both of which play a key role in the malignant transformation of squamous cells.

Poor oral health has also been linked to pancreatic, intestinal, and esophageal cancers. A reduction in tobacco consumption delays the clinical manifestations of chronic inflammation, and smoking cessation enhances gingival health [44].

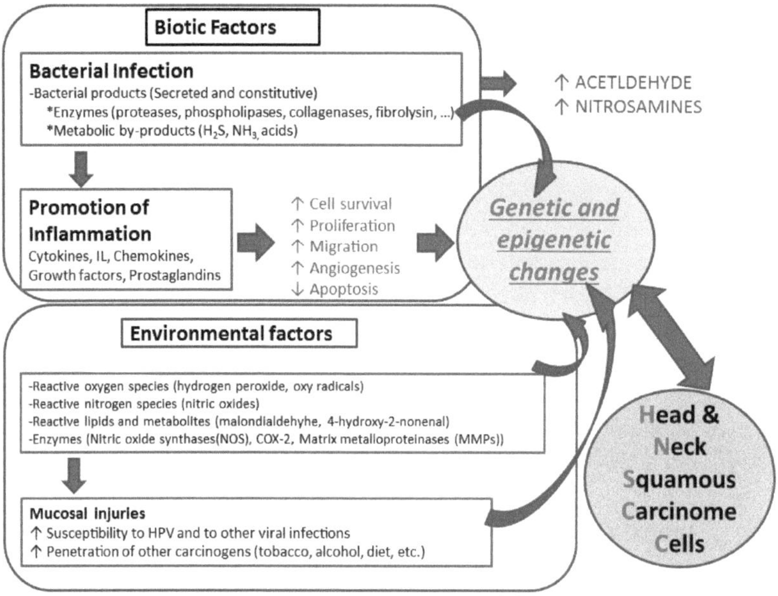

Figure 12.2 Pathways involved in the relationship between chronic periodontal disease and the induction of head-and-neck cancer. Adapted from [43].

Apart from bacteria other microbes, such as yeasts, have been also more or less implicated in some kinds of cancer. There is a lack of evidence to support the relation between chronic candidiasis and cervix cancer. Concerning oral chronic candidiasis, it has been shown that in immunocompromised patients, esophagus cancer is frequently associated with chronic mucocutaneous candidiasis and infrequently with autoimmune polyendocrinopathy-candidiasis-ectodermal dystrophy [45].

In fact, it has been suggested that the participation of nitrosamine compounds produced by chronic *Candida* infections could be a risk factor for esophageal cancer [45]. *Candida albicans* is the most typical *Candida* species present in leukoplakia and chronic hyper plastic candidiasis (CHC) [42, 46, 47]. Moreover, it has been reported that oral carriage of *Candida albicans* is higher in patients with OSCC or leukoplakia than in patients without oral pathology; and that the degree of epithelial dysplasia present in these patients also correlates with higher titles of yeasts in the oral cavity [48, 49].

12.4 Bacteria and Bacterial Products in Cancer Treatment

While bacteria have been implicated as causative agents in several cancers, they and their products have also been used to therapeutic effect. Over the last decade, there has been an explosion in the discovery and development of small organic molecule as anticancer drugs. Several gram-negative aerobes have been shown to exert inhibitory effects on cancer cells and are being explored as promising anticancer agents. For example, *Pseudomonas aeruginosa* fragments (mannose-sensitive fimbriae) inhibit pancreatic cancer growth [50] by inducing apoptosis and inhibiting tumor cell proliferation. This activity is mediated by hindering epidermal growth factor receptor signaling and by activation of the caspase pathway.

A diverse resource for new anticancer drugs is the marine environment, with its abundance of aquatic plants and animals, many of which have been screened for antifungal, antimicrobial, anti-inflammatory, anticancer, and analgesic properties. Among the more than 13,000 molecules described thus far, active properties were determined for ~3000 [51]. Of these, >590 are currently in the pipeline of pharmaceutical-discovery programs or phase III clinical trials [51–53].

Ionophores promote ion transport across lipid bilayers and include a large number of naturally occurring molecules. External disruption of the ion permeability of membranes disturbs the normal ion balance, a property that can be exploited in the induction of cell death (apoptosis, autophagy, or necrosis), including that of tumor cells, or the elimination of harmful microorganisms. While anion-selective ionophores (anionophores) are much less common than cationophores, they have attracted intense interest over the last two decades. Anionophores are natural products that facilitate transmembrane anion transport across phospholipid bilayers [54]. This capability is crucial for the maintenance of the concentration gradients that form the basis for signaling and cellular regulation.

A few examples of anionophores with anticancer activity are provided below.

12.4.1 Prodiginines

One of the first microorganisms to be used in cancer therapy was *Serratia marcescens,* a microorganism characterized by the production of prodigiosin [55]. The microbe and its secondary metabolites were first assayed to experimentally treat cancer in studies performed almost 70 years ago [56]. Soon thereafter, studies on the effect of bacterial polysaccharide fractions on tissue cultures of normal chicken fibroblasts and mouse sarcoma cells showed that while these fractions are not directly toxic for the tissues, they enhance the areal increase of both tissue types [57]. These results provided slight evidence that *Serratia marcescens*, while in principle useful as an anticancer agent, is also able to induce the abnormal growth of human cells. More recently, however, prodigiosin has been extensively tested in experimental oncology (for a review, see Ref. [58]).

One of the most important families of anionophores consists of prodiginines, produced by microorganisms such as *Streptomyces* sp. and *Serratia marcescens* [59]. Prodigiosin (2-methyl-3-pentyl-6-methoxyprodiginine), within the red-pigmented prodiginines family, is an alkaloid secondary metabolite synthesized by *Serratia marcescens*, among other microorganisms [55], and located in the bacterial inner membrane [60]. The structure of prodigiosin (Fig. 12.3a) ($C_{20}H_{25}N_3O$) was clarified in the early 1960s, when partial and total chemical synthesis revealed a pyrrolyl-dipyrromethene core skeleton. Prodigiosin occurs in solution in interconverting cis (or β) and trans (or α) conformations. The equilibrium between the two is dependent on the solution pH. The biological role of prodigiosin in producer organisms remains unclear [61], although the alkaloid is a very efficient anion exchanger that facilitates $Cl^-/HCO3^-$ exchange across lipid bilayers. The antifungal, immunosuppressive, and anticancer activities of prodigiosin have been described in several studies [62, 63]. Its structural analog obatoclax mesylate (GX15-070MS) is currently in phase II clinical trials to test its efficacy in combination with first-line drugs for the treatment of hematological malignancies and solid tumors [64–66].

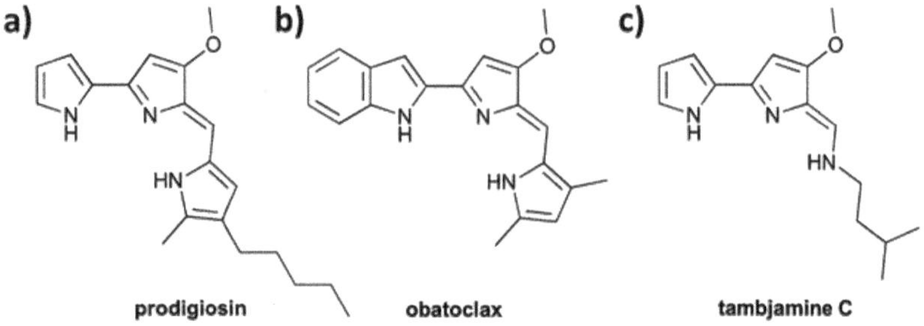

Figure 12.3 Molecular structure of three natural anionophores.

12.4.1.1 Properties and mechanism of action of prodigiosin

The wide-ranging pharmacological activities of the tripyrrole prodigiosin have been the focus of increasing interest, including as a potent antimalarial drug with high toxicity against the causative agent *Plasmodium falciparum* [67]; as an inhibitor of the growth of gram-positive and gram-negative bacteria [68] as well as fungi [69]; and as an immunosuppressive agent, based on the ability of prodigiosin to block T lymphocyte activation, primarily by inhibiting IL-2-receptor-α expression [70]. Of relevance to this review, however, is the capacity of prodigiosin to trigger apoptosis in malignant cancer cells. This small molecule is now generally recognized as an anticancer compound, an activity demonstrated both *in vitro* and *in vivo* [71, 72].

The mechanism of action by which prodigiosin exerts its cytotoxicity in cancer cells has yet to be fully elucidated, but it being a small molecule multiple processes are likely to be involved. Indeed, prodigiosin has multiple cellular targets, summarized in Fig. 12.4. The induction of cell stress is one of the mechanisms that may account for the anticancer activity of prodigiosin, specifically, uncoupling of the vacuolar-type ATPase by promoting H^+/Cl^- symport in lysosomes and subsequent disruption of the pH gradient [73, 74]. This can lead to cell-cycle blockage or cell death by apoptosis [75, 76] (Fig. 12.5). In addition, prodigiosin intercalates within double-stranded DNA, leading to the latter's copper-mediated cleavage. Prodigiosin also inhibits topoisomerases I and II activity, resulting in DNA rupture and therefore apoptosis [58, 76, 77].

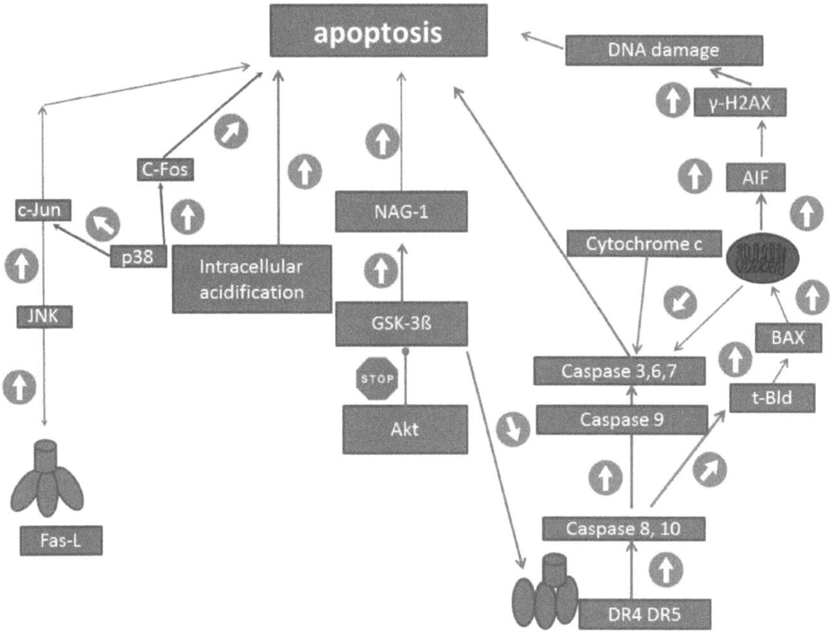

Figure 12.4 Prodigiosin activates pathways that promote the inhibition of cancer development.

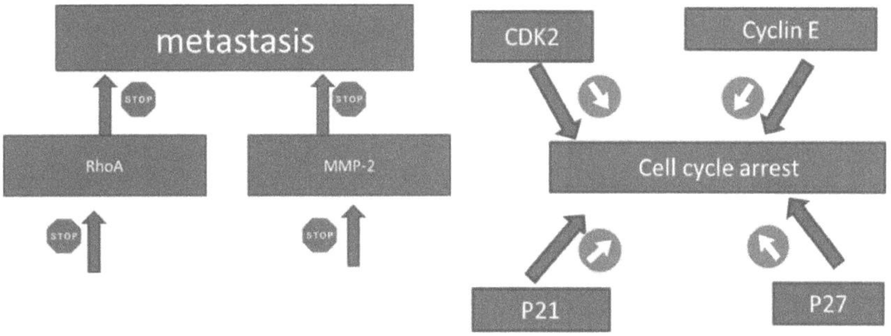

Figure 12.5 The inhibition of RhoA and MMP-2 has a result of inhibition of metastasis. The activation of cyclin E, CDK2, P27 leads to the arrest of cell cycle. In both cases these constitute anticancer mechanisms.

GX15-070MS inhibits the binding of antiapoptotic Bcl-2 to the proapoptotic proteins Bax and Bak, thus triggering the apoptosis pathway in Bcl-2-overexpressing cancer cells [78]. It also promotes other forms of programmed cell death, including autophagic cell death [79–82] and necroptosis [83].

12.4.2 Tambjamines

Tambjamines are derived from bacteria of the genus *Pseudoalteromonas* and from a large group of marine invertebrates, including bryozoans, nudibranchs, and ascidians [84]. In the latter group, they serve as chemical defense compounds that protect against predators. The 4-methoxy-2,2′-bipyrrolenamine structure (Fig. 12.6) of tambjamines is clearly related to the structure of prodiginines, including prodigiosin (Fig. 12.3a). Like these compounds, tambjamines are alkaloids with intriguing biological activities, including as antimicrobial, cytotoxic, and antitumor agents [85–88].

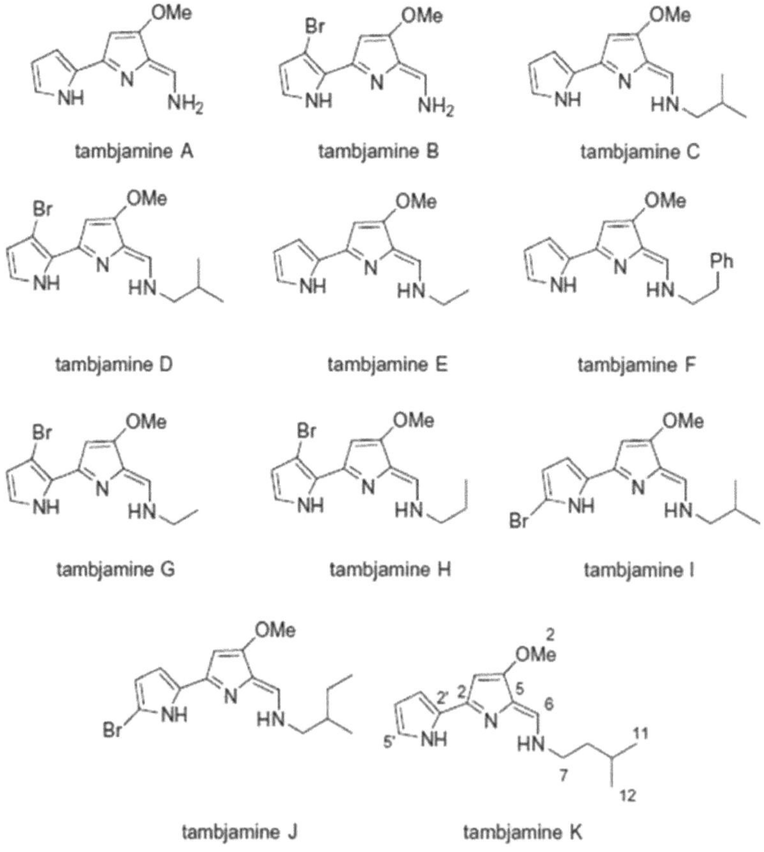

Figure 12.6 Structures of the tambjamines.

12.4.2.1 Properties and mechanism of action

The biological potential of tambjamines was confirmed in studies of tambjamines A–D, which demonstrated their antimicrobial effect [89].

As natural anionophores tambjamines facilitate the permeabilization of cell membranes and thus upset the normal intracellular ionic balance. Spectroscopic analysis of the structure of tambjamines revealed strong hydrogen bonding between these compounds and the chloride anion [87]. The two heterocycles and the enamine moiety are essentially coplanar. A chloride anion interacts with the pyrrole and enamine N–H groups, whereas the indole moiety is rotated 180° and interacts with a second chloride anion. However, in their preferred conformation tambjamines bind with the anion through the hydrogen bond cleft involving the three N–H groups of the molecule [90].

12.4.2.2 Synthetic analogs of tambjamines

In the search for compounds with efficient transport capacity, 11 derivatives of naturally occurring tambjamines have been synthesized (Fig. 12.7).

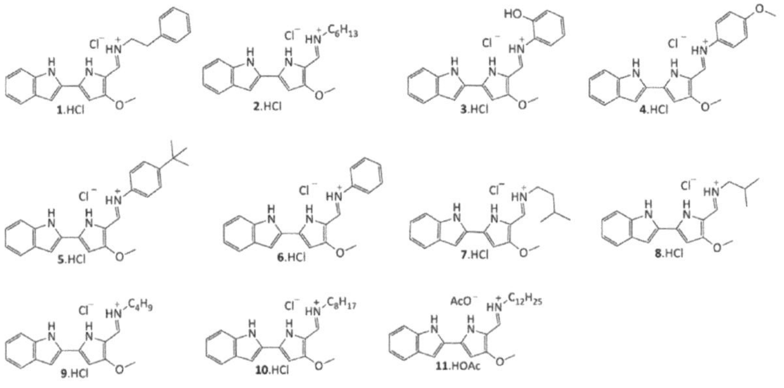

Figure 12.7 Tambjamine analogs.

These indole-based tambjamine analogs have been used to demonstrate that anion transport induces cell membrane hyperpolarization and cell death in cancer stem cells [91]. The mechanisms responsible for the cytotoxicity of these tambjamine analogs have been studied by one of the authors (Ricardo Pérez-Tomás). The results revealed both a decrease in the intracellular pH (acidification) and the induction of apoptosis through p38 mitogen-activated protein kinase activation [92].

References

1. Marshall B. J., Warren J. R. Unidentified curved bacilli in the stomach of patients with gastritis and peptic ulceration. *Lancet*, **16** (1984) 1311–1315.
2. Zhu R. M., Qin T. S., Jin X. X., Xu W. A., Wang Z. K., Wang L. *Helicobacter pylori* typing and upper digestive tract disease relationship. *Yixue Yanjiusheng Xuebao*, **18** (2005) 911017.
3. Shen J., Lu M., Feng C. W. *Helicobacter pylori* infection and diseases of liver and gall of progress. *Gastroenterology Hepatology Journal*, **22** (2013) 123–125.
4. Venkateshwari A., Krishnaveni D., Venugopal S., Shashikumar P., Vidyasagar A., Jyothy A. *Helicobacter pylori* infection in relation to gastric cancer progression. *Indian Journal of Cancer*, **48** (2011) 94–98 [PMID: 21248438 DOI: 10.4103/0019-509X.75840].
5. Sachs G., Wen Y., Scott D. R. Gastric infection by *Helicobacter pylori*. *Current Gastroenterology Reports*, **11** (2009) 455–461 [PMID: 19903421 DOI: 10.1007/s11894-009-0070-y].
6. Michaud D. S. Role of bacterial infections in pancreatic cancer. *Carcinogenesis*, **34** (2013) 2193–2197.
7. Pisani S., Gallinelli C., Seganti L., Lukic A., Nobili F., Vetrano G., Imperi M., Degener A. M., Chiarini F. Detection of viral and bacterial infections in women with normal and abnormal colposcopy. *European Journal of Gynaecological Oncology*, **20** (1999) 69–73.
8. Gulumian M. The role of oxidative stress in diseases caused by mineral dusts and fibres: current status and future of prophylaxis and treatment. *Molecular and Cellular Biochemistry*, **196** (1999) 69–77.
9. Balkwill F., Mantovani A. Inflammation and cancer: Back to Virchow? *Lancet*, **357** (2001) 539–545.
10. Ekbom A., Helmick C., Zack M., Adami HO. Increased risk of large-bowel cancer in Crohn's disease with colonic involvement. *Lancet*, **336** (1990) 357–359.

11. Ye Z., Petrof E. O., Boone D., Claud E. C., Sun J. *Salmonella* effector AvrA regulation of colonic epithelial cell inflammation by deubiquitination. *American Journal of Pathology*, **17** (2007) 882–892.

12. Wu S., Ye Z., Liu X., Zhao Y., Xia Y., Steiner A., *et al. Salmonella typhimurium* infection increases p53 acetylation in intestinal epithelial cells. *American Journal of Physiology. Gastrointestinal and Liver Physiology*, **298** (2010) G784–G794.

13. Nardone G., Compare D. The human gastric microbiota: Is it time to rethink the pathogenesis of stomach diseases? *United European Gastroenterology Journal*, **3** (2015) 255–260 doi: 10.1177/205064061 4566846.

14. Vázquez-Salas R. A., Torres-Sánchez L., López-Carrillo L., Romero-Martínez M., Manzanilla-García H. A., Cruz-Ortíz C. H., *et al.* History of gonorrhea and prostate cancer in a population-based case-control study in Mexico. *Cancer Epidemiology*, **40** (2016) 95–101 doi: 10.1016/j.canep.2015.12.001.

15. Rubinstein M. R., Wang X., Liu W., Hao Y., Cai G., Han Y. W. *Fusobacterium nucleatum* promotes colorectal carcinogenesis by modulating E-cadherin/β-catenin signaling via its FadA adhesin. *Cell Host & Microbe*, **14** (2013) 195–206.

16. DeStefano Shields C. E., Van Meerbeke S. W., Housseau F., Wang H., Huso D. L., Casero R. A. Jr., *et al.* Reduction of murine colon tumorigenesis driven by enterotoxigenic bacteroides fragilis using cefoxitin treatment. *Journal of Infectious Diseases*, **214** (2016) 122–129.

17. Gao S., Li S., Ma Z., Liang S., Shan T., Zhang M., *et al.* Presence of *Porphyromonas gingivalis* in esophagus and its association with the clinicopathological characteristics and survival in patients with esophageal cancer. *Infectious Agents and Cancer*, **11** (2016) 3 doi: 10.1186/s13027-016-0049-x. eCollection 2016.

18. Melkamu T., Qian X., Upadhyaya P., O'Sullivan M. G., Kassie F. Lipopolysaccharide enhances mouse lung tumorigenesis: A model for inflammation-driven lung cancer. *Veterinary Pathology*, **50** (2013) 895–902.

19. Takahashi H., Ogata H., Nishigaki R., Broide D. H., Karin M. Tobacco smoke promotes lung tumorigenesis by triggering IKKbeta- and JNK1-dependent inflammation. *Cancer Cell*, **19** (2010) 89–97.

20. Balkwill F., Charles K. A., Mantovani A. Smoldering and polarized inflammation in the initiation and promotion of malignant disease. *Cancer Cell*, **7** (2005) 211–217.

21. Sutcliffe S., Platz E. A. Inflammation and prostate cancer: A focus on infections. *Current Urology Reports*, **9** (2008) 243–249.

22. Pauly J. L., Waight J. D., Paszkiewicz G. M. Tobacco flakes on cigarette filters grow bacteria: A potential health risk to the smoker? *Tobacco Control*, **17**(Suppl 1) (2008) i49–i52.

23. Merlos A., Rodríguez P., Bárcena-Uribarri I., Winterhalter M., Benz R., Vinuesa T., *et al.* Toxins secreted by bacillus isolated from lung adenocarcinomas favor the penetration of toxic substances. *Frontiers in Microbiology*, **6** (2015) 1301.

24. Holla S., Ghorpade D. S., Singh V., Bansal K., Balaji K. N. Mycobacterium bovis BCG promotes tumor cell survival from tumor necrosis factor-α-induced apoptosis. *Molecular Cancer*, **13** (2014) 210 doi: 10.1186/1476-4598-13-210.

25. Wade W. G. The oral microbiome in health and disease. *Pharmacological Research*, **69** (2013) 137–143 doi: 10.1016/j.phrs.2012.11.006. Epub 2012 Nov 28.

26. Duran-Pinedo A. E., Chen T., Teles R., Starr J. R., Wang X., Krishnan K., *et al.* Community-wide transcriptome of the oral microbiome in subjects with and without periodontitis. *ISME Journal*, **8** (2014) 1659–1672 doi: 10.1038/ismej.2014.23.

27. López-López J., Omaña-Cepeda C., Jané-Salas E. Oral precancer and cancer. *Medicina Clinica* (Barc), **145** (2015) 404–408 doi: 10.1016/j.medcli.2014.11.014.

28. Chimenos-Küstner E., Font-Costa I., López-López J. Oral cancer risk and molecular markers. *Medicina Oral Patolologia Oral Y Cirugia Bucal*, **9** (2004) 377–384.

29. Sahingur S. E., Yeudall W. A. hemokine function in periodontal disease and oral cavity cancer. *Frontiers in Immunology*, **6** (2015) 214 doi: 10.3389/fimmu.2015.00214.

30. Albuquerque R. P., López-López J., Jané-Salas E., Rosa-Santos J., Ibrahim C. A pioneering epidemiological study investigating the incidence of squamous cell carcinoma of tongue in a Portuguese population. *Medicina Oral Patologia Oral Y CirugíaBucal*, **17** (2012) e550–e554.

31. Meurman J. H. Oral microbiota and cancer. *Journal of Oral Microbiology*, **2** (2010) 5195 doi: 10.3402/jom.v2i0.5195.

32. Pereira A. C., Dias do Carmo E., Dias da Silva M. A., Blumer Rosa L. E. Matrix metalloproteinase gene polymorphisms and oral cancer. *Journal of Clinical and Experimental Dentistry*, **4** (2012) e297–e301.

33. Hajishengallis G. Immunomicrobial pathogenesis of periodontitis: Keystones, pathobionts, and host response. *Trends in Immunology,* **35** (2014) 3–11 doi: 10.1016/j.it.2013.09.001.

34. Gholizadeh P., Eslami H., Yousefi M., Asgharzadeh M., Aghazadeh M., Kafil H. S. Role of oral microbiome on oral cancers, a review. *Biomedicine & Pharmacotherapy,* **84** (2016) 552–558 doi: 10.1016/j.biopha.2016.09.082.

35. Ha N. H., Woo B. H., Kim D. J., Ha E. S., Choi J. I., Kim S. J., *et al.* Prolonged and repetitive exposure to *Porphyromonas gingivalis* increases aggressiveness of oral cancer cells by promoting acquisition of cancer stem cell properties. *Tumor Biology,* **36** (2015) 9947–9960.

36. Zhou Y., Sztukowska M., Wang Q., Inaba H Potempa J., Scott D. A., Wang H., *et al.* Noncanonical activation of β-catenin by *Porphyromonas gingivalis. Infection and Immunity,* **83** (2015) 3195–3203 doi: 10.1128/IAI.00302-15.

37. Binder Gallimidi A., Fischman S., Revach B., Bulvik R., Maliutina A., Rubinstein A. M., *et al.* Periodontal pathogens *Porphyromonas gingivalis* and *Fusobacterium nucleatum* promote tumor progression in an oral-specific chemical carcinogenesis model. *Oncotarget,* **6** (2015) 22613–22623.

38. Hamada S., Koga T., Nishihara T., Fujiwara T., Okahashi N. Characterization and immunobiologic activities of lipopolysaccharides from periodontal bacteria. *Advances in Dental Research,* 2 (1988) 284–289.

39. Yu T., Wu Y., Helman J. I., Wen Y., Wang C., Li L. CXCR4 promotes oral squamous cell carcinoma migration and invasion through inducing expression of MMP-9 and MMP-13 via the ERK signaling pathway. *Molecular Cancer Research,* **9** (2011) 161–172 doi: 10.1158/1541-7786.MCR-10-0386.

40. Mager D. L., Haffajee A. D., Devlin P. M., Norris C. M., Posner M. R., Goodson J. M. The salivary microbiota as a diagnostic indicator of oral cancer: A descriptive, non-randomized study of cancer-free and oral squamous cell carcinoma subjects. *Journal of Translational Medicine,* **3** (2005) 27.

41. Hooper S. J., Wilson M. J., Crean S. J. Exploring the link between microorganisms and oral cancer: A systematic review of the literature. *Head & Neck,* **31** (2009) 1228–1239 doi: 10.1002/hed.21140.

42. Dwivedi P. P., Mallya S., Dongari-Bagtzoglou A. A novel immuno-competent murine model for *Candida albicans*-promoted oral

epithelial dysplasia. *Medical Mycology*, **47** (2009) 157–167 doi: 10.1080/13693780802165797.

43. Han Y. W., Houcken W., Loos B. G., Schenkein H. A., Tezal M. Periodontal disease, atherosclerosis, adverse pregnancy outcomes, and head-and-neck cancer. *Advances in Dental Research*, **26** (2014) 47–55 doi: 10.1177/0022034514528334.
44. Nair P., Sutherland G., Palmer R. M., Wilson R. F., Scott D. A. Gingival bleeding on probing increases after quitting smoking. *Journal of Clinical Periodontology*, **30** (2003) 435–437.
45. Domingues-Ferreira M., Grumach A. S., Duarte A. J., De Moraes-Vasconcelos D. Esophageal cancer associated with chronic mucocutaneous candidiasis. Could chronic candidiasis lead to esophageal cancer? *Medical Mycology*, **47** (2009) 201–205 doi: 10.1080/13693780802342545.
46. Jepsen A., Winther J. Mycotic infection in oral leukoplakia. *Acta Odontologica Scandinavica*, **23** (1965) 239–256.
47. Van der Waal I. Potentially malignant disorders of the oral and oropharyngeal mucosa; terminology, classification and present concepts of management. *Oral Oncology*, **45** (2009) 317–323.
48. McCullough M., Jaber M., Barrett A. W., Bain L., Speight P. M., Porter S. R. Oral yeast carriage correlates with presence of oral epithelial dysplasia. *Oral Oncology*, **38** (2002) 391–3.
49. Spolidorio L. C., Martins V. R., Nogueira R. D., Spolidorio D. M. The frequency of *Candida sp.* in biopsies of oral mucosal lesions. *Pesquisa Odontologica Brasileira*, 17 (2003) 89–93.
50. Cheng X., Wang B., Jin Z., Ma D., Yang W., Zhao R., *et al. Pseudomonas aeruginosa*-mannose-sensitive hemagglutinin inhibits pancreatic cancer cell proliferation and induces apoptosis via the EGFR pathway and caspase signaling. *Oncotarget*, (2016) doi: 10.18632/oncotarget.12844.
51. Harshad M. Exploring the ocean for new drug developments: Marine pharmacology. *Journal of Pharmacy and Bioallied Sciences*, **8** (2016) 83–91.
52. Mayer A. M., Glaser K. B., Cuevas C., Jacobs R. S., Kem W., Little R. D., *et al.* The odyssey of marine pharmaceuticals: A current pipeline perspective. *Trends in Pharmacological Sciences*, **31** (2010) 255–265.
53. Montaser R., Luesch H. Marine natural products: A new wave of drugs? *Future Medicinal Chemistry*, **3** (2011) 1475–1489.

54. Davis J. T., Okunola O., Quesada R. Recent advances in the transmembrane transport of anions. *Chemical Society Reviews*, **39** (2010) 3843–3862.

55. Williams R. P. Biosynthesis of prodigiosin, a secondary metabolite of *Serratia marcescens. Applied Microbiology*, **25** (1973) 396–402.

56. Creech H. J., Hamilton M. A., Diller I. C. Comparative studies of the immunological, toxic and tumor-necrotizing properties of polysaccharides from *Serratia marcescens* (*Bacillus prodigiosus*). *Cancer Research*, **8** (1948) 318–329.

57. Lasfargues E. Y., Wharton D. R., Difine J. C. Some effects of polysaccharide preparations from *Serratia marcescens* and *Aerobacter aerogenes* on cells in tissue culture. *Cancer Research*, **11** (1951) 425–427.

58. Pérez-Tomás R., Viñas M. New insights on the antitumoral properties of prodiginines. *Current Medicinal Chemistry*, **17** (2010) 2222–2231.

59. Bennett J., Bentley R. Seeing red: The story of prodigiosin. *Advances in Applied Microbiology*, **47** (2000) 1–32.

60. Viñas M., Loren J., Guinea J. Particulate-bound pigment of *Serratia marcescens* and its association with the cellular envelopes. *Microbios Letters*, **93** (1983) 19–26.

61. Darshan N., Manonmani H. K. Prodigiosin and its potential applications. *Journal of Food Science and Technology*, **52** (2015) 5393–5407.

62. Soto-Cerrato V., Llagostera E., Montaner B., Scheffer G. L., R. Pérez-Tomás. Mitochondria-mediated apoptosis operating irrespective of multidrug resistance in breast cancer cells by the anticancer agent prodigiosin. *Biochemical Pharmacology*, **68** (2004) 1345–1352.

63. Davis J. T., Gale P. A., Okunola O. A., Prados P., Iglesias-Sanchez J. C., Torroba T., *et al.* Using small molecules to facilitate exchange of bicarbonate and chloride anions across liposomal membranes. *Nature Chemistry*, **1** (2009) 138–144.

64. Chiappori A., Williams C., Northfelt D. W., Adams J. W., Malik S., Edelman M. J., *et al.* Obatoclax mesylate, a Pan–Bcl-2 inhibitor, in combination with docetaxel in a phase 1/2 trial in relapsed non–small-cell lung cancer. *Journal of Thoracic Oncology*, **9** (2014) 121–125.

65. Schimmer A. D., Raza A., Carter T. H., Claxton D., Erba H., DeAngelo D. J., *et al.* A multicenter phase I/II study of obatoclax mesylate

administered as a 3- or 24-hour infusion in older patients with previously untreated acute myeloid leukemia. *PLOS One*, **9** (2014) e108694.

66. Langer C. J., Albert I., Ross H. J., Kovacs P., Blakely L. J., Pajkos G., *et al.* Randomized phase II study of carboplatin and etoposide with or without obatoclax mesylate in extensive-stage small cell lung cancer. *Lung Cancer*, **85** (2014) 420–428.
67. Castro A. J. Antimalarial activity of prodigiosin. *Nature*, **213** (1967) 903–904.
68. Darah. I., The, F., Jain K., Sheh-Hong L. Prodigiosin-an antibacterial red pigment produced by *Serratia marcescens* IBRL USM 84 associated with a marine sponge *Xestospongia testudinaria*. *Journal of Applied Pharmaceutical Science*, **4** (2014) 1–6.
69. Berg G. Diversity of antifungal and plant-associated *Serratia plymuthica* strains. *Journal of Applied Microbiology*, **88** (2000) 952–960.
70. Han S. B., Kim H. M., Kim Y. H., Lee C. W., Jang E. S., Son K. H., *et al.* T-cell specific immunosuppression by prodigiosin isolated from Serratia marcescens. *International Journal of Immunopharmacology*, **20** (1998) 1–13.
71. Manderville R. A. Synthesis, proton-affinity and anti-cancer properties of the prodigiosin-group natural products. *Current Medicinal Chemistry–Anti-Cancer Agents*, **1** (2001) 195–218.
72. Pérez-Tomás R., Montaner B., Llagostera E., Soto-Cerrato V. The prodigiosins, proapoptotic drugs with anticancer properties. *Biochemical Pharmacology*, **66** (2003) 1447–1452.
73. Ohkuma S., Sato T., Okamoto M., Matsuya H., Arai K., Kataoka T., *et al.* Prodigiosins uncouple lysosomal vacuolar-type ATPase through promotion of H^+/Cl^- symport. *Biochemical Journal*, **334** (1998) 731–741.
74. Sessler J. L., Eller L. R., Cho W. S., Nicolaou S., Aguilar A., Lee J. T., *et al.* Synthesis, anion-binding properties, and in vitro anticancer activity of prodigiosin analogues. *Angewandte Chemie International Edition*, **44** (2005) 5989–5992.
75. Montaner B., Pérez-Tomás R. The Prodigiosins: A new family of anticancer drugs *Current Cancer Drug Targets*, **3** (2003) 57–65.
76. Castillo-Avila W., Abal M., Robine S., Pérez-Tomás R. Non-apoptotic concentrations of prodigiosin (H^+/Cl^- symporter) inhibit the acidification of lysosomes and induce cell cycle blockage in colon cancer cells. *Life Sciences*, **78** (2005) 121–127.

77. Montaner B., Pérez-Tomás R. Prodigiosin-induced apoptosis in human colon cancer cells. *Life Sciences*, **68** (2001) 2025–2036.

78. Montaner B., Martinell M., Öllinger E., Giralt E., Pérez-Tomás R. DNA interaction and dual topoisomerase I and II inhibition properties of the antitumor drug prodigiosin. *Toxicological Sciences*, **85** (2005) 870–879.

79. Goard C., Aaron D. An evidence-based review of obatoclax mesylate in the treatment of hematological malignancies. *Core Evidence*, **8** (2013) 1.

80. Pan J., Cheng C., Verstovsek S., Chen Q., Jin Y., Cao Q. The BH3-mimetic GX15-070 induces autophagy, potentiates the cytotoxicity of carboplatin and 5-fluorouracil in esophageal carcinoma cells. *Cancer Letters*, **293** (2010) 167–174.

81. Heidari N., Hicks M., Harada H. GX15-070 (obatoclax) overcomes glucocorticoid resistance in acute lymphoblastic leukemia through induction of apoptosis and autophagy. *Cell Death & Disease*, **1** (2010) e76.

82. McCoy F., Hurwitz J., McTavish N., Paul I., Barnes C., O'Hagan B., *et al.* Obatoclax induces Atg7-dependent autophagy independent of beclin-1 and BAX/BAK. *Cell Death & Disease*, 1 (2010) e108.

83. Espona-Fiedler M., Soto-Cerrato V., Hosseini A., Lizcano J. M., Guallar V., Quesada R., *et al.* Identification of dual mTORC1 and mTORC2 inhibitors in melanoma cells: Prodigiosin vs. obatoclax. *Biochemical Pharmacology*, **83** (2012) 489–496.

84. Basit F., Cristofanon S., Fulda S. Obatoclax (GX15-070) triggers necroptosis by promoting the assembly of the necrosome on autophagosomal membranes. *Cell Death & Differentiation*, **20** (2013) 1161–1173.

85. Soliev A., Kakushi H., Keiichi E. Bioactive pigments from marine bacteria: Applications and physiological roles. *Evidence-Based Complementary and Alternative Medicine*, (2011) 670349.http://dx.doi.org/10.1155/2011/670349.

86. Carbone M., Irace C., Costagliola F., Castelluccio F., Villani G., Calado G., *et al.* A new cytotoxic tambjamine alkaloid from the Azorean nudibranch Tambjaceutae. *Bioorganic & Medicinal Chemistry Letters*, **20** (2010) 2668–2670.

87. Pinkerton D. M., Banwell M. G., Garson M. J., Kumar N., de Moraes M. O., Cavalcanti B. C., *et al.* Antimicrobial and cytotoxic activities of synthetically derived tambjamines C and E-J, BE-18591, and a

related alkaloid from the marine bacterium *Pseudoalteromonas tunicata*. *Chemistry & Biodiversity*, **7** (2010) 1311–1324.

88. Iglesias P., Moreno D., Javier A. A., Torroba T., Pérez-Tomás R., Quesada R. Tambjamine alkaloids and related synthetic analogs: Efficient transmembrane anion transporters. *Chemical Communications*, **48** (2012) 1556–1558.

89. Hernando E., Soto-Cerrato V., Cortes-Arroyo S., Pérez-Tomás R., Quesada R. Transmembrane anion transport and cytotoxicity of synthetic tambjamine analogs *Organic & Biomolecular Chemistry*, **12** (2014) 1771–1778.

90. Carte B., Faulkner J. Defensive metabolites from three nembrothid nudibranchs. *The Journal of Organic Chemistry*, **48** (1983) 2314–2318.

91. Gale P., Perez-Tomas R., Quesada R. Anion transporters and biological systems. *Accounts of Chemical Research*, **46** (2013) 2801–2813.

92. Soto-Cerrato V., Manuel-Manresa P., Hernando E., Calabuig-Farinas S., Martinez-Romero A., Fernandez-Duenas V., *et al.* Facilitated anion transport induces hyperpolarization of the cell membrane that triggers differentiation and cell death in cancer stem cells. *Journal of the American Chemical Society*, **137** (2015) 15892–15898.

Index